Fleshing out surfaces

MANCHESTER
1824
Manchester University Press

rethinking
art's histories

SERIES EDITORS
Amelia G. Jones, Marsha Meskimmon

Rethinking Art's Histories aims to open out art history from its most basic structures by foregrounding work that challenges the conventional periodisation and geographical subfields of traditional art history, and addressing a wide range of visual cultural forms from the early modern period to the present.

These books will acknowledge the impact of recent scholarship on our understanding of the complex temporalities and cartographies that have emerged through centuries of world-wide trade, political colonisation and the diasporic movement of people and ideas across national and continental borders.

Also available in the series

Art, museums and touch Fiona Candlin

The 'do-it-yourself' artwork: Participation from fluxus to relational aesthetics
Anna Dezeuze *(ed.)*

The matter of miracles: Neapolitan baroque sanctity and architecture Helen Hills

The face of medicine: Visualising medical masculinities in late nineteenth-century Paris
Mary Hunter

Glorious catastrophe: Jack Smith, performance and visual culture Dominic Johnson

Otherwise: Imagining queer feminist art histories Amelia Jones and Erin Silver (eds)

After the event: New perspectives in art history Charles Merewether and John Potts *(eds)*

Photography and documentary film in the making of modern Brazil Luciana Martins

Women, the arts and globalization: Eccentric experience
Marsha Meskimmon and Dorothy Rowe *(eds)*

Flesh cinema. The corporeal turn in American avant-garde film Ara Osterweil

After-affects|after-images: Trauma and aesthetic transformation in the virtual feminist museum Griselda Pollock

Vertiginous mirrors: The animation of the visual image and early modern travel Rose Marie San Juan

The paradox of body, building and motion in seventeenth-century England
Kimberley Skelton

The newspaper clipping: a modern paper object Anke Te Heesen, *translated by* Lori Lantz

Screen/space: The projected image in contemporary art Tamara Trodd *(ed.)*

Art and human rights: Contemporary Asian contexts Caroline Turner and Jen Webb

Timed out: Art and the transnational Caribbean Leon Wainwright

Performative monuments: Performance, photography, and the rematerialisation of public art
Mechtild Widrich

Fleshing out surfaces

Skin in French art and medicine, 1650–1850

Mechthild Fend

Manchester University Press

Published by Manchester University Press
Altrincham Street, Manchester M1 7JA
www.manchesteruniversitypress.co.uk

British Library Cataloguing-in-Publication Data
A catalogue record for this book is available from the British Library

Library of Congress Cataloging-in-Publication Data applied for

ISBN 978 0 7190 8796 7 *hardback*

First published 2017

Typeset in Minion with Myriad display
by Koinonia, Manchester

Contents

Illustrations

Plates

The plates can be found between *pages* xvi and 1

Figures

Acknowledgements

This book has been very long in the making. The project – from when I started thinking about skin as an art historical topic to the writing of the final manuscript – accompanied me to many places, from Hamburg and Frankfurt to Berlin, via Princeton to London, and it changed language along the way. What started as a post-doctoral project in Germany finally became an English-language book in London. The various institutions and scholarly frameworks in which I conducted my research have all contributed to shaping it. I am grateful to the following people and institutions: a post-doctoral fellowship by the Deutsche Forschungsgemeinschaft (DFG) got me started, and I would like to thank Klaus Herding, also my former PhD supervisor, for his initial support. This was followed by a Getty Postdoctoral Fellowship, a two-month Fellowship at CRASSH (Centre for Research in the Arts, Social Sciences and Humanities), Cambridge in 2005, and in 2005–6 a membership at the Institute for Advanced Studies at Princeton. In 2010, an AHRC research leave grant enabled me to draft the chapter on skin colour. The years (2001–4), during which I worked as a research scholar at the Max Planck Institute for the History of Science in Berlin, were truly transformative for my understanding of skin as a scientific object; I learned a lot from many colleagues there but would especially like to thank Lorraine Daston for being such an exceptionally supportive director and intellectual model. The Graduiertenkolleg *Psychische Engergien Bildender Kunst* facilitated my co-operation with Daniela Bohde; it has been enjoyable and rewarding to co-organise a conference and workshop on skin and flesh tones in art with her, and jointly to edit the volume *Weder Haut noch Fleisch: das Inkarnat in der Kunstgeschichte* (2007) which became the stepping stone for chapter 2 of this book.

The UCL History of Art department which I joined in autumn 2006 has been an amazing place finally to turn this research into a book. I would like to thank all my colleagues for being so amicable and inspiring, and am particularly indebted to conversations with Tamar Garb, Maria Loh, Rose Marie San Juan and Richard Taws. Besides the colleagues in my department, Adrian Rifkin, Katie Scott, Bronwen Wilson and Joanna Woodall have been important interlocutors since moving to London. Friends and colleagues in Germany, France and America – Anke te Heesen, Andrea Klier, Melissa Hyde, Marianne Koos, Anne Lafont, Mary Sheriff, Abigail Solomon-Godeau, Bettina Uppenkamp – have each been important in their own way.

Besides the peer reviewers for Manchester University Press, to whom I am very grateful, a number of people have read drafts of this book or parts of it. Daniela Bohde and Rose Marie San Juan made constructive comments on the introduction; Richard Taws contributed ideas and suggestions for the chapter on the revolutionary period; and Anne Lafont motivated me by her response to the chapter on skin colour. I am especially grateful to Joanna Woodall for her generosity and friendship; she read the entire manuscript, and some chapters more than once, and made countless knowledgeable and encouraging comments. Last but not least I would like to thank Amelia Jones and Marsha Meskimmon for including this book in their series, and Manchester University Press and their staff for their patience and careful editing.

I dedicate this book to the memory of my friend Anne Hoormann, who died far too young in 2003, and whom I will never stop missing. It was from her that I first learnt the word 'Inkarnat', when we were working on a student presentation on Titian's *Sacred and Profane Love*.

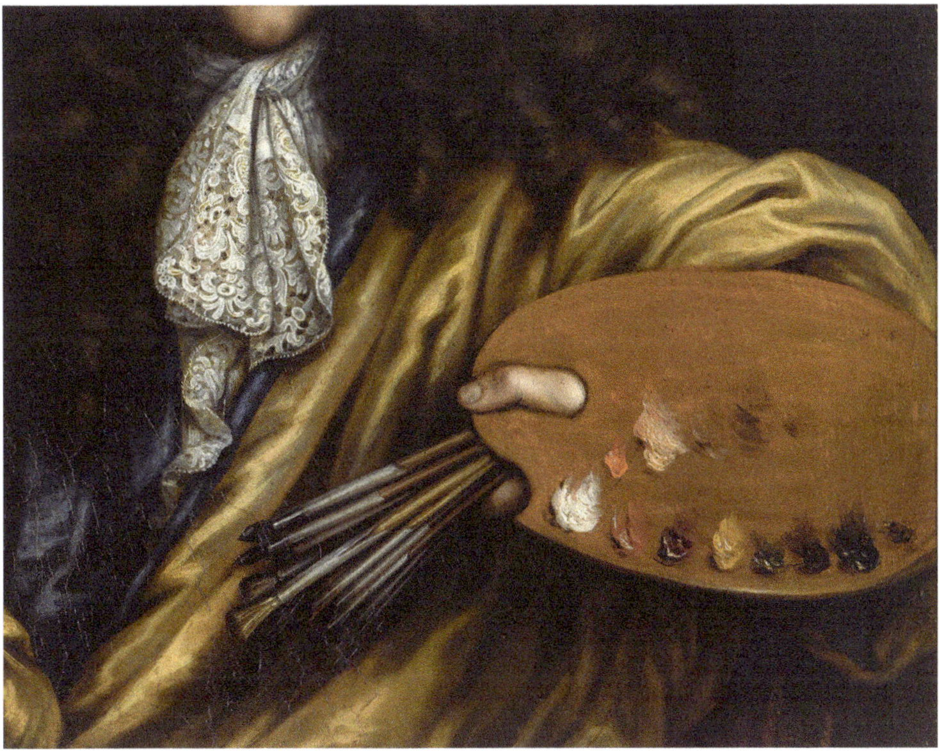

Florent de La Mare-Richart, *Noël Coypel père* (detail: palette and brushes), 1677, oil on canvas, 117 x 98 cm. **Plate 1**

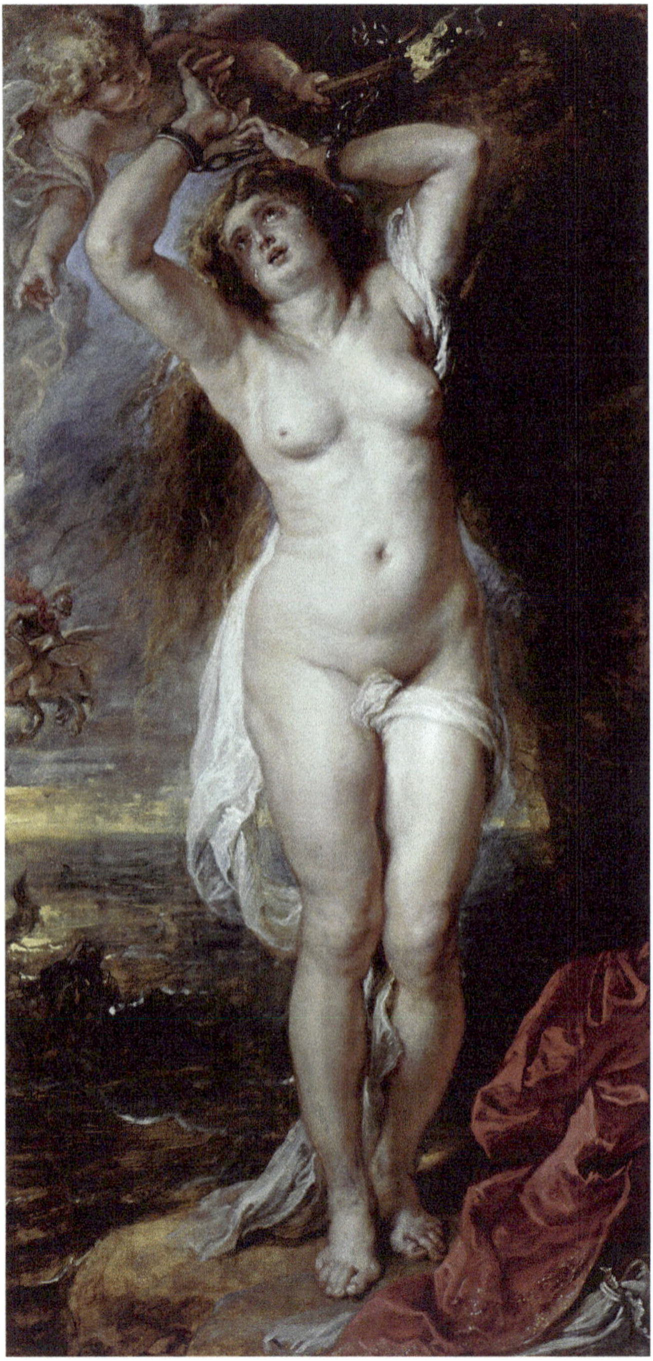

Plate 2 Peter Paul Rubens, *Andromeda*, ca 1638, oil on canvas, 188.6 x 93.8 cm.

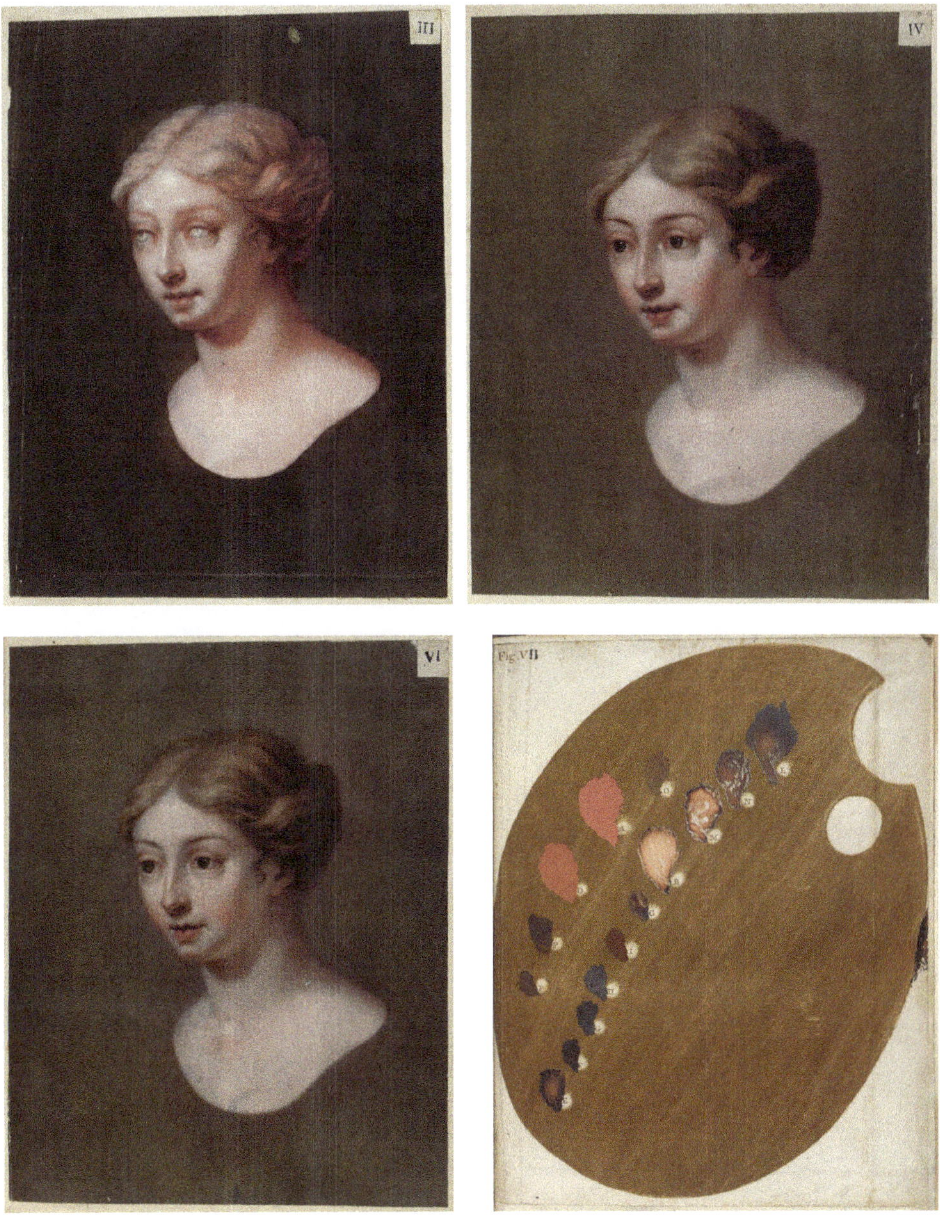

Jacob Le Blon, female head in various stages of colouring, palette, from *Coloritto; or the Harmonie of Colouring* (1725), Figures 3, 4, 6, 7, colour mezzotints, 28 x 22 cm each.

Plate 3a–d

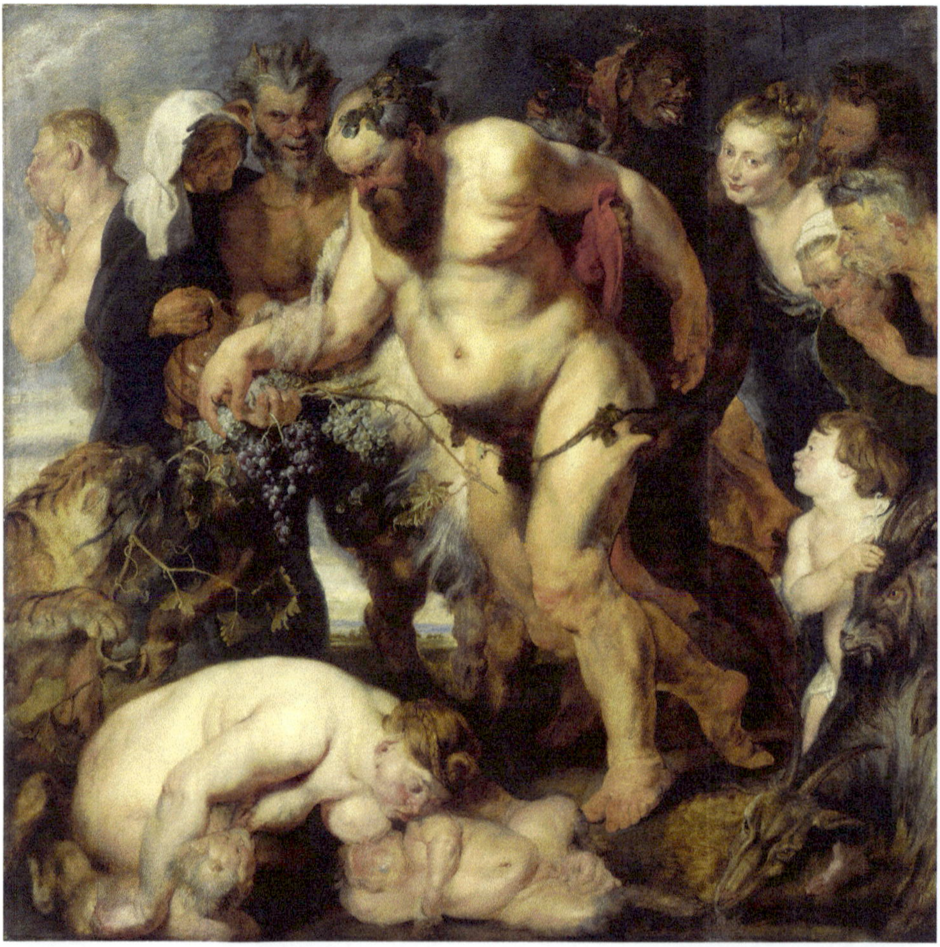

Plate 4 Peter Paul Rubens, *Bacchanal* (*Drunken Silenus*), ca 1616/25, oil on wood, 212 x 214.5 cm.

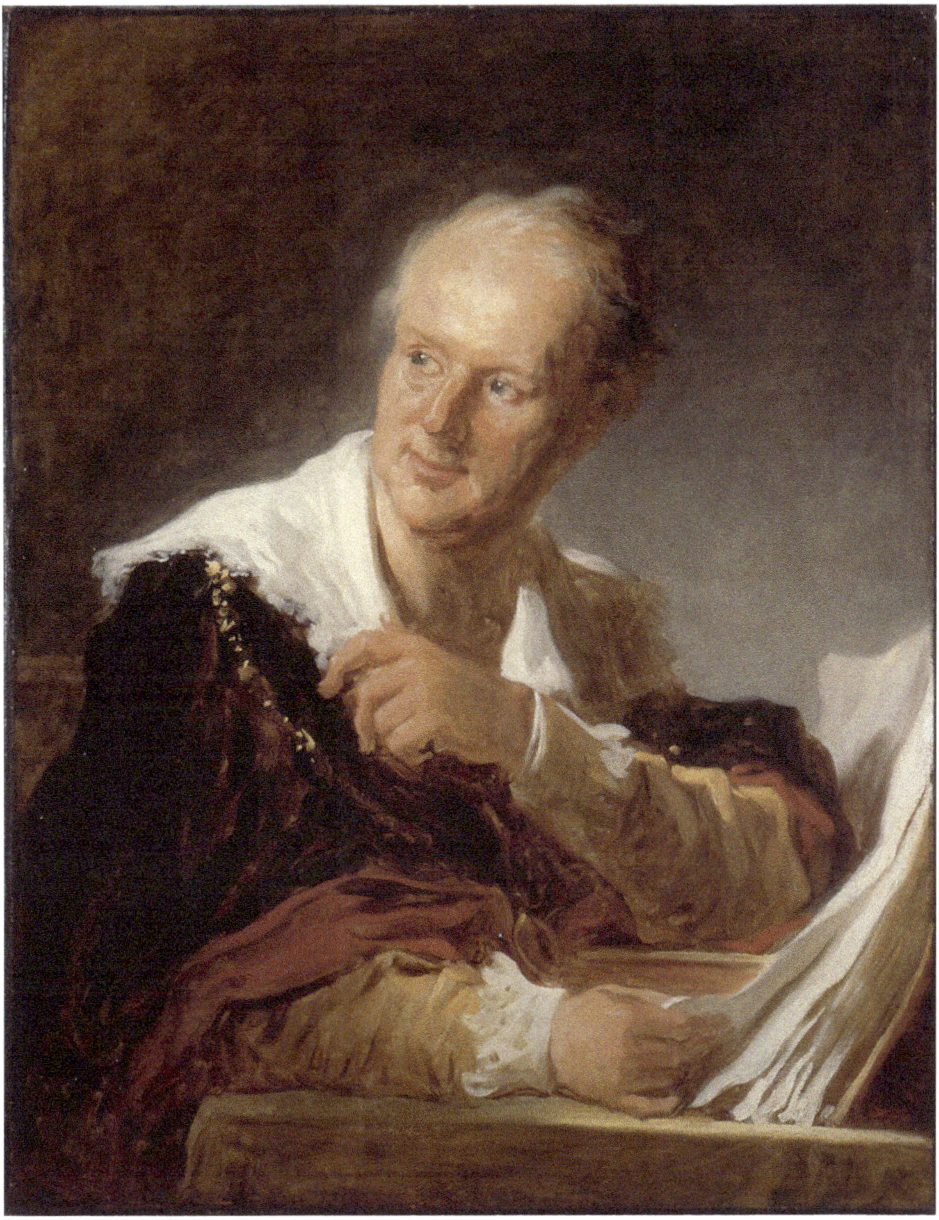

Jean-Honoré Fragonard, *Portrait of a Man of Letters* (formerly identified as Diderot), ca 1769, oil on canvas, 81 x 65 cm.

Plate 5

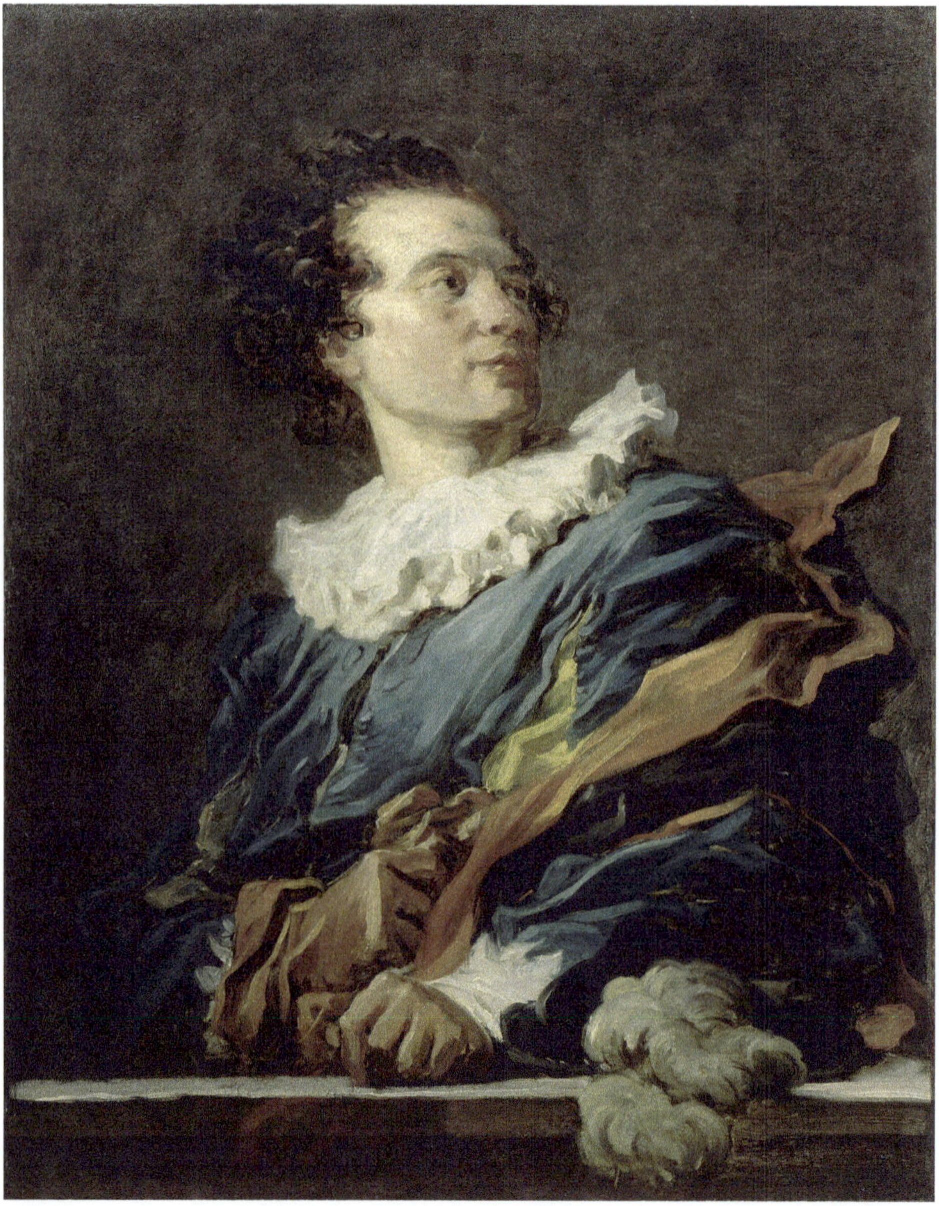

Plate 6 Jean-Honoré Fragonard, *Portrait of a Man* (identified as the Abbé de Saint-Non), ca 1769, oil on canvas, 80 x 65 cm.

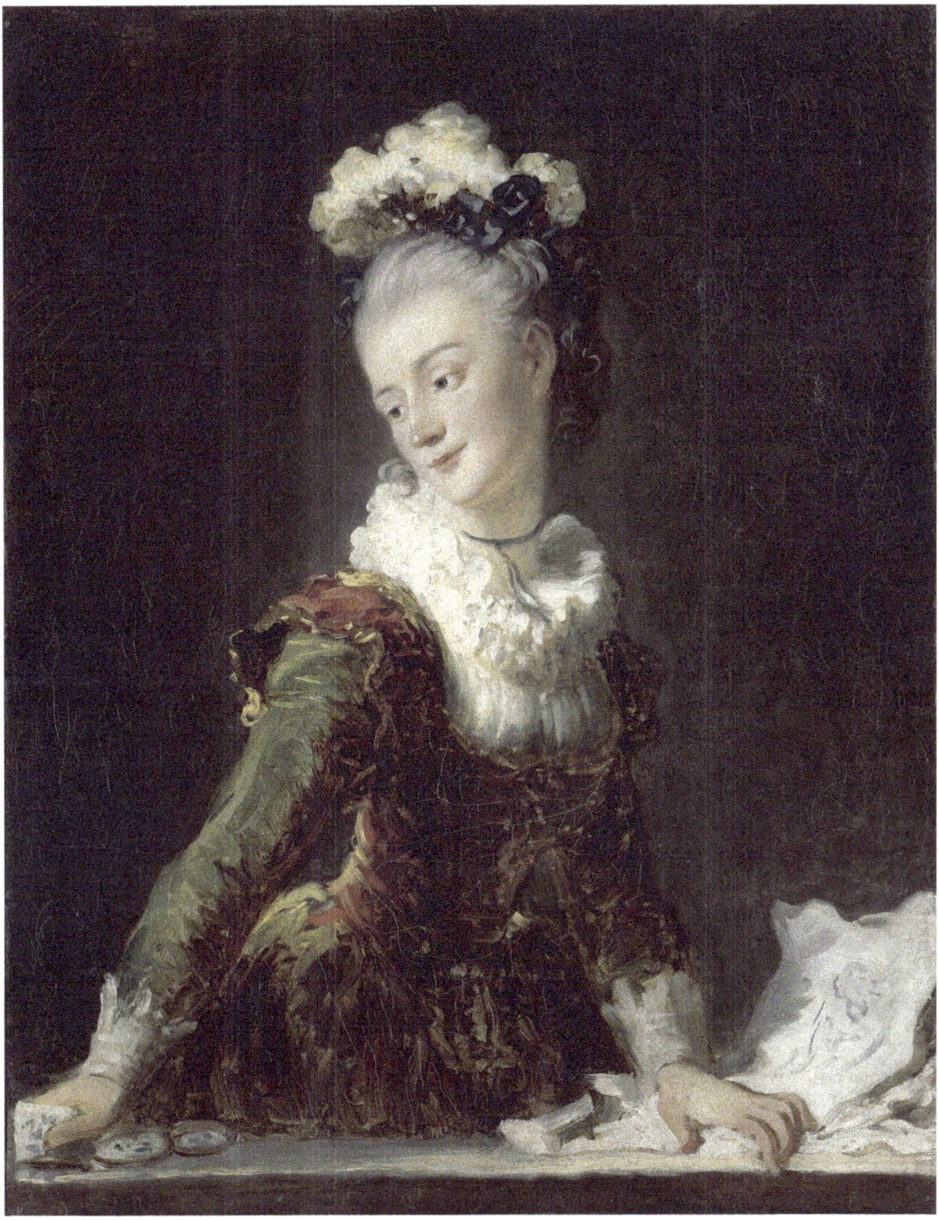

Jean-Honoré Fragonard, *Portrait of a Woman* (formerly identified as Marie-Madeleine Guimard), ca 1769–70, oil on canvas, 81.5 x 65 cm.

Plate 7

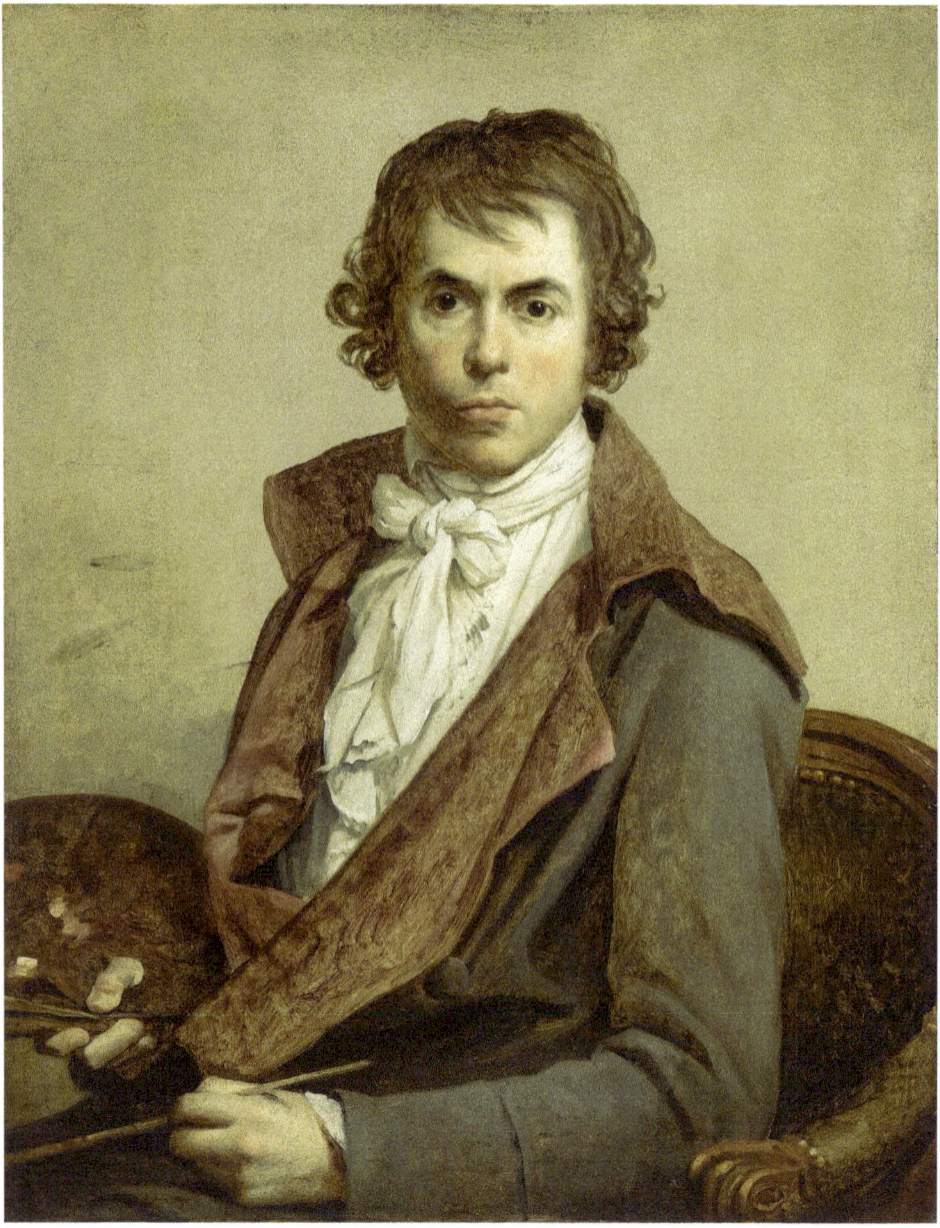

Plate 8 Jacques-Louis David, *Self-Portrait in Prison*, 1794, oil on canvas, 81 x 64 cm.

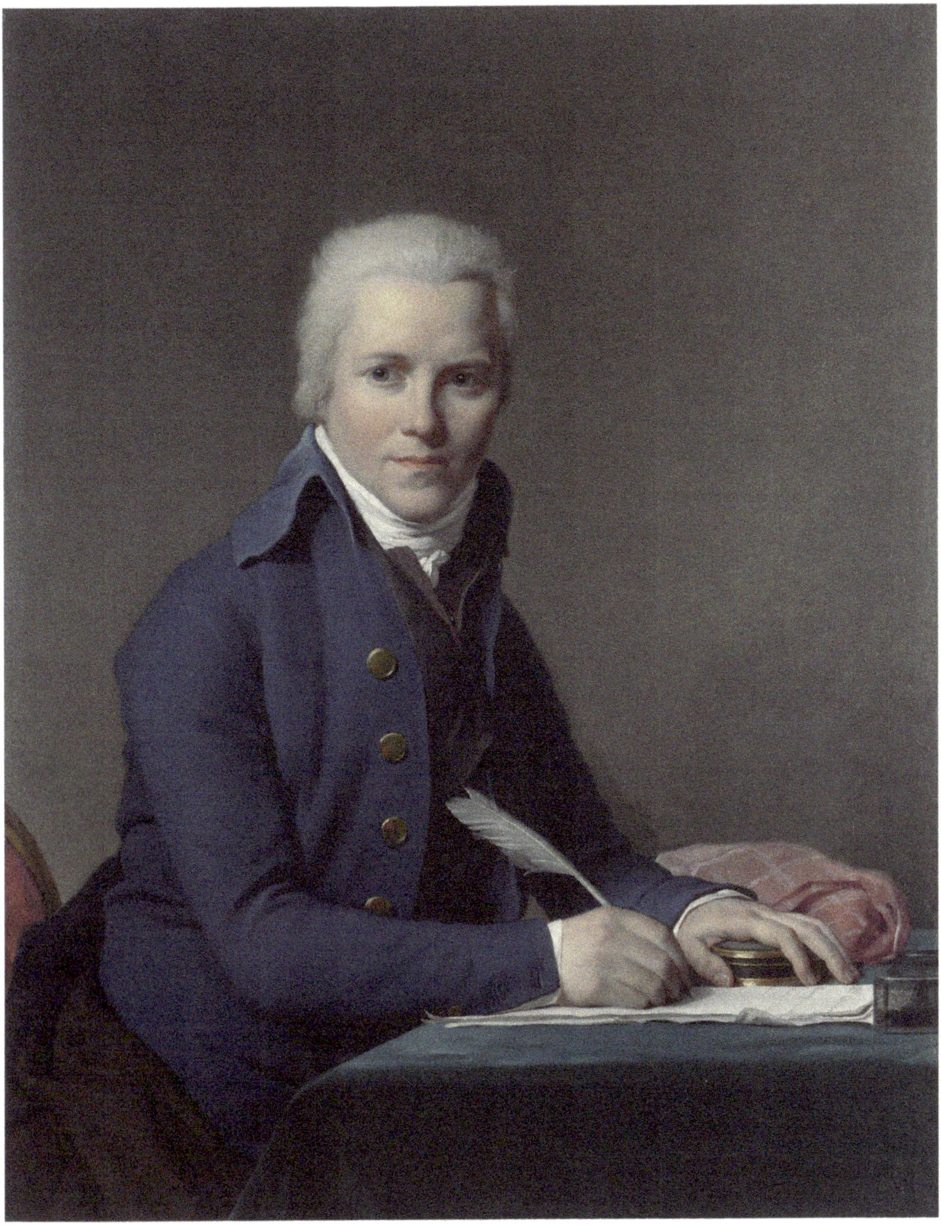

Jacques-Louis David, *Jacobus Blauw*, 1795, oil on canvas, 92 x 73 cm. **Plate 9**

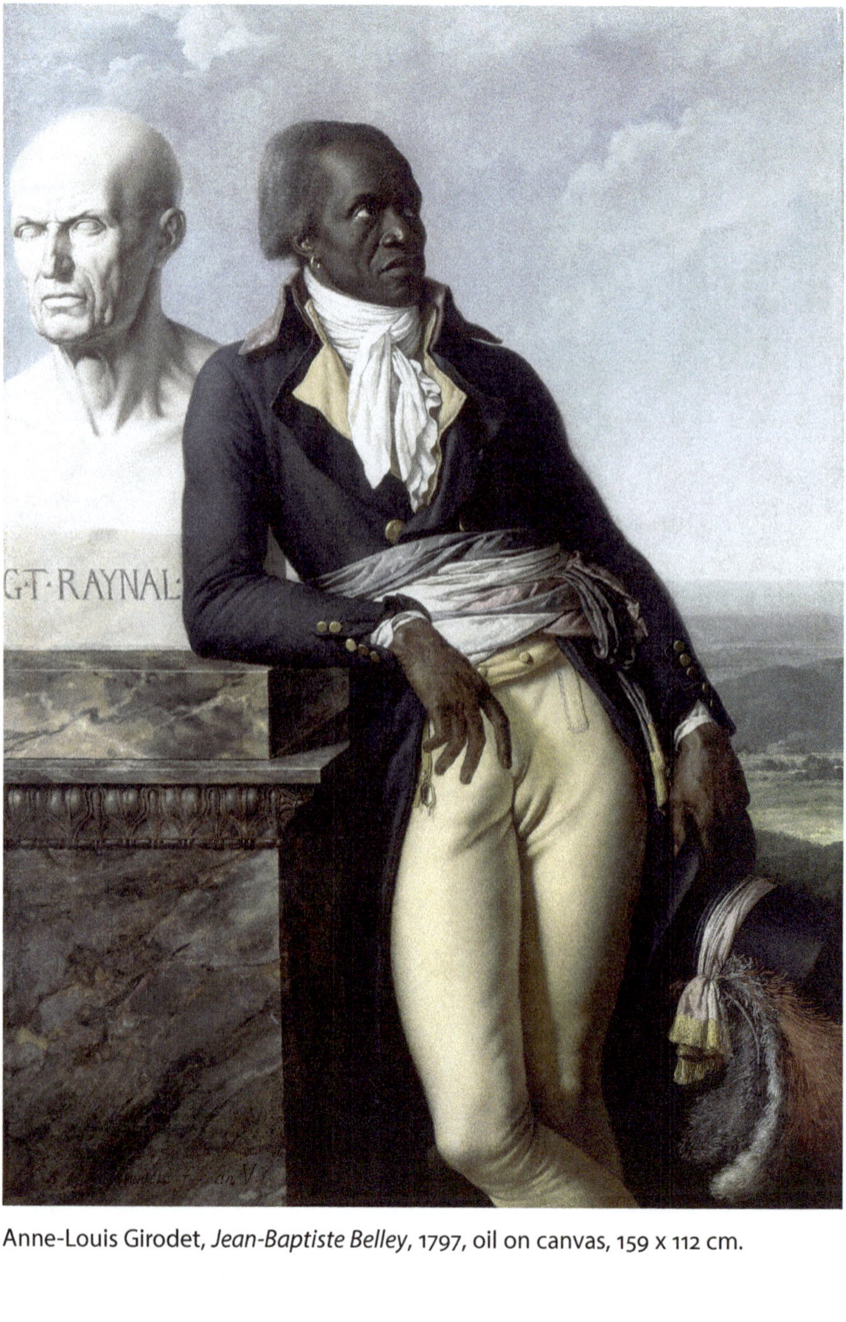

Plate 10 Anne-Louis Girodet, *Jean-Baptiste Belley*, 1797, oil on canvas, 159 x 112 cm.

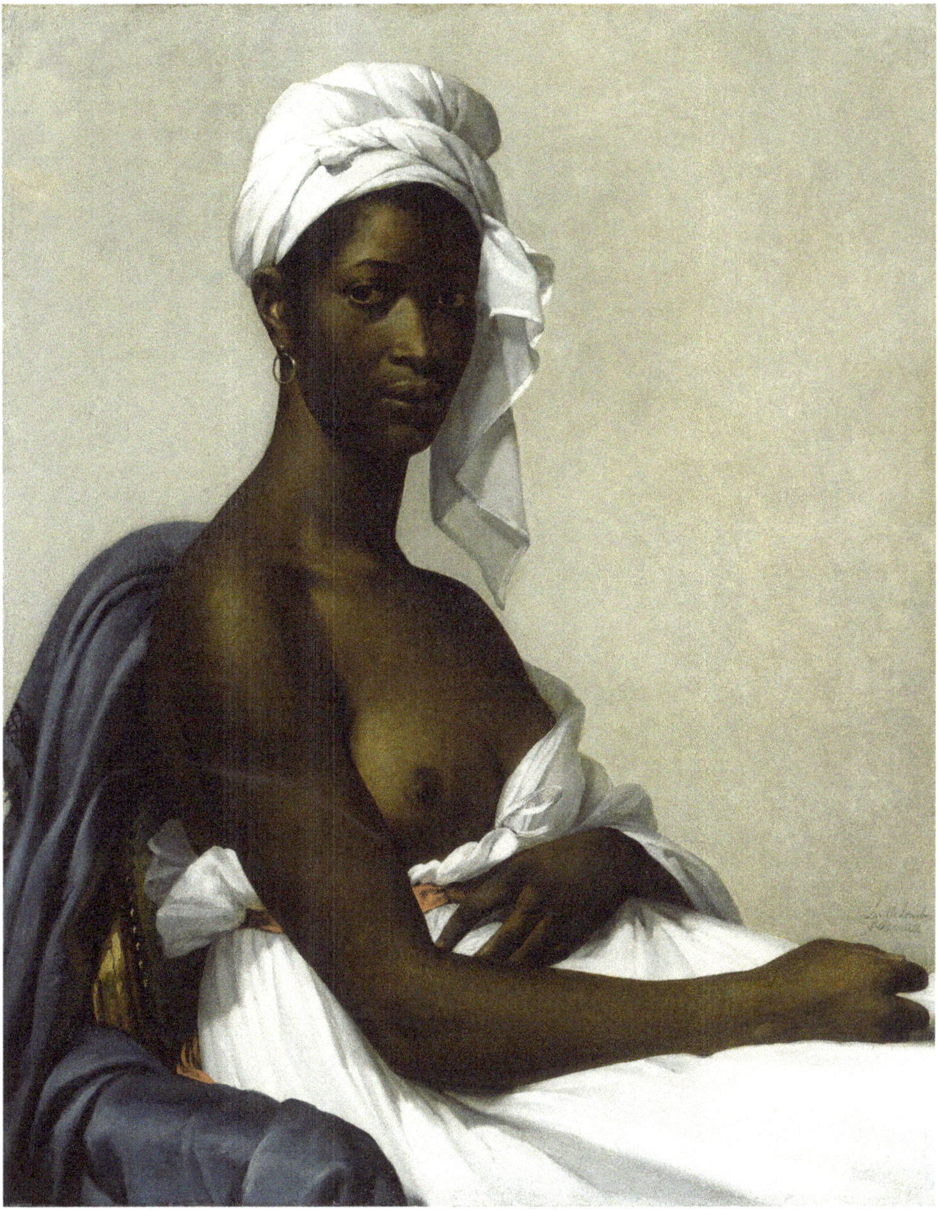

Marie-Guillemine Benoist, *Portrait of a Negress*, 1800, oil on canvas, 81 x 65 cm. **Plate 11**

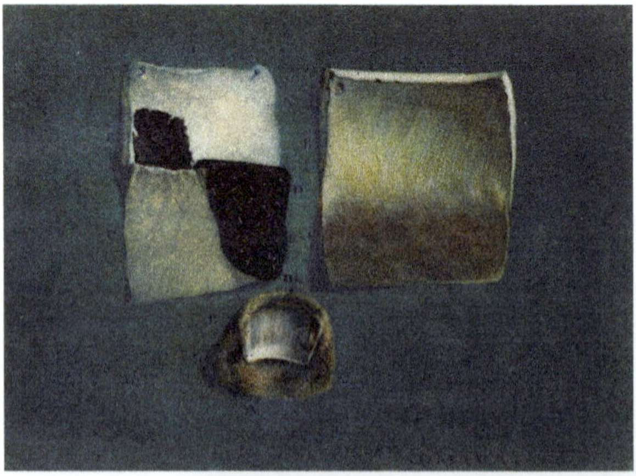

Jan Ladmiral, Fragments of skin and thumb, from Bernhard Siegfried Albinus, *Dissertatio secunda de sede et caussa coloris Aethiopium et caeterorum hominum*, 1737, colour mezzotint with etching, 11.7 x 16.3 cm.

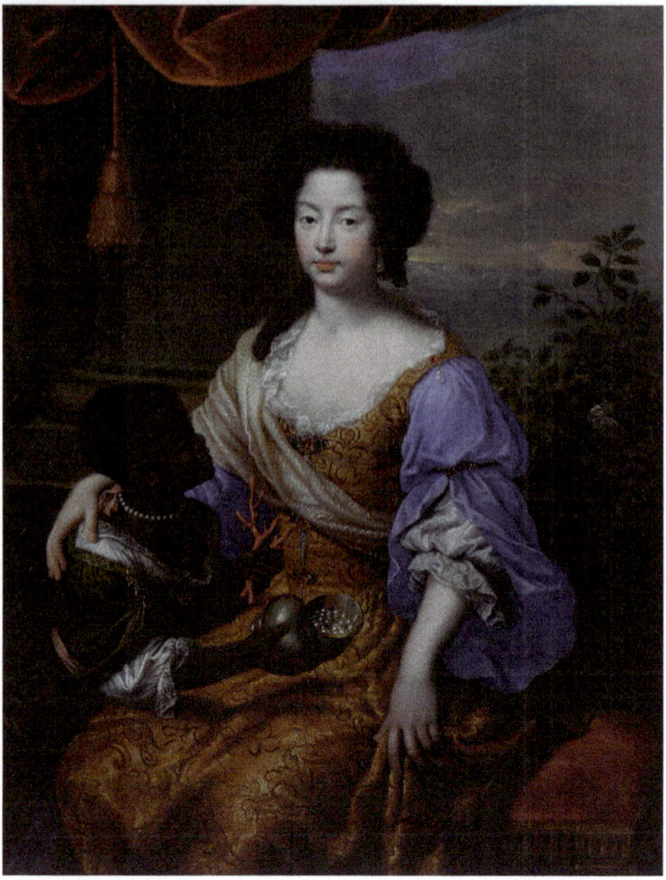

Plate 13 Pierre Mignard, *Louise Renée de Penancoët de Kéroualle, Duchess of Portsmouth*, 1682, oil on canvas, 120.7 x 95.3 cm.

a

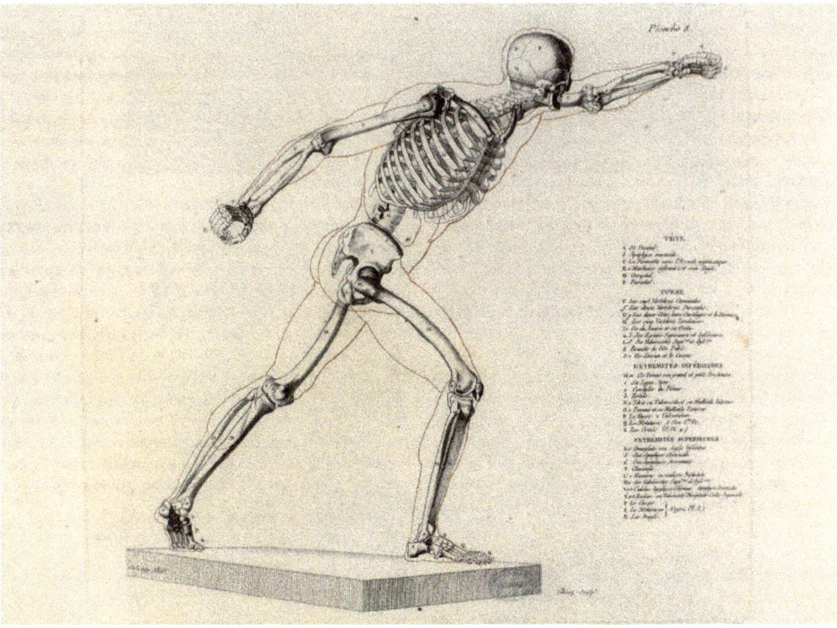

b

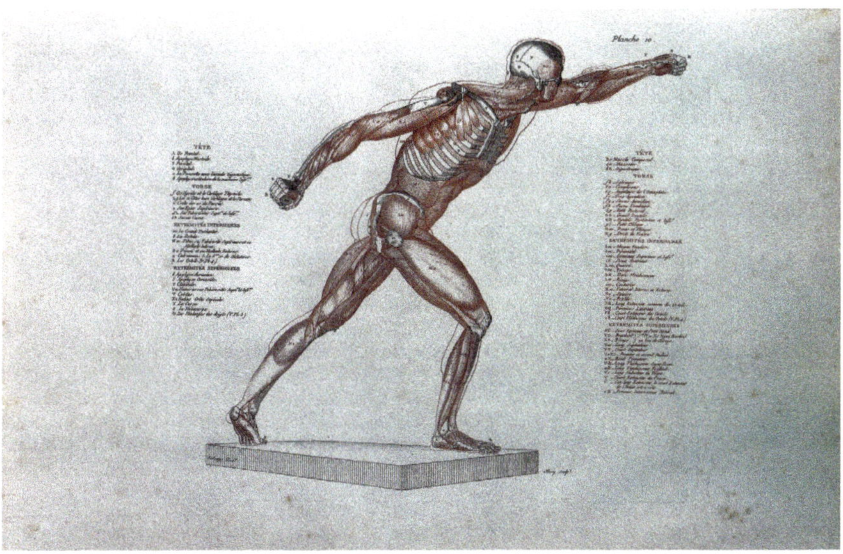

a Bosq after Jean-Galbert Salvage, skeleton drawn after the *Borghese Gladiator*, from *Anatomie du Gladiateur combattant*, 1812, plate 8, engraving printed in red and black ink, 31.5 x 35.5 cm (platemark).
b Bosq after Jean-Galbert Salvage, internal muscles, drawn after the *Borghese Gladiator*, from *Anatomie du Gladiateur combattant*, 1812, plate 10, engraving in red and black ink, 32.5 x 35.5 cm (platemark).

Plate 14

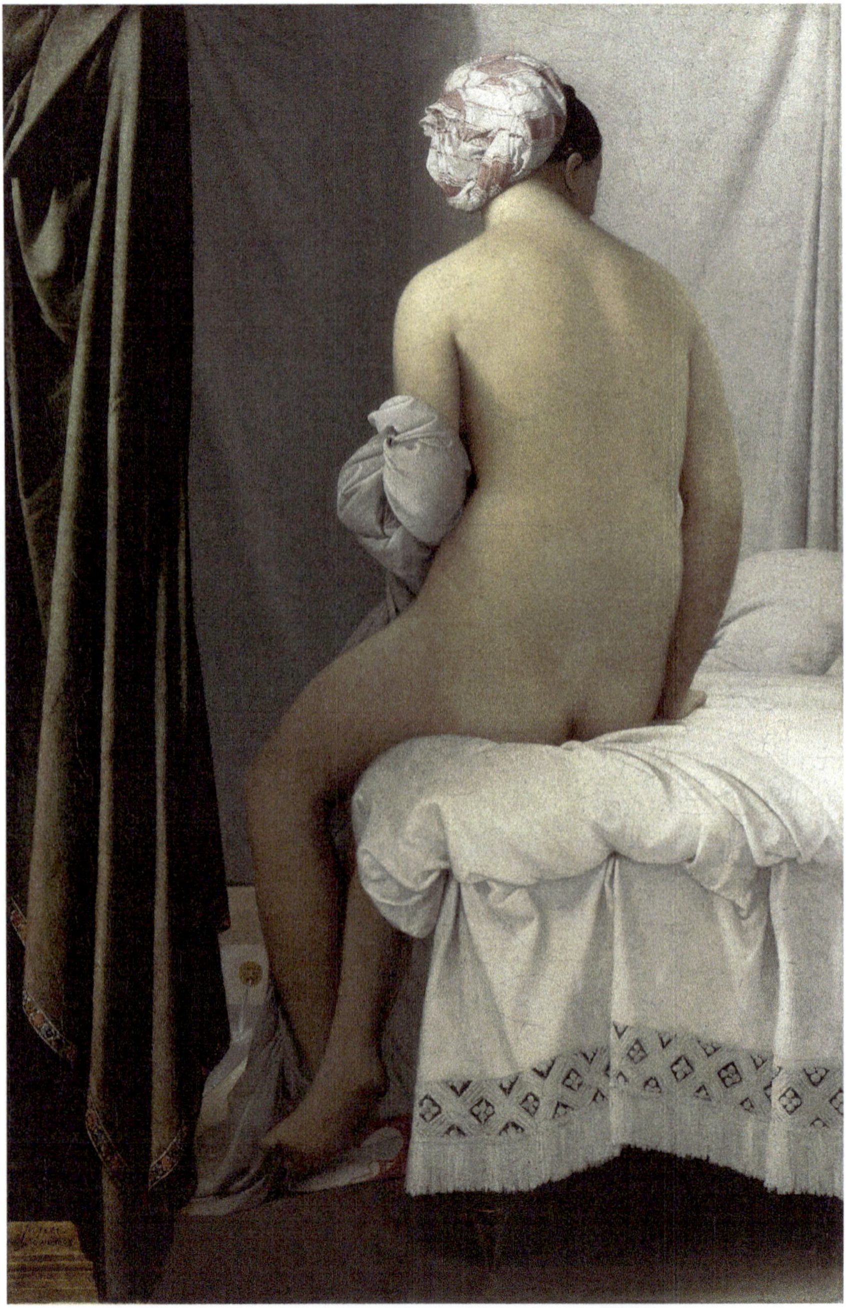

Plate 15 Jean-Auguste-Dominique Ingres, *Baigneuse de Valpinçon*, 1808, oil on canvas, 146 x 97 cm.

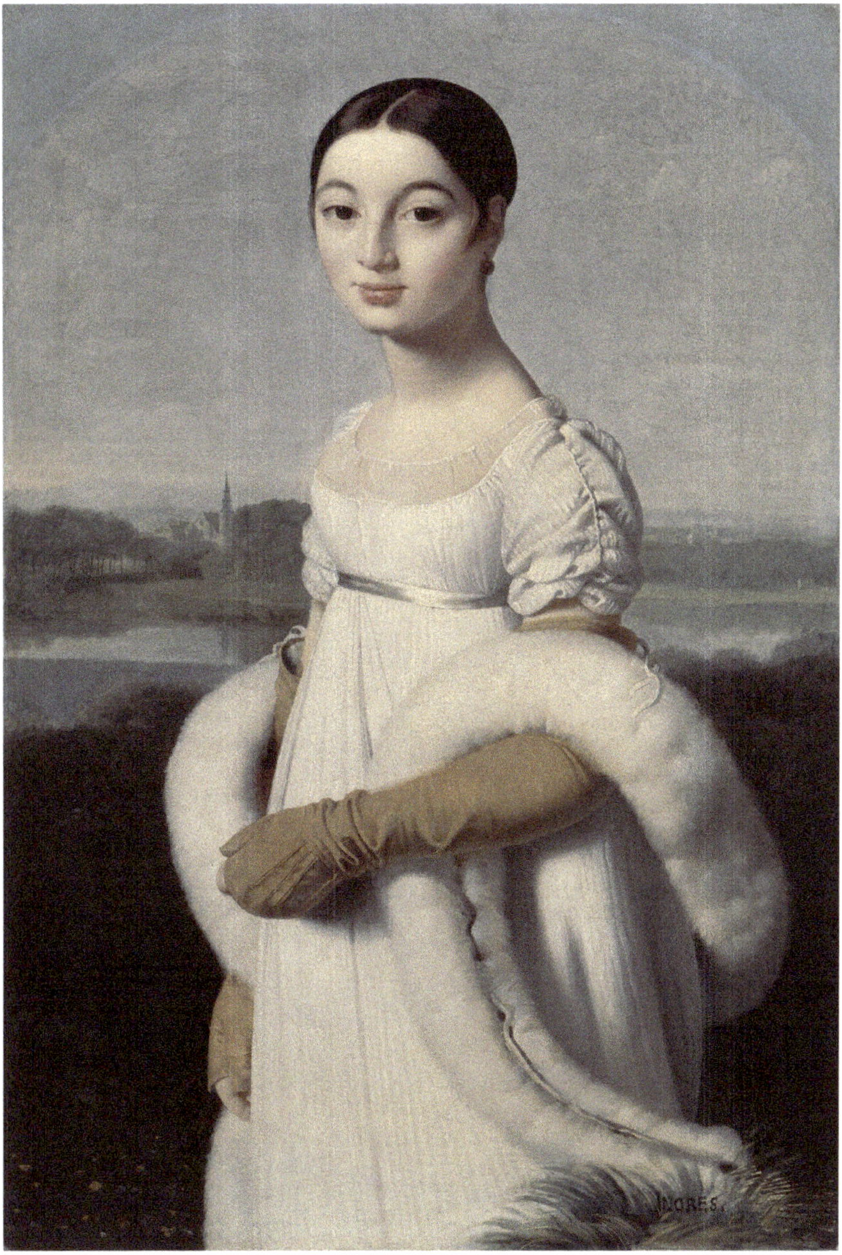

Jean-Auguste-Dominique Ingres, *Caroline Rivière*,
oil on canvas, 100 x 70 cm.

Plate 16

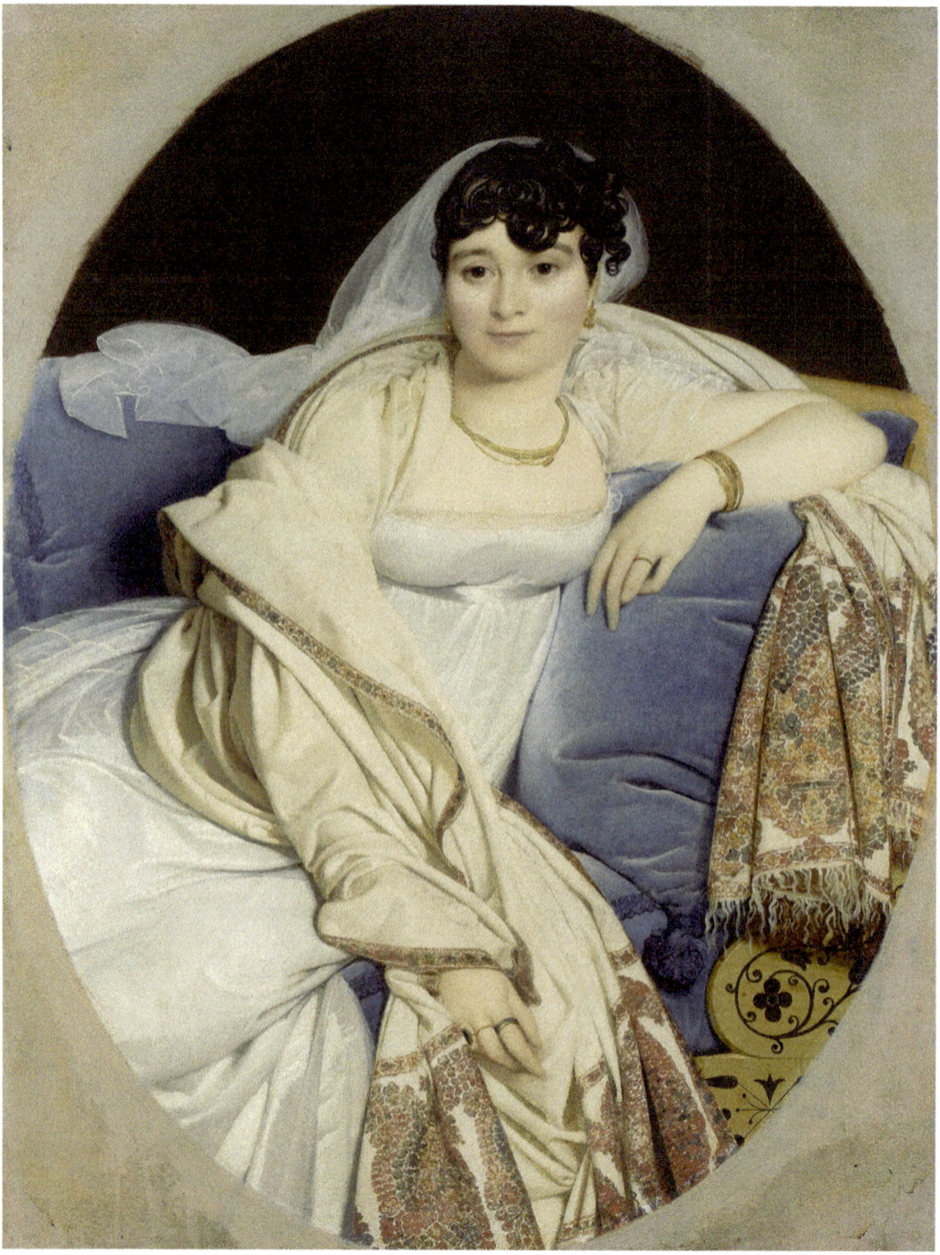

Plate 17 Jean-Auguste-Dominique Ingres, *Marie-Françoise Rivière* (detail), 1805, oil on canvas, 116 x 90 cm.

Introduction 1

Pedro Almodóvar's 2011 film *La piel que habito* (*The Skin I Live In*) is about a person who does not live in their own skin. The title itself distances the 'I' from 'the skin' inhabited. It disconnects the metonymic association of a person's skin with their life or identity made in many languages, for example in English when a person is called a 'good skin'. Almodóvar's film suggests a number of themes around skin that are pertinent to this book: skin and identity; the relations between inside and outside; the nude and its colour; artificial skin and fantasies of the human creation of life; skin, touch and the haptic potential of vision; finally, the relationship between skin's role as a medium and the mediality of the image.

The film starts with views of a well-gated country estate near the town of Toledo in Spain, and quickly moves to images of incarceration and surveillance: walls, grids, modern home security technology and an electronic eye monitoring a woman doing yoga exercises in a beige body suit that fits like a second skin. In a second sequence skin is addressed from a different angle: a physician is lecturing on face transplantation, and Almodóvar announces the disturbing topic of his film by referencing George Franju's 1960 classic *Les yeux sans visage* (*Eyes Without a Face*), a thriller about an obsessed surgeon who in order to reconstitute the disfigured features of his daughter's face resorts to murder and the harvesting of faces. The two main characters of *The Skin I Live In* – the plastic surgeon Dr Ledgard (Antonio Banderas) and his involuntary subject named Vera (Elena Anaya) – are brought together just a few moments later, at first indirectly. On a life-size plasma screen the surgeon watches Vera in a pose of a reclining nude seen from the back. He sees her as an image and her immaculate skin as a surface to be slowly sampled with the eye. This mediated encounter has already been prepared by shots of a number of paintings featuring female nudes. As the surgeon climbs the staircase to access his living room, he passes full-size reproductions of two paintings by Titian: *The Venus of Urbino* (Uffizi) and *Venus and Organ Player* (Prado) (Figure 1.1). The choice is hardly accidental: Titian's nudes are classic manifestations of the reclining female body in paint and were copied many times.[1] Almodóvar's

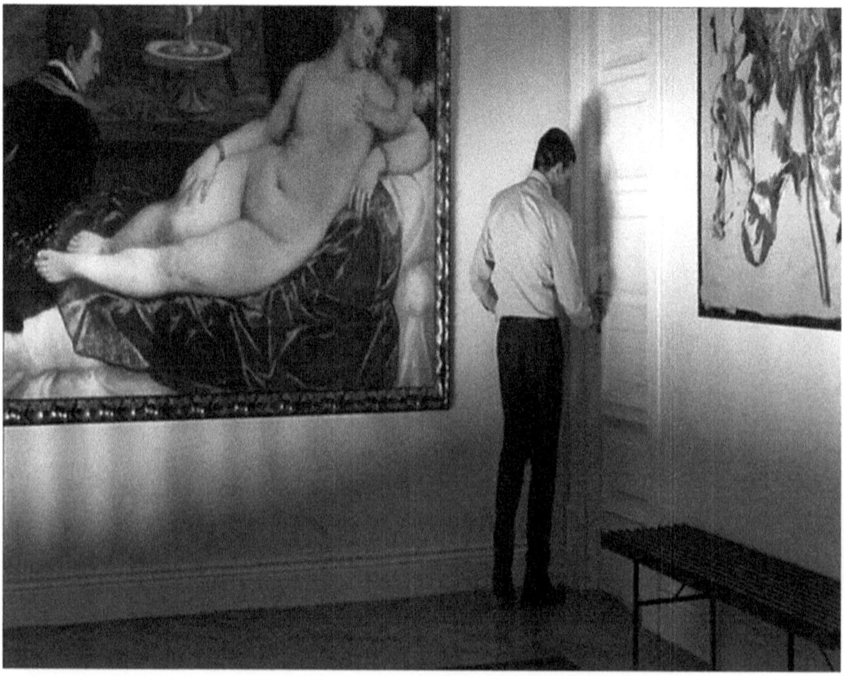

1.1 Screen shot from Pedro Almodovar, *The Skin I Live In*, 2011, 1:38:00.

film continues this chain of repetitions, as Dr Ledgard's surgical subject will mimic and perform reclining nudes throughout the film as she lies on her couch reading, fully aware of being watched, and pretending to turn herself into the persona the surgeon desired to create and wishes to see in her (Figure 1.2). Moreover, Titian's painting, celebrated for the soft and lifelike rendering of the body, is also pertinent to the overall theme of the film, the artificial making of skin. As Daniela Bohde elaborates, Titian was often praised for his quasi mystic ability to transform paint into flesh.[2] Vera's skin, the viewer will learn step by step, is as artificial as painted skin, fabricated by the surgeon and grafted on to the body of a young man.

The film weaves a network of relations between skin, flesh and painted or screened images and, later on, analogies are drawn between skin and the medium of film itself. Most of the time, Vera is quite explicitly seen through the eye of a camera. Kept in a luxurious cage, she interacts with the external world only through architectural orifices and technological interfaces: a vacuum cleaner tube installed in a wall, a dumb waiter, an interphone and, most importantly, two surveillance cameras. One of the latter projects black and white images into the kitchen that are monitored by the housekeeper, the other projects high resolution colour images on to the large screen contemplated by the surgeon.

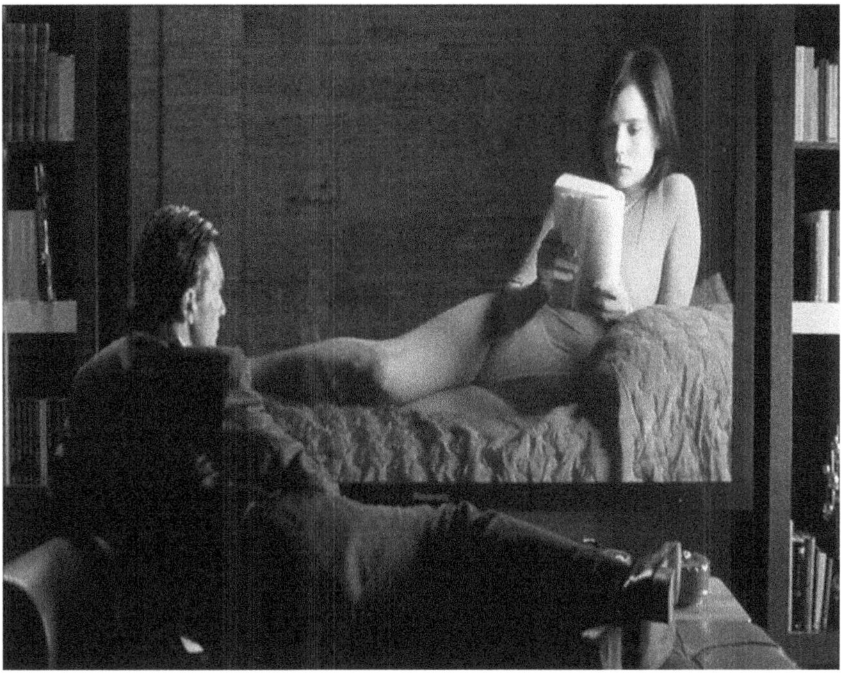

Screen shot from Pedro Almodovar, *The Skin I Live In*, 2011, 1:46:56. 1.2

This controlled life experiment is interrupted when another person in a different kind of artificial hide enters the scene: the housekeeper's delinquent and violent, yet beloved, son Zeca who, taking advantage of the carnival season, hides from the police in a tiger costume. He smuggles himself into the secluded estate by sticking out his naked behind to the camera of an intercommunication system thus identifying himself to his mother via a birth mark. The skin underneath the fake fur seems still able to tell the truth, but ends up being the entry ticket for betrayal. Immediately upon entering the house, Zeca is attracted by the image on the monitor showing Vera doing her exercises, and asks 'What's that?' Trying to hide the existence of the captive skin-patient the housekeeper just says 'it's a film', thus suppressing the content by referring to the medium. But it proves an impossible elusion; in Spanish her words are 'es una película', employing an expression for film that, deriving from the Latin *pelle*, literally means little skin. In Roman languages, the thin celluloid membrane coated with photosensitive material and used since the late nineteenth century as a negative film in analogue photography and later for motion pictures took on the name of the organic skin. And though a video such as that produced by the surveillance camera or a digitally produced film like Almodóvar's is not a film in this strict sense, the word – and with it the analogy with skin – is still present.

This connection has already been made by psychoanalyst Didier Anzieu in his 1985 *Skin Ego*, which has been crucial to numerous subsequent studies on skin:

> In its first sense, the French term '*pellicule*' designates a fine membrane which protects and envelops certain parts of plant or animal organisms; by extension, the word denotes the layer, also fine, of a solid matter on the surface of a liquid or on the outer surface of another solid. In its second sense, '*pellicule*' means the film used in photography, i.e. the thin layer serving as a base for the sensitive coating that is to receive the impression.[3]

The psychoanalyst continues that 'a dream is a "*pellicule*" in both these senses. It constitutes a protective shield which envelops the sleeper's psyche and protects it from the latent activity of the diurnal residues and … and from the excitation' of sensations and physical processes active during sleep. But the *película* produced by the surveillance camera in Almodóvar's film fails to serve as a protective shield, and the displacement only hints to what it seeks to conceal. Unwittingly the housekeeper conflates 'the skin of the film'[4] and the skin in the film: the carefully crafted and monitored skin that wraps Vera. The mother can't stop 'the tiger's' interest in his prey, since he soon sees Vera and thinks he recognises in her features the surgeon's late wife whom the artificial body uncannily resembles. Driven by a wild attraction that befits his animal costume, he violates all boundaries, breaks into the barred room and rapes Vera. This incursion and multiple penetration of screen, doors and a body triggers a series of flashbacks through which the viewer learns about the history of Vera as well as the surgeon's late wife and daughter. Gal, the wife, had an affair with Zeca; and, when trying to run away, the couple had a car accident that left Zeca unharmed but Gal barely alive with serious burns. Dr Ledgard – compensating, it seems, with obsessive care and fantasies of surgical omnipotence – makes every attempt to heal his wife. But having made a humble recovery, and unexpectedly seeing her own distorted features reflected in a glass pane, Gal kills herself by jumping out of a window. The suicide leaves its witness – the couple's little daughter Norma – so traumatised that she needs to be hospitalised and undergo long-term psychiatric treatment. Grown to a pretty teenager and showing signs of improvement, the father takes the unworldly girl to a party where she is approached and raped by a young man himself spaced out by party drugs. The daughter – traumatised again – hides even from her father and returns to hospital. Seeking revenge, the surgeon kidnaps the culprit – Vicente (Jan Cornet) – and uses him for a gruesome experiment: he completely remodels his body, castrating him in a sex change surgery, and grafting an artificial skin made from a mixture of animal and human genes, thus effectively turning Vicente into an artificially engineered body. Ironically, Vicente is renamed Vera, the 'true one'. From Dr

Ledgard's perspective the experiment is a stunning success: Vera is beautiful, resembles the late wife and has an immaculate skin that looks and feels soft while also being, after a series of improvements, flame proof and pain free. This is the skin the surgeon contemplates on the screen, while stretching on his couch mimicking Vera's pose, watching her in empathy and admiration for his own work. But that is precisely the trap. Vera is not as docile as Pygmalion's sculpture Galatea in the well-known story from Ovid's *Metamorphoses*, a myth of godlike artistic creation. The surgeon's product – the person with Vera's features and Vicente's mind (who never gives up his will to return home) – uses the attraction of their body and the narcissistic pride of their creator to foster his desire. Dr Ledgard imprudently trusts Vera's love and allows her to live with him, until s/he seizes the occasion to shoot those who held her/him captive.

Skin and identity are explicitly addressed in an early sequence of the film in which Dr Ledgard lectures on new possibilities of face grafts for victims of disfiguring accidents. The surgeon stresses the significance of this kind of surgery because of the crucial role face and facial skin play to a person's identity. Skin, forming the body's envelope, demarcation and visible aspect, has indeed often been understood as a safeguard of identity. However, any essentialist notion of identity is undermined in the film, as the surgical proposition is to restore identity via a transplant, with someone else's face. Still, Dr Ledgard insists on identity in pointing out that the face is a major means of human non-verbal communication and that skin is attached to the muscles that are responsible for facial expression. He thus addresses the function of skin as an interface for transmitting muscular activity and by extension emotions. The ways in which the face can express feelings, or what early modern writers call passions, through movement and colour change (as in blushing or blanching) have also been a major concern for artists aiming to convey psychological motion through outer appearance. The face's potential to signify has often led to the metaphoric association with canvas and paintings – both face and canvas are surfaces on which colour and line work and produce meaning. Beginning with the French seventeenth-century painter Charles le Brun, artists and physiologists have attempted to codify the passions by aligning specific muscular movements with particular emotions. However, these efforts to manage expression and its pictorial representation could not do away with the challenge that the mobility and transformative character of skin and face brought to artists.

Whether it is about the relatively fixed or rather volatile aspects of the body's surface, skin serves as a mediator between interior and exterior, as a membrane that communicates and filters physiological and psychological processes located inside. It provides, as Elizabeth Harvey suggests, a 'complex border between inside and outside, one that emphasises the shifting, dynamic relation between the two'.[5] Skin's role in negotiating the relation between the physical interior and exterior is particularly pertinent in the context of anatomy, where skin has to be literally removed or at least cut open to grant access to the body's physical interior. In both anatomical texts and images, the skin often becomes a symbol for the practice of anatomy and its way of gaining knowledge through dissection; indirectly however skin also points to anatomy's conundrum of understanding the living body by studying the corpse. In the practices of artistic anatomy, the skin's role remains especially ambivalent, as it hides immediate access to the interior while being the medium and instrument of its revelation.

Skin, the body's tegument, is often conceived as a veil (and vice versa), the physical or symbolic removal of which results in the revelation of an 'inner truth' or essence. The removal of the veil stands in for an act of knowledge production that tends to establish what is often a gendered hierarchy between inside and outside that values interiority at the cost of outer appearance. But, as Jacques Derrida reminds us, it is impossible to do away with the veil, especially through an act of revealing: 'finishing with the veil will always have been the very movement of the veil: un-veiling oneself, reaffirming the veil is unveiling'.[6] In his essay 'A silkworm of one's own', Derrida engages instead with the textility of the veil, and any other wrap or woof. In a similar vein, most recent studies of the cultural history of skin have challenged a hermeneutics that seeks to find hidden meanings, and have resisted the assumption that surfaces are invariably superficial.[7] From an art historical perspective, looking at skin means looking at surfaces of images, and keeping the materiality of skin as surface and part of the body in play. And it also entails factoring in the materiality of the fabricated surfaces of images.

In Almodóvar's film the viewers' customary attempts to read faces and surfaces are frustrated. Vera's exterior is no faithful expression of the inside. As the story of a person who couldn't save their own skin, the film can be interpreted as raising the question of what happens when the mind and inner body inhabit a remodelled envelope. The smooth and even skin most people desire to watch and have for themselves turns out to be monstrous. But rather than reiterating the platonic model of the soul trapped in a body, *The Skin I Live In* leaves its viewers puzzled and even disturbed as to what has become of the I that inhabits the immaculate skin and constitutes its interiority.

Whether the artificial skin still enables Vera/Vincente to have sensory feelings is a question the film leaves, somewhat frustratingly, open. It is the perfect protective barrier, but does it serve as the sense of touch, as is usually the case? Be that as it may, the film certainly activates the sense of touch through the cinematic images of the skin. In one of the scenes in which Dr Ledgard watches Vera on the screen, the camera takes the position of his eyes, and moves towards and across the reclining body. A soft light bathes the skin, and as the film turns more grainy it emphasises the curves and eroticises the body. Such images prompt an embodied kind of viewing, in which, as Laura Marks points out, the eyes seem to touch the film and, in turn, the skin it shows. The images of skin can recall a double sensation of touching and being touched. In *The Skin I Live In* the evocation of touch works in the rather conventional mode of the erotic film as – unlike in the more experimental films Marks analyses in her book – evocation of touch does not coincide with an explicit foregrounding of the materiality of the film. This corresponds with the fact that in the above-mentioned reproductions of Titian's paintings, which are seen from a distance, the materiality of paint and the traces of the painter's brush are completely effaced.

Marks discusses cinematic images that 'appeal to a haptic, or tactile, visuality',[8] and does so without distinguishing between the haptic and the tactile, as the two words – one of Greek, the other of Latin origin – are in fact often used synonymously. For my purposes, however, I propose to make a distinction in order to approach the different ways in which the sense of touch can be mobilised via two-dimensional images and the relationship between seeing and touching can operate. I will thus refer to the 'haptic' in the sense that art historian Alois Riegl and following him Gilles Deleuze and Felix Guattari have defined it, as a quality of smoothly rendered, clearly circumscribed forms that create the illusion of three-dimensionality and thus seem graspable, a 'becoming-haptical of the optical'.[9] Riegl, writing around 1900, contrasted it with the 'painterly',[10] a quality he aligned with the optical. But as an effect produced by the visible traces of the artist's hand, it also has the potential of stimulating tactility via the sight of the materiality of paint and brushstroke. I will address this latter form of touch in my chapter on eighteenth-century philosophical and art theoretical debates on the sense of touch and the artist's touch (both referred to as *la touche* in French), and the significance of brush-strokes in Fragonard's *portraits de fantaisie*. In contrast, the manner in which smooth surfaces can evoke the haptic will be an issue in relation to painted skin in works by Ingres (addressed in chapter 7).

Even though the protagonists of Almodóvar's film would be considered as 'white' in current modes of categorising skin, all skin, and in particular Vera's skin, has by no means a uniform or stable colour: it is honey-coloured when softly lit, and pale in the bright light of the operating theatre. Mostly though, Vera's skin remains covered under her jump suit, which looks like a tailored full body bandage as it has the standard colour of medical plaster. It is a shade that the fashion industry often labelled 'nude', a designation that has recently become contested as much as the biased neutrality of the colour of bandages. 'Nude' became an issue when Michelle Obama wore an evening dress described by its designer as 'nude strapless gown', and by an Associate Press journalist as 'flesh-coloured'.[11] 'Whose nude?' or 'whose flesh?' some rightly asked, and pointed out that Crayola, the American manufacturer of crayons and pencils, had changed the name of their 'flesh colour' to 'peach' by the 1960s.[12] 'Nude' and 'flesh colour' (and equivalents in other European languages) were designations for the colour of the body throughout the period considered in this book. They remain variable as long as they are attached to actual bodies and their colour, rather than being transferred to the systems of colour charts that abstract from the ties that colours and their names once had with the materiality of things and bodies.

Skin, flesh and colour have been a long-standing conglomerate. The ancient Greek notion of colour (*chrôma*) derives from *chrôs* – skin.[13] In contrast to *derma*, which is closer to the English word 'hide' and can also refer to animals and to skin that has been removed, *chrôs* specifically designates the visible surface of the living human body. In the vocabulary of the Homeric epics it is delicate and vulnerable, but also linked with beauty, and transformative in relation to emotions' change of colour. Because skin could be tinted it became a synonym for colour, and the intimate relation between the two outlived the emancipation of the notion of colour during the classical period.[14] Colour kept its alliance with the changeable complexions of the living in the medical theories of the Hippocratic Collection.[15] Early modern notions of flesh tones remain close to the Greek *chrôs* in the sense that they relate simultaneously to the visible body, including its coloration, and to its living substance, to the 'fleshy body with depth and surface fused together'.[16] Both in ancient culture and medieval Europe the words for colours were generally tied to the materials and objects which were of that colour (as is, for instance, still the case for gold or orange). It is however with flesh and skin that this way of linking colour and materiality was particularly persistent: notions like flesh tones – or *carnazione* in Italian or *carnations* in French – continued to be used in the art literature to designate both the tone of flesh and the imitation made from it. What is special about 'flesh' or 'nude' as a tone is that one doesn't know what shade it actually is, unless it refers to a particular person or a particular painted flesh. Of course, recipes for mixing flesh tones in artists' manuals, typically talk about mixtures that would produce some shade of rose, thus privileging people and ideals of beauty prevalent in Europe. Still, the proportions of pigments can always vary, and flesh tones are variable mixtures that are understood – as I will argue – in analogy to complexions. According to the Hippocratic theory of humours, developed in classical Greece and relevant in Europe until well into the nineteenth century, a person's colour or complexion is produced by varying compositions of four main bodily saps. Unlike the modern notion of skin colour, which has since the eighteenth century been tied to the classification of humans into races, complexions and flesh tones are open to transformation.

Vera's skin, to return one more time to Almodóvar's film, is both breathing and artificial, as lifelike and man-made as flesh tones painted on a canvas.

The Skin I Live In can be seen as playing on multiple levels with the crucial association of human skin and the image or medium in which it is represented: the skin of the film and the skin of the body are aligned with each other and with the painted skin of Titian's female nudes. The film thus takes up long established traditions of skin as a medium and of skin and flesh as the site in which artificial bodies are made lifelike. Skin has been called the oldest human medium, and the *longue durée* material history of skin as a medium dates back to pre-historic times when practices such as body painting or tattooing were used to decorate, inscribe or modify the body.[17] Beyond the living human body, skin has also been a regular support for images and letters. Books were initially made of animal hide – parchment – after the Roman codex, the earliest form of the book with pages bound together, had gradually replaced scrolls and other writing media. The material, typically the de-haired and limed skin of a calf (usually called vellum), goat or sheep, was valued for its durability. As is well known, medieval manuscripts and illuminations were generally also written and painted on parchment. But even though paper mostly superseded parchment as a material for books with the invention of the printing press, there is still a metaphorical linkage of skin and paper.[18]

The skin's capacity to be the human body's surface and to also form its outer appearance makes it comparable to images, whether photograph and film, or the media considered in this book: paintings, prints and drawings. It is a surface to be looked at, and a ground on to which images can be painted, drawn, incised or projected. This makes skin a very specific object, a privileged surface to be represented in film or other visual media. Skin variously blends with the ground of the image, its surface, or its crafted texture. It is the shared quality of skin and the visual image that gives imitations or reproductions of skin a self-referential quality, or to put it in Victor Stoichita's terms, they are the site where images have the potential to become self-aware.[19]

Skin is not only a medium, it is also matter. This has been especially stressed in recent art historical studies on skin, flesh and art, notably those by Daniela Bohde, Marianne Koos and Anne-Sophie Lehman.[20] It is in this vein that this book aims to 'flesh out surfaces'. It takes its starting point from the fact that the painting of the naked parts of the living human body is traditionally referred to in terms of flesh rather than skin, in terms of its materiality and coloured substance. But the book also looks at skin as thick and multilayered, as part of the body as well as its surface; and it studies the ways in which skin connects with the materiality of media and processes of image making, in which it is not only represented but also mimicked, made or re-enacted.[21] For example, the tissue of skin can be mimicked with the cross hatching of an engraving or the texture of the artist's brushwork. The complexion can be re-enacted with the mixture of dyes in colour printing, and skin colour is literally made in paintings. In all these ways images from both the medical and artistic realms not only embed pre-existing knowledge but also produce knowledge of the human's outermost organ, and thus contribute to the changing understanding of the physiology and substance of the body and its envelope.

This book will thus explore the multiple relations between skin and the image, between colour and nakedness, between paint and flesh. And even though it assumes that certain phenomenological qualities of skin as the surface, and of flesh as the substance of the human body, result in long-lasting affiliations between these organic matters and the media in which they are rendered, I aim to make historical rather than ontological arguments. Hence, while Anzieu's book has been very productive for thinking about the significance of skin, about the multiple symbolic meanings the human envelope can take on, and about the interconnectedness of body and psyche, I question its normative aspects, including the 'need to set limits'[22] that a study by a practising psychoanalyst may need to insist upon. Like many other cultural historians and historians of the body or the skin, I assume that there was a gradual shift in the understanding and the lived experience of the body and its contours between the early modern and modern period. And, I agree with anthropologist Mary Douglas that the human body is a 'complex structure' that can take on multiple, but culturally specific, meanings and can stand for a variety of boundary systems.[23] Following up on the work by scholars such as Michael Bakhtin, Claudia Benthien, Barbara Duden, Michel Foucault, Dorinda Outram, Philippe Sarasin, Barbara Stafford and Paul Vigarello, my argument is that there is – from the late eighteenth century onwards – a new focus on the surface and the borderlines of the body and a new understanding of the skin as physical demarcation of the self. This shift is also played out in a discourse so far barely considered for histories of the body: art literature. As this book will show, the word 'skin' rather than 'flesh' is used with increasing frequency when referring to the surface or substance an artist imitates when painting the naked parts of a human body. This process runs parallel, and is connected with, the medicalisation of skin that has emerged since the seventeenth century, when the organ of touch and its colour came under intensified medical, including microscopic, scrutiny.

While these historical shifts are significant for early modern Europe more widely speaking, my study focuses on France and the specific transformations of the concepts of flesh, skin and epidermis in the French art literature since the foundation of the Académie royale in 1648 and in the debates prompted by it. Further on it takes into account the emerging genres of art criticism and specialised dictionaries that bring art and the reasoning about it to broader audiences. And it is within a discursive constellation specific to mid-eighteenth-century France – characterised by intense interaction between the discourses of art literature, medicine and philosophy – that the ties between new notions of skin as tissue and the fabricated surface of paintings, as well as between the sense of touch and *la touche*, the painterly brushwork, become uniquely close. Likewise, the context of the French Revolution with its promise and violence puts particular pressure on the variously interconnected notions of the self and portraiture, on neoclassicism and its obsession with whiteness and on the problems of skin colour. Furthermore, artistic anatomy, to which one of my chapters is dedicated, develops specific practices in nineteenth-century France and in relation to the École des beaux-arts in Paris. The idiosyncratic new genre of publications called 'Anatomy of exterior forms' allocated to skin a newly defined role as interface. Ingres' manner of hermetically sealing the painted body is – I will argue – both in line with this novel focus on surfaces and a rejection of artistic anatomy and the relationship between interior and exterior it establishes.

Engaging with the interrelations between artistic practices, and the discourses of art and medicine, this book aims to understand the historically specific terms in which artists could think of the body, its substance and surface. If I am talking about 'thinking' in this context, it is in the sense Michael Baxandall has given it in his *Patterns of Intention* where he stresses:

> 'Thought' can mean a range of things, and it seems important not to suggest that philosophy or science are more or better thought than what a painter does as he paints … the typical form of thought in a picture is something more like 'process', the attention to a developing pictorial problem in the course of activity in a pictorial medium.[24]

Baxandall's work has recently regained pertinence due to its early interest in materials and materiality, and the ways artists think pictorially. His *Patterns of Intention* provides astute methodological propositions for relating images and discourses in meaningful ways. Thus keeping the question in mind of how one can 'move from a vague sense of affinity towards something critically useful and historically sustainable',[25] my study seeks to show that questions of the texture, substance and colour of flesh or skin are as much of painterly as they are of medical concern, and to elaborate on the relations and mediations between these fields. While taking a historical approach, this book does not construct a seamless, mono-directional historical narrative nor does it provide a comprehensive history of flesh and skin in art. The six chapters are roughly organised in chronological order – ranging from a discussion of seventeenth- and early eighteenth-century art theoretical, medical and philosophical discourses to a study of skin and surfaces in the nineteenth-century female nudes and portraits by Jean-Auguste-Dominique Ingres. Several sections take their own *longue durée* perspective, and each chapter takes a slightly different angle and theme: flesh and flesh tones; tissue, textures and the sense of touch; complexions and skin colour; skin as sensitive limit; as semi-transparent veil in artistic anatomy; and finally skin as hermetic surface and borderline. All of them deal with the multiple exchanges between the world of images and medical discourse; they demonstrate the role of art theory and anatomical publications dedicated to artists as intermediaries, while highlighting simultaneously that the exchange is no one-way street. A number of words used in colloquial and medical language today derive from the area of the arts and the crafts: the word 'pigment' for example derives from the Latin *pingere* – to paint – and only moved into medical language around 1800. 'Tissue' referred to a man-made woven fabric before it entered the parlance of natural philosophers and physicians to describe organic material. And, as chapter 2 elaborates, one particular image had a role to play in the establishment of this metaphor, which first appears in medical language in relation to skin. To mobilise the migration of metaphors between art and medicine, two chapters 'Nervous canvas' and 'Sensitive limit' take up medical designations of skin to provide a model for thinking about the rendering of skin in contemporary paintings. Overall, the images discussed range from seminal medical images of skin and skin colour via the illustrations for nineteenth-century artistic anatomies to paintings by Fragonard, David, Girodet, Benoist and Ingres. The focus in the latter field is (with a few exceptions) on portraits, and not on nudes despite the abundance of skin and flesh displayed there. Portraits are images of the body after all, and the usually disclosed facial skin is a special site for testing painterly skills and one where the body (for example in blushing or the display of emotions) and the image made of it become particularly expressive. What is more, from Cennino Cennini's late medieval artist's manual, via Le Blon's introduction to the techniques of colour printing, to the art criticism of Denis Diderot, the head and face (most often a woman's head) are frequently the model employed to explain the making and difficulties of skin and flesh tones in colour images.

The choice of artists and specific works is based on my view that these images do not only depict skin, but are *about* skin and skin colour. Each set of portraits brings a particular aspect of skin via distinct painterly procedures to the fore: skin as colourful sense organ full of nervous energy in Fragonard's *Portraits de fantaisie*; as sensitive limit and semi-transparent screen in David's post-revolutionary portraits; or the interconnected political and painterly issues of skin colour in Girodet's *Jean-Baptiste Belley* and Benoist's *Portrait d'une négresse*. The book ends with a chapter on a selection of nudes and portraits by Ingres and the artist's radical manner of sealing the painted surface. Human nakedness painted by Ingres is about skin rather than flesh. Flesh had been written out of medical discourse by the end of the nineteenth century and been replaced by differentiated tissues defined via their specific structure and function. This does not mean though that flesh is a disappearing matter in the modern world. It becomes the body's undisciplined substance and as the *informe* it continues to be associated with paint. The objective of this book is thus to discuss embodiment in images as an ongoing problem and contested issue.

Notes

1 Maria Loh, *Titian Remade: Repetition and the Transformation of Early Modern Italian Art* (Los Angeles/Cal.: Getty Publications, 2007).
2 See in particular her book on skin, flesh and colour in Titian – Daniela Bohde, *Haut, Fleisch und Farbe: Körperlichkeit und Materialität in den Gemälden Tizians* (Emstetten: Edition Imorde, 2002); and '"Le tinte delle carni": zur Begrifflichkeit von Haut und Fleisch in italienischen Kunsttraktaten des 15.–17. Jahrhunderts', in Daniela Bohde and Mechthild Fend (eds), *Weder Haut noch Fleisch: das Inkarnat in der Kunstgeschichte* (Berlin: Gebr. Mann, 2007), pp. 41–63.
3 Didier Anzieu, *The Skin Ego* [1985], trans. Chris Turner (New Haven; London: Yale University Press, 1989), p. 210.
4 Laura Marks, *The Skin of the Film: Intercultural Cinema, Embodiment, and the Senses* (Durham/N.C.; London: Duke University Press, 2000).
5 Elizabeth D. Harvey, 'The touching organ: allegory, anatomy, and the Renaissance skin envelope', in Elizabeth D. Harvey (ed.), *Sensible Flesh: On Touch in Early Modern Culture* (Philadelphia: University of Pennsylvania Press, 2003), pp. 81–102 (p. 85).
6 Jacques Derrida, 'A silkworm of one's own', in Hélène Cixous and Jacques Derrida, *Veils*, trans. Geoffrey Bennington (Stanford/Cal.: Stanford University Press, 2001), p. 25.
7 See in particular Claudia Benthien, *Skin: On the Cultural Border Between Self and the World* [1999], trans. Thomas Dunlap (New York; Chichester: Columbia University Press, 2002); and with particular regard to early modern images of flaying Daniela Bohde, 'Skin and the search for the interior: the representation of flaying in the art and anatomy of the cinquecento', in Florike Egmond and Robert Zwijnenberg (eds), *Bodily Extremities: Preoccupations with the Human Body in Early Modern European Culture* (Ashgate: Aldershot, 2003), pp. 10–47.
8 Marks, *The Skin of the Film*, p. 2.
9 Gilles Deleuze and Felix Guattari in their chapter 'The smooth and the striated' of *A Thousand Plateaux: Capitalism and Schizophrenia*, trans. Brian Massumi (Minneapolis/Minn.: University of Minnesota Press, 1987), pp. 492–3; see for a critical discussion of it Jacques Derrida, *On Touching, Jean-Luc Nancy*, [2000], trans. Christine Irizarry (Stanford/Cal.: Stanford University Press, 2005), pp. 123–6; see further Laura Marks, *Touch: Sensous Theory and Multisensory Media* (Minneapolis; London: University of Minnesota Press, 2002), pp. 4–9.
10 See in particular his theoretical overview in Alois Riegl, *Historical Grammar of the Visual Arts*, trans. Jacqueline E. Jung (New York: Zone Books, 2004). The text was initially written between 1897 and 1899, but published only in 1966; see in particular the introduction to the chapter on 'Form and Surface', pp. 395–400. On Riegl and haptic vision see Mechthild Fend, '"Körpersehen": über das Haptische bei Alois Riegl', in Andreas Mayer and Alexandre Métraux (eds), *Kunstmaschinen: Spielräume des Sehens zwischen Wissenschaft und Kunst* (Frankfurt a. M.: Fischer, 2005), pp. 166–202.
11 Morvenna Ferrier et al., 'The trouble with nudity in fashion', *Guardian*, 10 May 2010, www.theguardian.com/lifeandstyle/2010/may/20/fashion-colour-nude-racist.

12 Samantha Critchell, 'What colour is "nude"? Fashion debates a loaded term', *Associated Press*, 17 May 2010, www.nola.com/fashion/index.ssf/2010/05/what_color_is_nude_fashion_deb.html.
13 Steven Connor, *The Book of Skin* (London: Reaktion Books, 2004), pp. 10–11.
14 Marcello Carastro, 'La notion de *khrôs* chez Homère: éléments pour une anthropologie de la couleur en Grèce ancienne', in Marcello Carastro (ed.), *l'Antiquité en couleurs: catégories, pratiques, représentations* (Grenoble: Jérôme Millon, 2009), pp. 301–13; Adeline Grand-Clément, *La fabrique des couleurs: histoire du paysage des Grecs anciens* (Paris: de Broccard, 2011), in particular pp. 33–42.
15 Carastro, 'La notion de *khrôs* chez Homère', p. 310.
16 Valeria Gavrylenko, 'The body without skin', in Manfred Horstmanshoff, Helen King and Claus Zittel (eds), *Blood, Sweat and Tears: The Changing Concepts of Physiology from Antiquity into Early Modern Europe* (Leiden: Brill, 2012), pp. 481–502 (p. 489).
17 Charles Grivel, 'Der siderale Körper: zum Prinzip des Kommunikation', in J. Hörisch and M. Wenzel (eds), *Armaturen der Sinne: literarische und technische Medien 1870 bis 1920* (München: Fink, 1990), pp. 177–99. I have further explored this aspect of skin in a study of Valie Export's *Body Sign Action*, see Fend, 'Zeichen in der Oberfläche: Valie Exports body sign action', *Psychoanalyse im Widerspruch*, 15:29 (2003), 51–9; see also Bernadette Wegenstein, *Getting Under the Skin: The Body and Media Theory* (Cambridge/Mass.: MIT Press, 2006).
18 The relationship between skin and the book has been explored by Ulrike Zeuch in *Verborgen im Buch. Verborgen im Körper: Haut zwischen 1500 und 1800*, exh. cat. Herzog Anton August Bibliothek Wolfenbüttel (Wiesbaden: Harrowitz, 2003).
19 Victor Stoichita, *The Self-Aware Image: An Insight into Early Modern Meta-Painting* [1993] (Cambridge: Cambridge University Press, 1997).
20 Bohde, *Haut, Fleisch und Farbe*; Marianne Koos, *Haut, Farbe und Medialität: Oberfläche im Werk von Jean-Étienne Liotard (1702–1789)* (Paderborn: Fink, 2014); Ann-Sophie Lehmann, 'The matter of the medium: some tools for an art theoretical interpretation of materials', in Christy Anderson et al. (eds), *The Matter of Art: Materials, Practices, Cultural Logics, c. 1250–1750* (Manchester: Manchester University Press, 2015), pp. 21–41; and 'Fleshing out the body: the "colours of the naked" in workshop practice and art theory, 1400–1600', in Ann-Sophie Lehmann and Herman Roodenburg (eds), *Body and Embodiment in Netherlandish Art. Nederlands Kunsthistorisch Jaarboek* 58 (Zwolle: Wanders, 2008), pp. 86–109.
21 Hanna Rose Shell has developed this productive notion for analysing the casting techniques Bernard Palissy used for his *rustiques figulines* as a re-enactment of processes of fossilisation' see her article: 'Casting life, recasting experience: Bernard Palissy's occupation between maker and nature', *Configurations*, 12 (2004), 1–40.
22 Anzieu, *Skin Ego*, p. 6.
23 Mary Douglas, *Purity and Danger: An Analysis of Concepts of Pollution and Taboo* (London: Routledge and Kegan Paul, 1966), p. 138.
24 Michael Baxandall, *Patterns of Intention: On the Historical Explanation of Pictures* (New Haven; London: Yale University Press, 1985), pp. 74–5.
25 Ibid., p. 75.

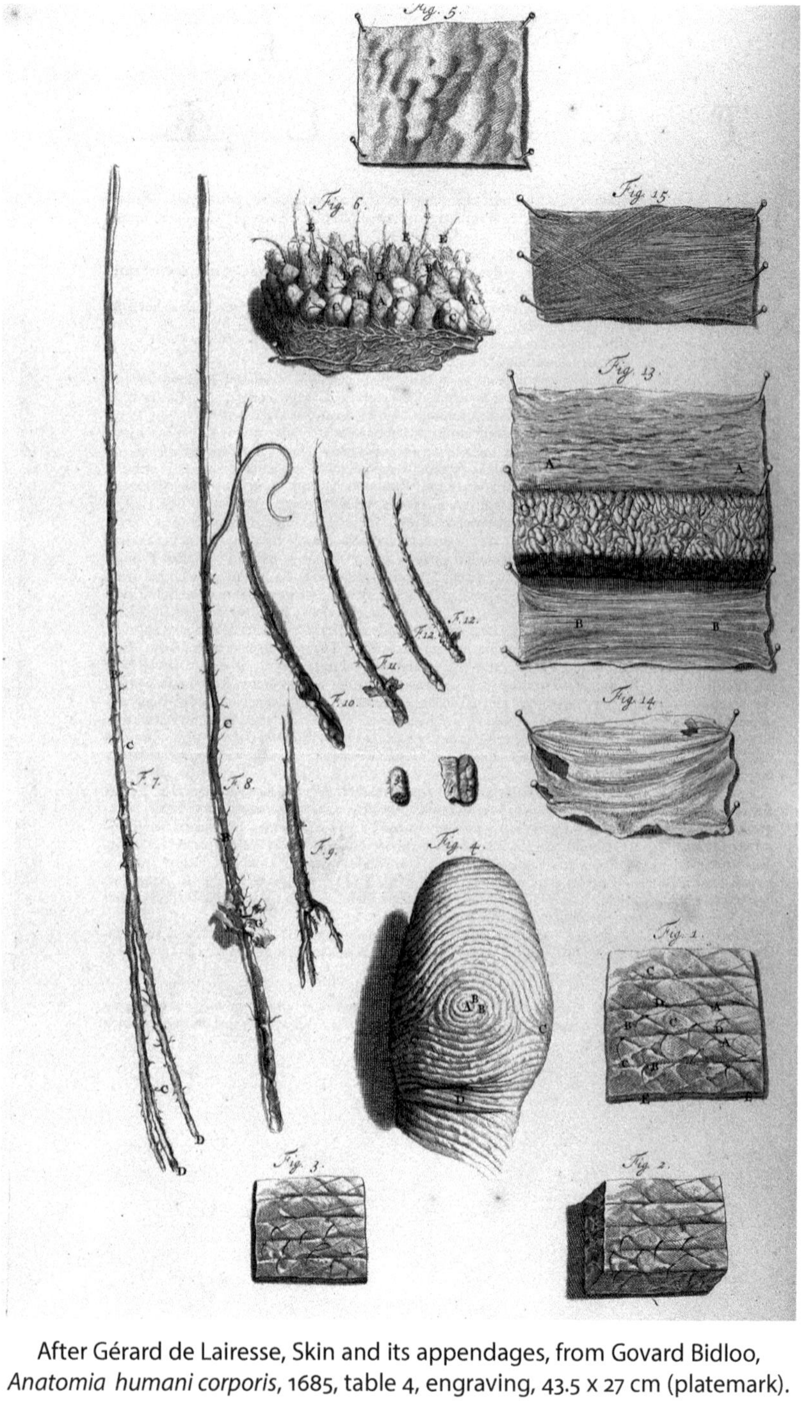

2.1 After Gérard de Lairesse, Skin and its appendages, from Govard Bidloo, *Anatomia humani corporis*, 1685, table 4, engraving, 43.5 x 27 cm (platemark).

The surface's substance 2

The naked areas an artist represents when painting a human body were traditionally not conceived of in terms of skin but of flesh. It was the body's substance, its living matter, rather than its surface that was meant to be brought on to the canvas (or any other support such as wood, or a wall in the case of frescoes). The medieval and early modern art literature referred to painterly imitations of the unclothed human body in terms related to flesh: the Italian *carnagioni* as well as the French *carnation* derived from the Latin word for flesh and meat. Skin was however not absent from art discourse: it was used as a metaphor to describe various kinds of crafted surfaces. Leon Battista Alberti in his famous treatise on architecture, *De re aedificatoria*, written around 1450, and first printed posthumously in 1486, described any architectural surface – walls, roofs, tiled floors or ceilings – or smoothly plastered or varnished surfaces as skins.[1] With respect to painting, both the support, in particular the canvas or the priming coat of a wall prepared for fresco painting, and the outer layers of a painting – a thin final membrane of paint or even the patina resulting from aging – could be considered as skin.[2] From this metaphoric use of the word 'skin', it can be concluded vice versa that this part of the body was generally considered a membrane, a garment-like envelope rather than an organ with a certain density itself. In what follows I will initially discuss notions of flesh and flesh tones in the European art literature, and then show how skin slowly made its entry into French art theory during the eighteenth century. As I argue throughout the next two chapters, skin came to be perceived as a different thing during the early modern period, both as a scientific object and an object of representation (Figure 2.1). In accordance with the new medical understanding of the dermis as a tissue built of interwoven layers, eighteenth-century art practice and discourse turned skin into a complex organ that was supposed to be rendered via an appropriately textured painterly brushwork.

Incarnation: painting as embodiment

In Christian culture, the genesis and the incarnation of Christ provided strong models for the generation of images, and the painting of the human figure could be literally understood as an embodiment.[3] Flesh – in the sense of the living substance of the body – was the aim of the imitation in paint. The Italian artist and writer Cennino Cennini described painting in his well-known late fourteenth-century treatise *Il Libro dell'Arte* explicitly as a process of embodiment. While earlier manuals, including ancient ones, had already treated the highly sensitive matter of the rendering of skin and flesh,[4] Cennini combined instructions for painters with theoretical reflections on painting as a medium for the simulation of nature. As has been convincingly argued by Christiane Kruse, he did so in choosing the notion of *incarnazione* for the process of the becoming of an image when a human being is frescoed on a wall.[5] Kruse's argument is that '*incarnazione* is a meta-pictorial metaphor, which describes painting as a process of embodiment'.[6] The term itself is of theological origins and designates the Christian mystery that God became flesh in the person of Christ, and most closely refers to the prologue of the Gospel according to John stating that the word was made flesh ('verbum caro facto est'), also interpreted as logos, the divine principle of reason that became flesh for the sake of men.[7]

Operating within a theological framework throughout, Cennini opened his treatise with a reference to the Christian genesis, and in particular to God's creation of man after his own image. From the outset, he thus related human art production to divine creation and quite originally expanded the idea that man was made in the visual likeness of God in his endowment with God's virtues. Adam, gaining insight into his failure after the fall, used his divine gifts to realise 'theoretically that some means of living by labour had to be found',[8] whereupon he and Eve found practical skills out of which other useful human occupations developed. Among those, Cennini singled out painting, as it couples manual skills with imagination (*fantasia*), enabling the artist to represent and fix 'what does not actually exist'[9] under the guise of natural objects. He thus foregrounded the non-mechanical aspects of art production and in the same vein likened the painter to the poet who equally uses his imagination to produce figures unknown in the natural world. The more striking aspect of this manual is, though, that Cennini sought to enhance the status of the visual arts not only by stressing their intellectual aspects, but more importantly by teasing out the transformative potential of the work of painting. The ability to embody a figure on a wall thus becomes crucial. Cennini mentioned this act of embodiment at various occasions in the text, most importantly in a chapter on the 'Red called cinabrese, for doing flesh (*incarnare*) on the wall',[10] stressing the significance of the red pigment for the lifelike rendering of the human body. Cinnabar or vermilion, a synthetic version of the former produced since the

Middle Ages, are both scarlet-coloured mineral pigments based on mercuric sulphide and were traditionally associated with blood; Cennini made this link specifically in his chapter on how to paint wounds.[11] This blood-red pigment containing quicksilver is a central ingredient of lifelikeness. In chapter 67 entitled 'The method and system for working on the wall, that is, in fresco; and on painting and doing flesh (*incarnare*) for a youthful face',[12] Cennini elaborated on how to render the face of a young woman (who is later specified as Virgin Mary) by paying close attention to the ways in which the painter should use three gradations of pink not only to make the flesh tone credible and to give the face a healthy, lifelike appearance by reddening checks and lips, but also for shading and to give the figure *reliefo*. It is thus the combination of the production of a plausible flesh tone with that of an illusion of three-dimensionality that ensures the incarnation on the wall. Written within the context of fourteenth-century Italian humanism, Cennini's treatise was part of a movement aspiring towards a new valorisation of the visual. The choice of the charged theological term *incarnazione* for the painting of a human figure is a major argument in this endeavour and by using it, Cennini imbued the (minutely described) painterly skills with a mystical component, understanding the transformation of paint into the image of a human body almost as a transubstantiation during which paint turns into flesh.

The term *incarnazione* remained specific to Italian art literature, had its historical momentum within the late medieval argument for the revaluation of the visual arts, and soon lost its significance. It was employed rarely in fifteenth-century Italian art treatises and was mostly replaced by the notion of *carnazione*, thus losing the magical 'in' with which embodiment was marked as a process.[13] However, as Bohde argues, *carne* and *carnazione* could take on the metaphysical dimension of the theological term,[14] and played a role in mystifying painting as creation of life on canvas. This is certainly the case in an early seventeenth-century French treatise on painting techniques, Étienne Binet's chapter on art from his *Essay des merveilles de nature* (1621), which was also taken up almost word for word in a slightly later manuscript compiled in Paris by the painter Pierre Lebrun. In Binet's account, the mixing of pigments is likened to procreation as the palette was literally described as 'mother of all colours' on which are placed the 'mother colours'. Out of the mixture of these colours the painter's 'pencil will create [*faire naistre*], and as it were, cause to flourish all kinds of colours'.[15] The mixing of colours performed by the artist's brush on the maternal palette is thus analogised to a generative act. While the 'mother colours' listed are the main ten pigments for an artist to use, the *palette de carnation* is specifically mentioned in this context, so that the mixing of the flesh colours becomes a creation of human flesh. Flesh tones are the paradigm of colour mixture and in many seventeenth- and eighteenth-century portraits of painters the palette is shown in the manner described by Binet and later by de Piles, among others, with the main colours organised separately along the border and some premixed shades of flesh tones in the centre, near where the artist's thumb reaches through the hole (Plate 1).

Flesh and fleshiness (*carne, carnositá*) became the favoured material and quality that determined an artist's capacity to establish lifelikeness in a painting. Imitating the tone and softness (*morbidezza*) of flesh correctly would guarantee that not only the painted bodies but the entire painting would look alive.[16] Beautiful and beautifully painted bodies were meant to be fleshy, not skinny. Not surprisingly then, the notion of skin never occurred in discussions of painted healthy young bodies. In contrast to flesh, skin had a rather negative connotation in this context and was used only whenever the human envelope is perceptible as an independent entity, as in representations of old or cadaverous bodies with folded skin.[17] Skin is also named as such when the integument is removed. Depictions of this gruesome act were particularly prominent in sixteenth-century art, for example in representations of the flaying of the satyr Marsyas or of Saint Bartholomew, in Titian's *Flaying of Marsyas* or Michelangelo's *Bartholomew* from the Sistine Chapel.[18] Another pertinent sixteenth-century rendition is an engraving produced in Italy by German printmaker Melchior Meier (Figure 2.2). It features Apollo triumphantly holding Marsyas' removed skin. The satyr, who was punished for his

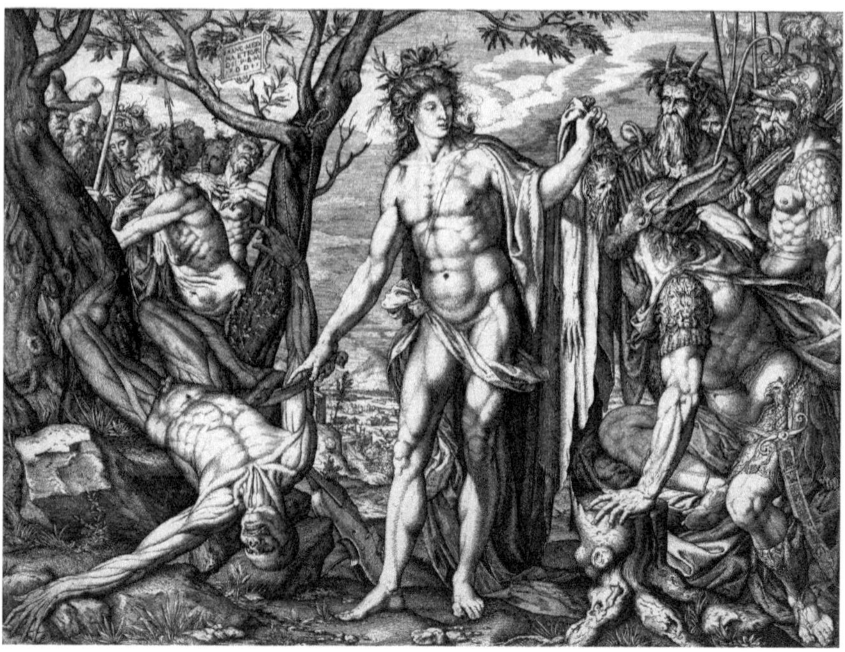

2.2 Melchior Meier, *The Flaying of Marsyas*, 1581, engraving, 23 x 31.2 cm.

hubris, is lying head upside down, half suspended in a tree with a terrified face and his inner body laid bare. With the exposed and clearly detailed muscles, the print makes a connection between the violent punishment and anatomical dissection, while simultaneously displaying the artist's own anatomical knowledge.[19] In turn, some anatomical imagery of the period references the iconography of flaying, staging dissection as a violent process of revelation, an aspect I will return to in chapter 6.

A structural element of the discourse on the lifelike image of the intact, fleshed human body – both in the Italian and Northern tradition – is the intertwining of the body, its colour and the image. The same word is frequently used for flesh or skin as a substance, for its colour and for the imitation made of it. As early as the twelfth century, the monk Theophilus Presbyter stated in his *De diversis artibus*, a comprehensive account of artists' working methods, that you need a colour called skin (*membrana*) to paint the basic tone of faces and naked bodies. It consists of lead white and vermilion, which the artist is meant to mix until 'it is like flesh'.[20] Besides *membrana* a variety of pigment mixtures are then used for the shades, and to indicate the facial features. Using the term *membrana* for the basic flesh tone, Theophilus emphasised the relationship between the painterly process of layering colours to imitate skin and the quality of the organ as a layer. Dedicating the first of the three books of his manuscript to the art of painting and the first chapter to 'The Mixture of Pigments for Nude Bodies' (*De temperamento colorum in nudis corporibus*), he explained in detail what mixture and layering of whites with cinnabar are needed to represent the naked part of bodies, but the result is not referred to as, let's say, light pink, but as *membrana*, a colour that thus merges with the material it depicts. While *membrana* suggests a film or skin and puts the focus on the layering of paint, most treatises refer to the entire body, its substance and hence volume along with colour when it comes to the painting of flesh. In tracts written between the late Middle Ages and the eighteenth century in Germanic languages, words such as body colour (*lybfarb*), human (*mensch*) and even life colour (*lebendfarb*) are to be found.[21] The same goes for Cennini: *incarnazion* is the colour with which to realise (incarnate) *incarnazione*. In a similar vein the anonymous author of an early fifteenth-century Bolognese manuscript suggests that the artist should use flesh tone to 'flesh figures' ('Ad fatiendum incarnatum pro incarnare figuras').[22] This entanglement of the terms should not be understood as simply redundant, or as a naïve inability to recognise the difference between representation and represented. After all, all of these authors wrote artists' manuals and could not have been more aware of the madeness of the painted skin or flesh. It rather testifies to an early modern mode of analogical thinking in which like is made with like. What is more, their use of the terms is in line with the ways colours were more generally referred to in antiquity and the Middle Ages: not with abstract designations (red, blue etc.), but with the names of the materials that embodied certain hues, and from which, in certain cases, pigments for painters were made. Beyond that, the employment of a single word for the hue of the paint, the hue the body, and the image made from it, is an indication of the complexity of the representational task given that the painting of flesh was regarded as the primary site of lifelikeness.[23] What is intriguing about these notions of *membrana*, *lybfarb* or *incarnazion* is that they are oblivious to the kinds of distinctions we are used to making today when talking about skin colour. We could dismiss Theophilus's or Cennini's mixtures of white with vermilion meant to represent generic flesh tones, as implicitly instating a supremacy of whiteness. But I propose (as I will further elaborate in chapter 5) to mobilise the potential of these terms for conceptualising a person's colour beyond classifications such as 'person of colour'.

In fifteenth-century France there was already an awareness of the complexity and significance of the vocabulary for flesh tones. Jean Lebègue, secretary to the French King Charles VI and a humanist with a keen interest in the arts, assembled a number of medieval art manuals and recipe books (including Theophilus's *De diversis artibus*) and compiled a dictionary of technical terms with a long list of words for flesh tones under the lemma *carnatura*.[24] By the beginning of the seventeenth century the term *carnation*, like the previously discussed terms that typically designate both the colour of the flesh and the imitation made of it, was firmly established in French art literature, and became an increasingly important art theoretical notion. André Félibien the historian, art theorist and chronicler of the Académie royale de peinture et de sculpture, included it in the glossary that concludes his 1676 *Principes de l'architecture, de la sculpture, de la peinture*. The dictionary is key to the *Principes* and comprises art theoretical as well as practical terms deriving from artisanal knowledge.[25] *Carnation* is explained as 'a general word used in painting to express the colour of the flesh and of all the naked or uncovered parts of a body'.[26] Another prime example of the new encyclopaedic endeavours of the seventeenth century, is the *Dictionnaire de l'Académie française*, the first authoritative dictionary of French language, published in 1694 by the institution that was founded under Louis XIII for the protection of the French language. It defines *carnation* very similarly as: 'Term of painting, colour of the flesh of men. *This carnation is beautiful, lively, natural.*'[27] While *carnation* is merely considered the colour of the flesh here, the initial restriction of the word's use to the area of painting suggests that it refers both to the flesh and its imitation. These aspects became more clearly separated from the second edition (1718) of the *Dictionnaire de l'Académie française* onwards. *Carnation* is now defined as the 'representation of human flesh by the means of colour'.[28] The inclusion of this single word marks a considerable shift: flesh tones (of the body) and flesh tones (in painting) are no longer likened through analogy, but distanced within the framework of representation. The definition of the adjective *incarnat* – 'kind of red colour that resembles that of living flesh'[29] – in the 1694 edition of the dictionary had already begun to separate means of representation and subject matter, as they are simultaneously bound together and divided by resemblance.

Incarnation on the other hand, was restricted by the *Dictionnaire* to the field of religion. Without much variation in the entries of the seventeenth to nineteenth centuries, it is defined as the 'Mystery by which the son of God, the eternal word made itself man.'[30] But, even if *incarnation* ceases to be a term for an embodiment by the means of painting, the term 'flesh' itself retained (here as much as in the Italian art literature) a strong religious connotation. Generally defined as a 'soft and sanguine substance that sits between the skin and bones of the animal' one of the first more specific usages listed is: 'one says, *the son of God has taken on human flesh* to say that he has made himself human.'[31] It is the religious context that also makes the notion of flesh highly ambivalent, since flesh denotes at the same time the living substance of the human – shared with Christ by grace of the mystery of incarnation – and the negative aspects of humanity, earthly in contrast to heavenly existence. In the latter sense it is associated with concupiscence, luxury and sin in general.[32]

In the art literature, however, both the terms *chair* (flesh) and *carnation* were imbued with a positive meaning as they referred to the successful lifelike painting of healthy human bodies. In assessments of specific paintings, most famously those delivered in the *conférences* of the Académie royale, *carnation* is employed mainly as a descriptive term for the appropriate representation of a human figure in accordance with their age, gender and particular action within the overall composition and colouring of a painting.[33] It was by no means as charged as in Cennini's *Libro dell'Arte*, but it was one of the terms, with its associated painterly techniques, the academicians had to come to grips with in their self-defining attempts to demonstrate that one can reason about art. The Académie royale de peinture et de sculpture, already formed in 1648 under the reign of Louis XIV (then still a child) and his prime minister Cardinal Mazarin, gradually consolidated its status and structures until 1664, and continued throughout the seventeenth century to negotiate its position against the *Maîtrise* (guilds).[34] It did so by making a claim for the intellectual component of the visual arts, modelling itself after its literary counterpart, the earlier founded Académie française, as well as claiming for the visual arts a rank equivalent to that of poetry. The *conférence*s, properly institutionalised in 1667 under Jean-Baptiste Colbert (*surintendant des bâtiments* since 1664) and Le Brun (then *chancelier* of the Académie), were minuted by the royal historiographer Félibien. Their rationale was to help the members of the Académie develop rules for the judgement, production and teaching of art alongside a discussion of art works (mostly paintings) from the royal collections at the

Louvre.[35] The fact that they were recorded and published by Félibien in the *Conférences* extended their reach far beyond the members of the Académie and the moments of their gatherings. What is more, rather than producing a coherent doctrine they brought controversy in judgement and opinion to the fore.[36] Recent accounts of the early history of the Académie and of the *conférences* thus highlight that it was not a monolithic institution with one single binding doctrine. The Académie lectures were an arena of debate and dissent since notions of art and rules for its production were – throughout the late seventeenth and the eighteenth century – far more flexible than has often been assumed.[37]

This became even more apparent later in the seventeenth century, especially in discussions around the significance of colour in painting – the so-called *Querelle du coloris*. Within these debates the *carnations* gained significance as a measure for the capabilities of imitation in paint. The famous French controversy about the supremacy of drawing or colour, also referred to as the quarrel between Poussinistes and Rubénistes,[38] has drawn considerable art historical attention following the re-editions of the *conférences* from the nineteenth century onwards. Often seen as an initial step in the apotheosis of modernism narrated as a history of the increasing dominance and autonomy of colour, the late seventeenth-century discussions seemed relevant only as far as they could be projected on to the nineteenth-century conflict between the avant-garde and the academic traditions (which was itself unduly polarised).[39] Tentative arguments for the significance of colour came from within the Académie itself and the academicians agreed, for example, with the traditional praise of Titian's (or generally the Venetian painters') mastery of colour. In a lecture on Titian's *Entombment of Christ* held in 1667, for example, Philippe de Champaigne lauded the artist as a champion in colouring, and detailed how Titian had used the overall colour scheme and the smooth transitions between tones to express the theme of mourning. Champaigne particularly highlighted the tints used for the flesh tones and considered how Titian foregrounded the deadness of Christ by juxtaposing his paleness with the colourful flesh tones of the disciples holding the corpse. According to Champaigne, Titian rendered the dead body in a way that enabled the viewer to tell that the 'privation of blood and of life turn [the members] pale and livid, so that the flesh and veins, muscles and nerves that make a living body firm and round, seem squashy, caved in and flattened'.[40] In describing what he deemed an appropriately painted dead body, Champaigne, by negation, also reaffirmed an attitude similar to that of Cennini according to which a living body in paint should be 'in living colour' and in full relief.

Félibien, who framed the lectures in his introduction to the *Conférences*, was more constrained in his appraisal of Titian's colouring, reminding readers that, while Titian excelled in the handling of colours and in giving an overall harmony of colours to his compositions, he was less good in other aspects of painting. The more powerful spokesmen of the Académie, most importantly Le Brun, are well known for promoting Raphael and among the more contemporary painters Nicolas Poussin as models for *all* aspects of painting, because they excelled both in drawing and in the appropriate and skilful use of colour. When Louis-Gabriel Blanchard held his lecture on the merits of colour in November 1671, the main provocation was not emphasising colour's significance as *one* element of painting, but arguing that it is *the* defining element of painting. 'One can,' he postulated, 'define painting in the following manner: an art that, by the means of form and colours, imitates all the objects that can be in front of our eyes on a flat surface. This definition seems to me quite right as it suits painting perfectly and distinguishes it from all the other arts.'[41] He further stressed that a painter's aim is 'to deceive the eye and to imitate nature' and that this is achieved by the means of colours.[42] With this intervention Blanchard took up arguments that had originally been voiced from outside the Académie by Roger de Piles, an amateur, art collector and diplomat, who would become the most prominent spokesman in favour of colour and who stressed the specific visual effects with which paintings attract their viewers.[43] Towards the end of the seventeenth century de Piles was admitted to the Académie, and his lectures became themselves part of the academic discourse.[44]

Roger de Piles and the seductions of colour and flesh

De Piles first entered the arena of art discourse with an introduction to an anatomical treatise by Tortebat (which will be discussed in chapter 6), and an annotated translation of the art theoretical poem *De arte graphica* by Charles-Alphonse Dufresnoy (1668) from which Blanchard drew many of the arguments of his 1671 lecture. In a 1673 re-edition of the book, de Piles augmented *De arte graphica* by his *Dialogue sur le coloris* which set out his ideas on painting more explicitly. The literary form of the dialogue, at the time a favoured format for art theoretical debate in print,[45] allowed him to sharpen his arguments against the objections of his adversaries. Both the *Dialogue sur le coloris* and his 1677 *Conversations sur la peinture* feature two main characters, Pamphilus and Damon, having a master-apprentice-like relationship, with Damon often naively bringing forward conservative criteria for the judgement of art which are then challenged by Pamphilus. Speaking through these two characters, de Piles not only inverted the traditional ranking of colour and design in arguing that colour is the distinctive and hence defining element of painting, but also used the traditional hierarchy of the senses (that considered sight the superior of the five senses) to make a claim in favour of colour. Since drawing mainly indicates the shape of things, it imitates a quality of objects just as perceptible by the sense of touch, while colour is only accessible to sight. This association

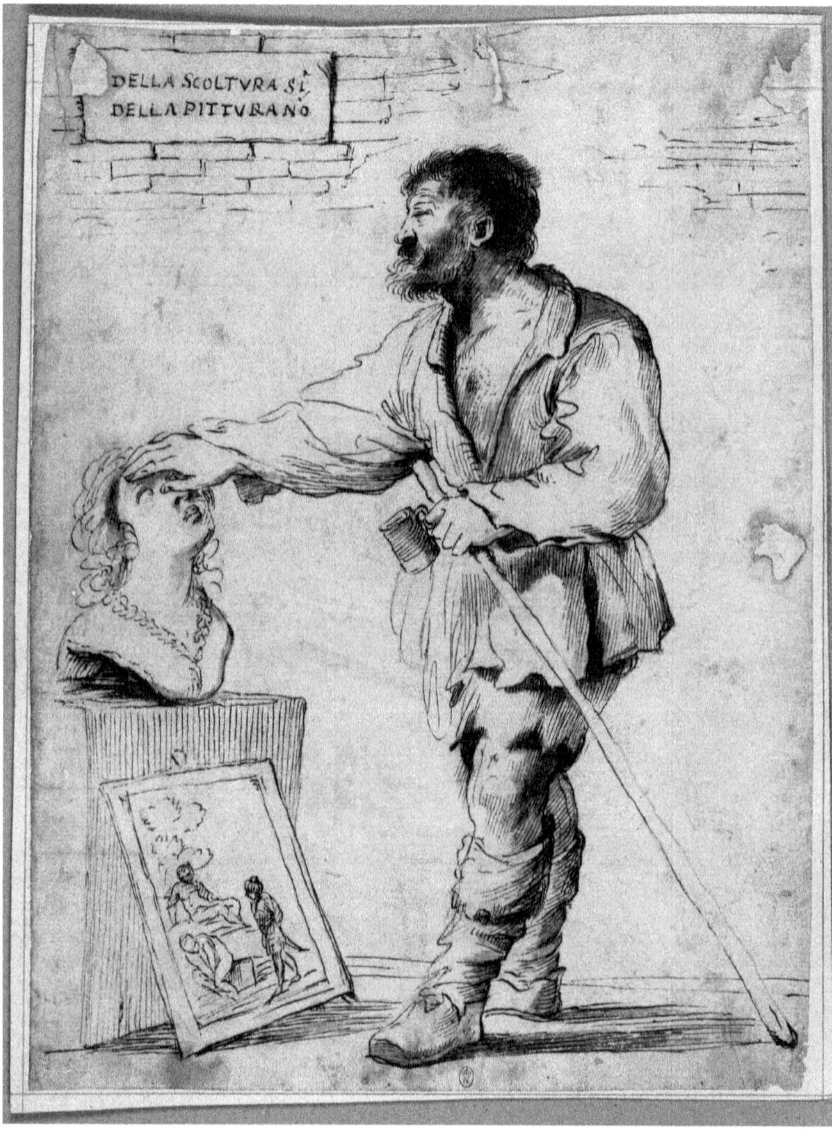

2.3 Il Guercino (school of), *Della scultura si, della pittura no*, black chalk, pen and brown wash on paper, 26.9 x 20.1 cm.

of sculpture and touch had already been made in the Italian *paragone* (the dispute about the rivalry of painting and sculpture) and in several art works, among them paintings by Jusepe de Ribera showing a blind man (also referred to as blind sculptor) experiencing a sculpture with his hands, and a drawing attributed to the school of Il Guercino that explicitly plays off sculpture against painting (Figure 2.3). De Piles first let Damon make the traditional argument for the primacy of drawing and sculpture. Damon reports his encounter with a blind artist, who was perfectly capable of making portraits with a good likeness in wax. Asked whether he did not at least see a little, the sightless sculptor 'reply'd he saw nothing at all, and that his Eyes were at his Fingers ends … I feel my Original again and again; I attentively examine the Dimensions, the Risings, and the Fallings; I imprint them in my Memory; then I take my Wax, and by the Comparison which I make of one and the other by carrying my Hand to and again several times, I finish my Work in the best manner I can.'[46] Unlike the form of things which the blind sculptor can perceive and reproduce perfectly well, their colour can only be sensed by the eye, as colour is 'only the Object of the Sight'.[47] Within this argument colour was understood as an accidental quality of objects and hence a secondary aspect of their imitation. Consequently, the apologists of *dessin* professed that colour is like make-up, only there to feign and arouse sensual pleasure and covering up the essential quality of things sufficiently indicated by outlines and shades. To this de Piles had his spokesman in the dialogue reply that painting is and should precisely be the art of make-up and visual seduction. Generally a promoter of the art of Rubens, de Piles made him counter the argument that there is not much truth in Rubens's paintings because the lights and colours are exaggerated, making his works 'only specious': 'Specious! cry'd Pamphilus, wou'd to God, Friend *Damon*, the Pictures that are drawn now-a-days were *So Specious*! Are you ignorant that Painting is nothing but *Speciousness*, that it is its Essence to deceive, and the greatest Deceiver in that Art is the greatest Painter.'[48]

De Piles claimed that the purpose of painting is to catch the spectators' eyes with its colourful appeal and to hold their attention through sensual pleasure. While he was in accord with probably any art theorist or painter of his time in postulating that the rationale of painting is to imitate nature, it was not generally concluded that successful imitation always leads to deception. De Piles praised colouring and make-up (*le fard*) as the essential means by which paintings attract their audience. If lifelike imitation of nature was the key to paintings' ability to deceive, perfectly rendered flesh tones were the most delicate form of deception. De Piles elaborated this in his comments on Rubens suggesting that *chair* and *carnations* are at the heart of what painting can achieve, the best applications for colour.[49] In the *Dialogue upon Colouring* flesh figures as *the* exemplary subject matter to argue for the potential of colour. Discussing the question whether colour is necessary to produce a beautiful painting, Pamphilus, speaking in favour of colour points out:

> I shall then say there's nothing wanting … but it is a true piece of Painting; since in the Design and Colour it will imitate a work of Sculpture which you suppose. The Beauty of Colouring does not consist in a multiplicity of different

> Colours, but in their just distribution, so that the painted Objects have the same Colour as the true; a painted Stone for example to resemble a natural one; Carnation to appear true Flesh [*que les carnations paroissent de véritables chairs*]; and in a word, that not only each particular Object do perfectly represent the Colour of those it imitates; but that they altogether make an agreeable Union throughout the whole Piece.[50]

Flesh and stone are of course not randomly chosen objects; they could not be more adverse in their relevance for narrative painting, and in their material qualities: hard and soft, organic and inorganic. Moreover, in the metonymic flow in which topics tend to meander through de Piles's texts (in particular in his dialogues and conversations), the juxtaposition of stone and flesh also refers to the *paragone* of painting and sculpture. It evokes the well-known critique of those painters (usually associated with the mastery of *disegno*) whose painted bodies look as if made of stone rather than flesh due to an excessive study of ancient sculpture instead of the life model. In his *Conversations* de Piles dismissed Poussin as having 'only seen Antiquity and surrendered to stone'.[51]

The quoted passage from the *Dialogue upon Colouring* concludes with the overall visual effect of a work. What counts for de Piles in addition to the skilful rendering of individual objects is the 'agreeable Union' that catches and holds the eye of the spectator. This concept of the harmonious disposition of a painting, of the economy of the *tout-ensemble*, was, for Thomas Puttfarken, far more original than the mere defence of colour, as de Piles formulated with it an art theory emancipated from its literary counterpart. Puttfarken stresses the relative autonomy de Piles accorded to the visual and argues that this is an aspect which got lost in the course of the eighteenth century, because the Enlightened pleas for a morally uplifting art were more concerned with the content than the form of art works.[52] With this, Puttfarken isolates not only de Piles from subsequent art theorists but also subject matter from the ways it is represented. However, as Mary Sheriff has pointed out, such a dissociation of the visual elements of painting is against the grain of art historical thinking of the time, and both Félibien and de Piles, despite disagreement in other respects, would have understood the appropriateness – *convenance* – of co-ordination of subject and pictorial means.[53] In fact, de Piles's idea of the visual effect and the attractions of colouring is inseparably bound to imitation, and more than anything else to a particular subject matter, deeply entangled with painting: flesh. Through the simulation of flesh, a painting most effectively deceives the spectator, and the slight difference in the choice of words in de Piles's aforementioned passage is telling: a painted stone shall '*resemble* a natural one' while carnation is meant to '*appear* true flesh'.

In his account of Rubens's works in the collections of the Duc de Richelieu, that forms part of his *Conversations sur la peinture*, de Piles praised the painter's mastery of colour, evoking in his discussion of an *Andromeda* again the *paragone* along the contrast of flesh and stone (Plate 2). The mythological subject of Andromeda's captivity and liberation by Perseus had been treated by Rubens several times. Featuring also in the decorations of the artist's house in Antwerp, it has been interpreted as a programmatic theme, that is, as a painted *paragone* in which the distinct qualities of sculpture on the one hand and painting on the other can be exposed.[54] This understanding of the topic is based on two aspects of the myth of Perseus and Andromeda in Ovid's version and its post-antique adaptations: upon first sight Perseus takes Andromeda, chained naked to a rock at the shore and watched by a sea monster, for a marble statue. Only Andromeda's tears and the fluttering of her hair in the wind betray the fact that she is a living human being. The challenge for the painter is thus to render the flesh of a figure petrified by fear, looking like a sculpture in her perfect nudity and enforced stillness. The figure of Andromeda can thus be understood as an allegory of painting that exposes the specific ability of the medium to imitate any material from stone to organic matter, and in particular its power to enliven flesh via the use of colour.

Given that the competitive comparison between painting and sculpture, often discussed along with the juxtaposition of flesh and stone, is a leitmotif throughout de Piles's writings, it seems sensible to consider it also as a subtext of his account of Rubens's *Andromeda*. The author himself gradually fills the painted female figure with emotions and life, paradoxically evoking colour by its very absence. He thus introduces yet another capacity of colour, that of expressing emotions on the body's surface. Describing the captured Andromeda, who is represented as a fully exposed standing nude, he particularly focuses on the physical and visible effects of her ambivalent feelings provoked by the situation in which a cupid announces to the captive that she is about to be liberated by Perseus: 'She reacts to this novelty with hope and fear, and her face expresses this uncertain state marvellously. Fear has made her blood retract to the interior, which shows in particular at the extremities that are very pale. Although there is almost no red in this figure, one can never see anything that is more of flesh, and this seems even more so as she is accompanied by a bluish background composed of sky and sea.'[55]

Further on in the *Conversations* de Piles more generally speaks about the relation between colour and soul, drawing the two very close together by first postulating that colouring is the 'soul of painting' in order to continue that 'the soul is the ultimate perfection of the living and what gives it life'.[56] For him, it is impossible to render a human figure lifelike without colour and to represent the expression of emotions in a drawing. Coming back to Rubens's *Andromeda*, he claims that her emotions are much better visible via the colour than through her facial features.[57] This remark is a direct riposte to Le Brun who proposed, with his influential 1668 lecture on the expression of passions, a codification of human emotions that was based almost exclusively on the movements of facial features. A set of drawings condensed the expression of single and mixed emotions to varying positions of a set of lines signifying eyes, eyebrows, nose and mouth (Figure 2.4).[58] According to Le Brun, colour is hardly needed to express a passion; and the actual body and the representation made of it are not distinguished here. In his response to Blanchard's lecture on the merits of colour, he explicitly stated that drawing (and he refers to *dessin pratique* in contrast to *dessin intellectuel où théorique*) 'can imitate everything visible including the passions of the soul without the need of colour, except for representing blushing and pallor'.[59] In his lecture on the expression of passions, although focusing on facial features, he thus describes the effects that the emotions have on the complexion in a variety of cases in terms of reddening and blanching. Regarding the traces of fear he states: 'The movements of Fear are expressed by the inner end of the eyebrow slightly raised; the mouth is open, drawn back, and the sides more open than the centre, and the under lip drawn further back than the upper. The complexion is redder than in Love or Desire, but not so beautiful, for it has a somewhat livid tint; the lips are of this same colour, and also dryer than in Love.'[60]

Speaking about the *Andromeda* de Piles inverts Le Brun's idea of the reddening of the body as an expression of fear. This might be an indication not only of his pleasure in contradicting an opponent in art theoretical debates, but also of the fact that he was aware of the significance of the topic for a painterly engagement with the *paragone* between painting and sculpture. De Piles himself used the painting to highlight the exceptional mastery of Rubens who is able to render a pale body lifelike despite the almost entire absence of red, usually an essential ingredient of the flesh tones. At the same time de Piles formulated a concept of the physical effects and expressions of passion in which the emotions act in the entire body becoming visible on its surface as a spectacle of colours. Recent scholarship on Rubens has confirmed de Piles's physiological account of his art, arguing that the artist, who was a member of neostoic circles around Justus Lipsius, developed a physiological method of painting. A regular reader of Seneca, Rubens shared the stoic idea of the physicality of affects and represented the various bodily effects of the passions via a highly differentiated use of colour.[61] In this particular understanding of the imitation of nature, the body expressing passions is likened to the way images communicate.

Despite the disagreements between Le Brun and de Piles regarding the particular impact of the passions on the body, both assumed in more general terms that they manifested themselves on the body's surface. Equally interested in the ways something invisible – the various states of the soul – can gain visibility, they shared a notion of representation in which the body expressing

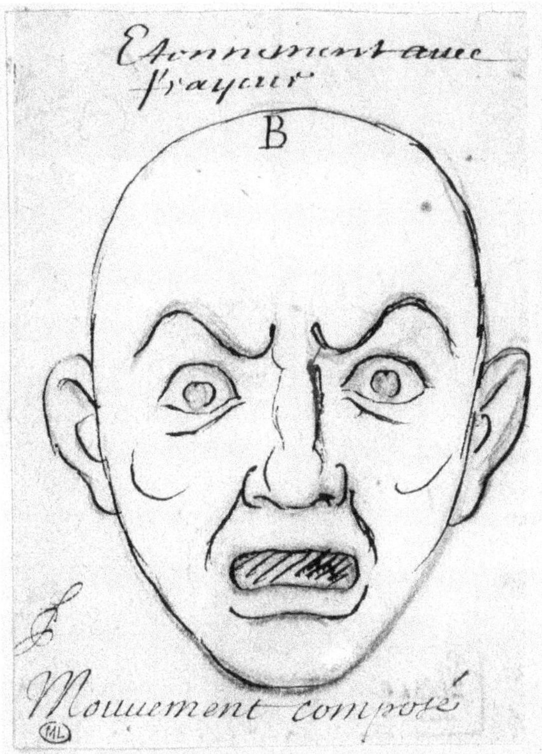

Charles Le Brun, *Surprise Mixed with Fear*, black chalk, pen and ink on paper, 13 x 9.5 cm. 2.4

passions becomes the model for the ways images enunciate and produce meaning. In turn, the body is understood like a canvas on which emotions paint or imprint themselves.[62] De Piles, using precisely this trope, argued for Rubens's *Lion Hunt* in a similar vein as for *Andromeda* that colour – even if it suggests the withdrawal of blood from the face – is the perfect means 'to imprint' fear on the body.[63]

If this sounds like a natural language of involuntary bodily expression that has just to be mimicked by the artist to render emotions faithfully, de Piles stressed elsewhere that exaggeration and artifice are needed to make things seem natural. Defending Rubens against those who 'find little truth' in the artist's works, and who argued that his colour and light are excessive, de Piles stated again that paintings should be made-up (*fardés*) and that the aim of painting is to deceive.[64] As Jacqueline Lichtenstein has pointed out, it is precisely around the intersection of deception, visual pleasure and persuasiveness that the representation of flesh becomes a crucial site for argument. Studying the history of the philosophical dismissal of colour and painting since Plato, her interest in de Piles lies not so much in him as a founder of a genuine and modern theory of art, but as a partisan in her critique of idealist philosophy and its ramifications in art theory. For her, de Piles, in describing the effects with which paintings catch the eye, employed the language of female seduction and envisaged the spectator as an art lover in the most literal sense.[65] He thus took up the notion of colour as feminine already implicit in Italian art theory (and that both in negative or positive accounts of colour)[66] in order to emphasise colour's seductive potential. Given these gender dynamics, it is not just *carnations* and *chair* as such, but more precisely the female flesh which is the site where the oscillation between illusion and deception, between the desire to touch and the awareness of the artificiality of the painting, arouses maximum pleasure. No other subject matter makes the contrast between illusion and disillusion be felt as deeply as female flesh. Regarding a female figure in Rubens's *Drunken Silenus* de Piles wrote for example: 'The flesh of this satyress and that of her children seem so real that you can easily imagine that if one reached out for them one would feel the warmth of the blood.'[67]

Everything is done in this description to evoke life, but at the same time de Piles expected nobody to actually confound representation and represented, and it is clear that the verisimilitude of the flesh tones activates an imaginary sense of touch. Actually reaching out and feeling the cold and flat paint, realising a deception, is held at bay by keeping a distance and enjoying the illusion. The pleasure of deception is bound to the spectator's ability to play with the confusion of representation and represented by being simultaneously aware of their distinction. There is no more potential transubstantiation of paint into flesh as had been evoked in the early Italian art literature when Cennini spoke of the act of painting as making flesh (*incarnazione*). And still in the sixteenth-century, the Venetian art theorist Lodovico Dolce not only generally praised Titian's mastery of the flesh tones, but even suggested that the painter had used flesh instead of paint to produce his *St. Sebastian*.[68] De Piles, despite the continuing use of the terms *chair* and *carnations* that tend to mingle the flesh tones and the painted flesh, and despite his quest for lifelikeness, always stressed the artifice with which it was achieved. In line with the shift in the dictionary entries discussed earlier, the art theorist thought of the flesh colours as representing flesh rather than being like flesh. Along with it, he understood the painted picture more explicitly as a two-dimensional medium that creates illusion as a surface effect. And, when body and image are aligned as expressive media, as in his account of Rubens's *Andromeda*, the association is rather with the skin as expressive surface than with the body and its substance as a whole.

This understanding of painting as a practice that operates on a picture plane and creates superficial effects also resonates in de Piles's association of painting and make-up. Praising the art of deception and the images' power to seduce, de Piles embraced the equation of colour and painting with *fard*. In the subsequent decades this conflation of paint and make-up or painting and cosmetics became an important art critical topos. By the mid-eighteenth century it was employed mostly in negative terms in the critique of the art of the so-called Rococo as a false and feminised product of a degenerate aristocratic culture.[69] Enlightenment critique, in a quest for transparency in visual language and physical expression, dismissed the concealment of the natural expressiveness of the facial skin along with the exaggerated artifice in painting. A moralising denunciation of make-up was certainly not an eighteenth-century novelty, but it took on a particular tone at the time. Medical professionals became an important voice in the debate distinguishing between the concealing *fard* and beneficial remedies that help to embellish skin by cleaning, polishing and softening it, as for example the article on cosmetics in the *Encyclopédie* put it.[70] Early skin specialists such as Anne-Charles Lorry, author of a treatise on skin diseases published in 1777, particularly cautioned against the use of products with metallic ingredients, most famously white make-up or bleaching remedies containing lead.[71] But the fact that the latter type of cosmetics, and generally products that altered the natural complexions and covered up sentimental skin reactions such as blushing, were increasingly critiqued, cannot be taken as an indicator that the use of make-up came out of fashion.[72] On the contrary, as has been demonstrated by French historian Catherine Lanoë in her analysis of the material culture of cosmetics in early modern France, the employment of powder, pomade and particularly of rouge became increasingly widespread in the later decades of the Ancien Régime. As part of a general development of consumer culture, a wider range of ready-to-use products – from luxury items to fairly inexpensive preparations – were available especially in urban centres like Paris, also reaching the lower classes such as merchants, artisans and servants.[73] In court culture, the use of make-up was a regular part of a model of self-representation and social exchange that expected men and women to control their faces.[74] But along with its growing use in the course of the eighteenth century, make-up developed from a distinctive sign of aristocratic identity into a cultural practice that provoked anxieties about the blurring of social and gender boundaries.[75]

Rouge became famously associated with personalities like Madame de Pompadour, who rose from non-noble origins to marquise and mistress of Louis XV. In this context, make-up was perceived as an instrument of social rise and self-invention. Melissa Hyde and Ewa Lajer-Burcharth have argued that this is made an issue in François Boucher's portrait of Madame de Pompadour at her toilet (Figure 2.5). Showing Pompadour with the brush in her hand and about to apply rouge to her cheeks, the portrait not only represents her literally

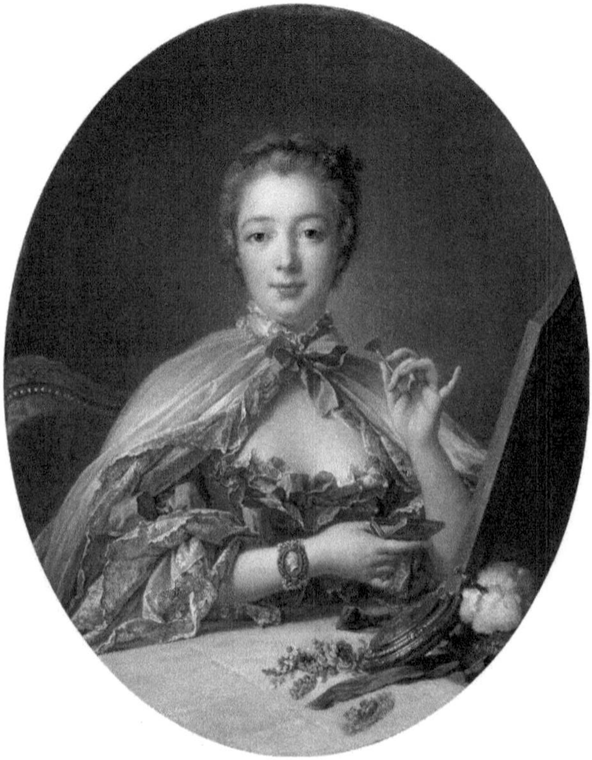

2.5 François Boucher, *Madame de Pompadour at Her Toilette*, 1758, oil on canvas, 81.2 x 64.5 cm.

as a self-made woman, but also turns her into an ally in the artist's activity of painting her face, hence presenting her image as the result of a co-production between Boucher and the sitter/patron.[76] Using a trope of artistic self-portraiture – in placing her in front of a mirror with the brush in her left hand (as if she had painted herself inverted from her mirror image) – the portrait embraces the association of painting with *le fard* as much as de Piles did in his writings. Where Boucher paints the rouge (in the box, on Madame de Pompadour's cheeks and on the tip of the powder brush), make-up and oil paint literally converge – the painter paints red pigment with red pigments. What is more, this association had a material base in the fact that some of the red pigments used for rouge were the same as those used by painters. Cinnabar and vermilion, as well as carmine, a crimson pigment derived from cochineal, a bug native in Middle and South America, were ingredients of rouges and an important component of flesh tones in painting.[77] But even though Boucher's portrait takes up de Piles's association of painting and *le fard*, of female attraction and a painting's seductiveness, the secret of the painting's appeal is not vividly rendered flesh tones. Rather than the warm, pulsating multi-coloured body that de Piles evoked in his account of Rubens's *Bacchanal* (Plate 4) or a figure whose complexion is determined by physical reactions to her emotions, as in Rubens's *Andromeda*, Boucher's painted Madame de Pompadour is all white surface on to which red (which does not refer to blood) is applied. The portrait is not so much about flesh as about her skin equated with the canvas as a surface to be painted.

Printing flesh tones: Le Blon's *Coloritto* and colouring as animation

The prominence de Piles allocated to flesh as *the* object to be represented with colour, also becomes apparent, and more surprisingly so, in a treatise today mainly known for having introduced the three-colour system into printing: Jacob Christoph Le Blon's *Coloritto; or the Harmony of Colouring in Painting* issued 1725 bilingually in English and French.[78] 'COLORITTO, or the *Harmony* of Colouring', Le Blon stated bluntly in the opening sentence of his prelimi-naries 'is the *Art* of *Mixing* COLOURS, in order to represent naturally, in all Degrees of painted Light and Shade, the same FLESH, or the colour of any other Object, that is represented in the true or *pure* Light'.[79] The author thus privileging flesh as the first and foremost object of representation in colour, was a painter and printer born into a Frankfurt-based Huguenot family of print-makers in 1667. He spent most of his life outside Germany seeking his fortune in various European capitals and centres of print making. Around 1710, while living in Amsterdam, he started to experiment with inks suitable for colour printing, and from 1717/18 onwards, he was active in London, where he ran a 'picture office' and received the first patent for the exploitation of colour printing; finally he moved his business to Paris where he received a patent for the technology in 1737.[80] The printing technique as such was the mezzotint, a method developed in the mid-seventeenth century enabling the production of prints with a large variation of tonal values between a saturated velvety black and sheer white. The painterly effect of the mezzotint was enhanced by the use of coloured inks, and the technique allowed gradual optical mixing of the three superimposed layers of yellow, red and blue inks when working with a set of three copperplates. Eventually a forth plate for black ink was used in order to reproduce outlines and enhance the variety of shades.[81]

The knowledge that one can produce virtually any colour shade by mixing varying amounts of red, blue and yellow was not new as such, and during the seventeenth century many painters had already made the primary colours the principle of their colour organisation.[82] Artists such as Rubens made them visibly the basis of their flesh tones,[83] and de Piles similarly recommended the use of these colours for the representation of flesh. Taking a head to be copied as his example, he explained that the bright areas should be painted in various mixtures of white and yellow, and of white and two red pigments (vermilion and *lacque*), while mélanges of different amounts of yellow, red or ultramarine with white are to be used for the half tones and the shades.[84]

When Le Blon referenced Newton's *Opticks* (first published in 1704) prominently in his book, this was not so much to indicate that he owed the recognition of the primary colours to the theorist of colour, but rather to use Newton's fame to propagate his idea. Le Blon was well aware of the difference between coloured light and material colours.[85] While the physicist was concerned with the seven distinct colours in the spectrum including the primary colours, artists dealt with pigments, the hues of which rarely matched the pure primary colours. Le Blon exploited the potential of mixing material primary colour to produce prints showing all colours of visible objects by using only three printing plates. While the principle as such has been the basis of colour printing up until today, producing coloured mezzotints was technically complex and expensive at the time, and did not prove a financial success for Le Blon. His treatise *Coloritto* itself was issued in a very small print run of twenty to thirty copies, but Le Blon made sure to advertise it in the right places. He sent a copy to the Académie royale in Paris, where it was read on October 1725 as one of the Académie lectures.[86] Half a century later, it was more widely disseminated in France via a reprint within a book entitled *L'Art d'imprimer les tableaux. Traité d'après les Ecrits, les Opérations & les Instructions verbales de J. C. Le Blon.*[87]

In the short but remarkable text of the original treatise Le Blon initially explained the principle of mixing colours stating that 'painting can represent all *visible* Objects with three Colours, *Yellow*, *Red*, and *Blue*; for all other Colours can be compos'd of these *Three*, which I call *Primitive*'.[88] He then discussed how light, shade and reflections add to the visible appearance of objects and continued with the issue of good colouring: 'When a Painter says, that such Artists make a good *Coloritto*, he means, that they represent truly and naturally the Nude or the naked human Flesh; supposing they can paint all other visible Objects well, and without Difficulty.'[89] A good colourist is again judged on their capacity to represent flesh true to nature, and anyone capable of rendering this most difficult of all objects is assumed to be able to paint anything else. Accordingly, this is the representational task chosen to demonstrate the technique and capability of colour printing: if the colour mezzotint can reproduce the most complicated painterly subject, then it is fit to reproduce any painting and the most complex shades faithfully.

Consequently, flesh, or what Le Blon also called 'a good nude', is the only subject matter he considered in his treatise and in the sample prints that accompany it (Plate 4a–c). Curiously, though, he assumed that a painter, before moving to the living human body, should first learn how to represent a white object. From a didactic perspective, the purpose of this verbal argument

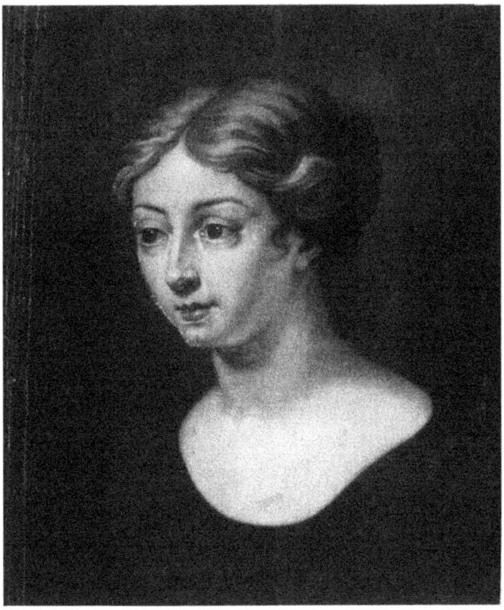

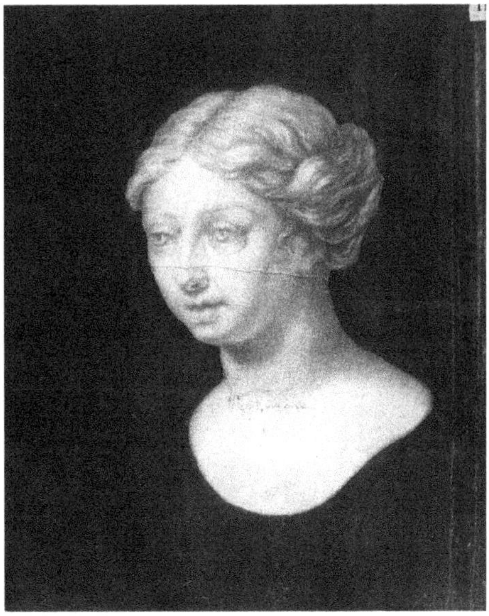

Jacob Le Blon, female head printed in black and white, female plaster head, from *Coloritto; or the Harmonie of Colouring*, 1725, figure 1–2, mezzotints, 28 x 22 cm each. **2.6–7**

and the two corresponding illustrations is to point out that representing an object in black and white is not the same as representing a white object, as even for the representation of the latter, colour is needed in order to indicate the coloured reflections on the white material (Figures 2.6 – 2.7). His series of illustrations thus begins with a female head represented in black and white, in other words by a black and white print standing in for itself. It is followed by the same head, now made of plaster and represented in a print. Emphasising the whiteness of the plaster, this mezzotint works with far less dark shading than the previous one; and, with none of the coloured reflexions mentioned in the text, it has a ghostlike appearance.[90] The plaster head is the degree zero of colour printing; made of a material often described as passive or dead, it provides a receptive figure, subsequently 'stain'd with the Colour of Flesh'.[91]

In the sequence of illustrations this looks like a figure to which life is gradually given. The first of the coloured heads mainly adds red and slight amounts of blue to the figure, exhibiting the shades of rose produced by red tincture printed in mezzotint on white paper: '*Vermilion* and *White* compose *Flesh-Colour*; yet *Vermilion* is the *Dye* of that *Flesh-Colour*; and *White* is the *Light*, which is dyed by the said *Vermilion*.'[92] While the print very well demonstrates the tonal gradations that can be produced in mezzotint, featuring only the basic component of a flesh tone, the effect is hardly that of a healthy complexion. A further figure aims to exhibit the complete effect of a natural head and includes colours beyond the flesh tone, such as the red of the mouth, the colour of eye and hair. An additional illustration represents a painter's palette organised to paint flesh (Plate 4d). Around a large patch of vermilion mixed with lake (A), further spots of paint are arranged, most importantly and immediately neighbouring it a mixture of the prominent red with white (B) labelled by Le Blon 'true *Flesh-Colour*'. The illustration of the palette unwittingly also proves the limitations of colour printing: while the wooden palette as such is printed, the various patches of paint were applied by hand.[93]

An appendix to *Coloritto* provides four additional illustrations: two prints of the same female plaster head coloured with yet different tints together with an accompanying palette for each. Le Blon thus further demonstrated that he could represent virtually any flesh tone by varying the pigments used for printing. The only tones considered, however, are variations of fair complexions that were within the range of shades that remained the ideal flesh tones in artists' manuals well into the nineteenth century. As in Cennini's *Libro dell'Arte* a female face represents the complexities of flesh tones and the process of recreating them. But whereas for Cennini the act of painting a face was a process of embodiment, in Le Blon the colouring of the face is more one of animating the dead matter of plaster. The sequence of Le Blon's figures 2 to 4, especially, proceeding from the ghostlike white plaster head to the increasingly tinted figure looks like an enlivenment, following less the Christian notion of divine incarnation than the mythical story of the sculptor Pygmalion whose sculpture, a female figure (made of ivory in Ovid's and of marble in eighteenth-century versions), becomes animated with the help of Venus.[94] This story (to which I will come back in more detail in the next chapter) was immensely popular in the eighteenth century and re-imagined in many paintings, sculptures and prints, as well as in literary texts and philosophical tracts.

Besides the reproduction of paintings, in particular portraits, the other application for colour printing Le Blon experimented with was anatomical illustration, an area where flesh was of equal importance. It is a different flesh though: unlike the rosy complexions of the body's surface, the anatomical images in coloured mezzotint dived into the deep red of the body's interior substance. Le Blon mentions this kind of work in the dedication to his *Coloritto*,[95] and one of his early colour prints was an illustration for a treatise by the King's anatomist Saint André representing male genitals infected with gonorrhœa. While Le Blon did not pursue the project of medical representations himself, some of the most luxurious coloured mezzotints produced in the eighteenth century were anatomical illustrations and for about half a century the colour print remained most closely linked to anatomy.[96] In France, Gautier Dagoty, who had studied with Le Blon for some weeks and later claimed for himself (unjustifiably so) the invention of colour printing, published between 1745 and 1775 a series of mostly large format, anatomical colour prints. Jan

Ladmiral, another former student of Le Blon, worked for Siegfried Albinus in Leiden and illustrated among other things the anatomist's treatise on the location and origins of colour in humans (an aspect that I will discuss in the chapter on skin colours).

Brushstrokes, textures and tissues

The association of flesh and colour was a major concern of writers with such different agendas as de Piles and Le Blon, and the lifelike rendering of flesh was generally considered the highest achievement of the arts of colouring. If the right mixture and distribution of colours were regarded as crucial for a lifelike effect, in the course of the eighteenth century a further element of painting, paint handling, would hold an increasingly important role in French painterly practice and art discourse. The focus on the visible traces of the painter's brush went along with a new attention to the making of art works and, as I will argue in what follows, gradually altered the rapport between the body's surface and the surface fabricated by the artist.

For de Piles, the handling of the brush (or the crayon in drawings) remained of lesser importance than the effects of colouring, but he occasionally talked about it in relation to manner (*manière*), to the style of paintings or when he dealt more explicitly with painterly practice. In the 1684 *Premiers élémens de la peinture pratique*, he generally praises the *facilité du pinceau*,[97] but mostly spoke about the handling with respect to drawing, arguing that the lack of colour in drawing has to be substituted by a 'spiritual expression of the traits' and a differentiating use of the crayon or pen for rendering each represented object distinct in a medium without colour.[98] In his remarks on Dufresnoy's *L'Art de Peinture* he highlighted that artists should not 'torment' the paint by blending the brush strokes, but leave the paint untouched once it has been put on the canvas. For him, artists such as Titian, Veronese, Rubens and Van Dyck mastered this technique that enabled them to preserve the freshness of their paintings, a conserved liveliness of the painting that goes along with the vivacity of the flesh tones.[99] In the praise of the 'astounding freshness' of the tint of the satyress in Rubens's *Bacchanal*, freshness of colouring as a painterly process and of the flesh imitated are inextricably mingled.[100] De Piles made similar observations with specific regard to portraiture in his later *Cours de peinture*. He generally recommended that a portrait should be worked in three different stages, as the painter should 'sketch, paint and retouch it'. While each step is of equal importance, it is with the final retouches of the flesh tones that the painter supplies the portrait with personality by giving it 'spirit, physiognomy and character'.[101]

The topos of the living image that has been traditionally linked to the lifelike rendition of flesh tones is taken up here, but the liveliness of the image has migrated on to the surface of the painting. Rather than via the building up of flesh – a literal embodiment – as in Cennini's *incarnare*, the vivacity of the image is achieved through an animation of lifeless matter. The power of the artist to imbue a painting with life was emphasised by the artist Antoine Coypel, director of the Académie since 1714. In a series of conferences initially held between 1712 and 1720 and reread several times over the course of the eighteenth century, he elaborated on the aesthetics of painting and specifically discussed, in one section, the significance of the brush. While praising the *facilité du pinceau* and critiquing a licked or laborious-looking paint handling, he equally pointed out (with the moderation of the representative of the Académie) that the seeming facility is the result of hard training and an awareness of the rules, warning that an excess of facility verges on the frivolous. He was less moderate though when rhapsodising about the operations of artistic inspiration:

> The original genius, carried away by a fortunate verve, spreads the fire that inflames him on everything he touches. In fact, it is with some kind of divine fire that one should animate the bodies that one has regularly formed via the art of drawing and the charms of colouring. Like a new Prometheus one has to inspire a celestial fire with the help of Minerva, just as he himself said in the tragedy by Thyeste: 'Humans were created like animals, without intelligence or spirit. I have tamed them with the celestial fire that I aspirated into their souls.'[102]

Taking up long established myths of artistic creation, Coypel likened the artist to Prometheus (thus also positioning him as male) and at the same time, art making to godlike creation capable of animating bodies with 'divine fire'. In French eighteenth-century art discourse 'fire' (*feu*) was generally associated with enthusiasm, a quality that was increasingly considered the driving force behind original artistic production. Moreover, Coypel used the word *touche* for describing the way the artist's 'fire' is transported into the work. Seen as the visual manifestation of the artist's enthusiasm, *la touche* became the predominant term in the discussion of paint handling and it had different connotations from *le pinceau* or *le faire* (the brush or the making). While the latter terms foreground the artist's tool and the skills with which it is used, *touche* fuses 'the manner with which the painter applies and layers the paint'[103] with the artist's touch. Referring both to the brushstrokes and to the sense of touch, the French words *la touche* and *toucher* have manifold meanings. The term not only highlights the tactile skills of the hand an adept artist needs, but also interprets painting or drawing as a mark making process.[104] The brushstrokes became traces of the brush touching the canvas, the brush a tool that mediates the physical movement of the artist's hand and, in an indirect way, also his psychological state. For Coypel the inspired artist ignites everything he touches, thus transforming the material activity of art making into an act of divine animation incited seemingly by a single moment of contact. This miraculous touch also evokes the healing and animating powers of saints and the magic powers of the French kings' touch.[105]

What is more, an understanding of *la touche* as voiced by Coypel contributed to the emergence of the modern myth of the genius as an inspired and exceptionally gifted personality that expresses his (the genius was almost by definition male) subjectivity in his work. A relationship between an artist's mental or emotional state and the touch was established, turning the utterances of the hand into natural signs, into immediate traces of his personality.[106] This emphasis on the brushstroke as a trace of the artist conceived artistic production as self-expression and placed it within new models of bourgeois subjectivity. In parallel, however, *la touche* and the facility with which it was uttered and displayed on the canvas was still linked to older models of aristocratic behaviour and physical expression, going back to the Italian ideal of *sprezzatura* as one of the major qualities of a courtier. Transported into France as *négligence* it was a performed ease of social and physical behaviour that did not show itself as the result of training and effort. In the same sense the *facilité du pinceau* meant the display of skilfulness without the signs of work. Needless to say, if it was supposed to show in a painting, this apparent ease of the brush demanded considerable previous exercise, as it did not allow for correction and reworking of the paint once placed on the canvas.[107]

During the eighteenth century, a sense of the technical aspects of the brushwork remained, in other words, an acknowledgement that it was a code to be learned. Some voices in the discussion around the visible brush took *le faire* and *la touche* mainly as pleasing surface effect which paintings should feature but were of lesser importance than elements like composition and colouring. Such a view was held for example by the Comte de Caylus who spoke to the Académie as an amateur in a series of lectures, and elaborated on the matter in his 1755 'Conférence sur la légèrté de l'outil'.[108] Others, such as the painter, engraver and theorist Charles-Nicholas Cochin (the Younger), valued it as a more substantial part of painterly practice and the main element for judging the perfection of art works. Cochin associated the brushwork (to which he referred mainly as *le faire*) with enthusiasm and confidence of the execution, considering it thus as an effect of both inspiration and training.[109]

However, *la touche* did not only refer to the artist, it was also seen as tool for the depiction of natural objects. Several art critics and theorists stressed that the manner of paint handling, far from just adding some inspired *touches* on an otherwise finished art work, was an important means of precise imitation. De Piles had already made this point with respect to drawing, when he argued that a differentiated handling of the crayon is necessary for an appropriate rendering of objects as different as landscapes, animals or human figures. Coypel similarly emphasised that a painter should 'vary his touch according to the character of the objects he is representing.'[110] How this was to be done was specified by later writers, with particular focus on the imitation of the flesh. Far from being a mere surface effect, some superficial *touches spirituelles* added at the last minute, the brushwork was meant to mimic the texture of the body. In the eyes of the portrait painter Louis Tocqué, the artist worked so close to the body that the act of painting flesh amounted to a penetration of visceral cavities:

> Vis-à-vis the *Dejaneira* by Guido Reni I ask myself: how did he find on his palette these apt pastes of colour the heaviness of which he took away? How, by the means of variety, does he manage to show blood through the skin, lending so much delicacy and freshness to the flesh? How by bluish tints does he make us imagine the veins so slightly covered that it seems as if a prick could make blood leak from them … One has, I dare say, to have a feeling in the brush that grubs for the muscles and discovers them neatly in order to show them with ease in the fleshy parts. That is what produces this appearance of movement that gives a soul to the figures. From early on, you should accustom yourself to be the master of your touch in order to operate effortlessly.[111]

In Tocqué's imagination the brush penetrates the body like an anatomist's knife. Rummaging through the inner parts while painting, the artist seems to feel his way with his brush, gaining insight into anatomical knowledge. This sensible brush leads the painter to 'discover the muscles neatly', to organise the amorphous flesh, and enables him to represent the body with ease and precision simultaneously. The inspired use of the artist's tool even makes thick paint smart and takes the weight from the matter. It is the combination of skill and inspiration that keeps the artist from being a mere worker: 'Take care first of all to grasp the spirit of nature, because, if you limit yourself to the material, you will lapse into this coldness and plain sleekness that reduces the artist to the rank of a worker.'[112] In the case of the human body, the 'spirit of nature' seems to be brought out via its fleshy surface. Knowing the body with the brush, the painter animates the flesh by feigning blood shining through the skin. Besides its visceral quality, this passage is highly interesting in the ways it redefines artistic knowledge. A century after the Académie's foundational moment, there is no more need to stress the intellectual dimension of art making. The artist's competence is now specialised and based on technical skills joined by inspiration;[113] the painter's knowledge of anatomy does not derive from learned texts but lies in their experience with brush or crayon.

Almost *en passant*, skin enters the art discourse here with a new connotation. It is not the skin of elderly persons that Le Brun had referred to when lecturing on Poussin's *Gathering of Manna*,[114] an envelope discernible as a discrete entity due to folds and looseness, which is contrasted with the *morbidezza* of young and healthy bodies. For Tocqué skin was a vital part of the body, a transparent membrane intermingled with the flesh. In a slightly later text, Antoine-Joseph Pernety's 1757 *Dictionnaire portatif de peinture*, skin not only has an equally positive connotation, but is linked even more than in Tocqué's writings with the artist's *touche*. The art dictionary, of which Félibien's aforementioned glossary was an early example, became a prominent genre during the eighteenth century along with the rise of art criticism,[115] and art criticism itself established a close relationship with artistic practices, using terms like *faire* and *touche*.[116] Under the heading 'touche' Pernety discussed various manners of paint handling which are for him first of all a means of 'imitating objects as they are in nature'. And again, much like Le Blon, the predominant objects he treated are *carnation*, flesh and flesh tones, but he also used the word 'skin' in this context: 'If the skin tissue is or at least seems uniform, the brush should be so too.'[117] Two fabrics are closely associated here, on the one hand the texture an artist produces with his tools and, on the other, the texture of the organic substance he is representing. This is remarkable from two angles: skin makes its entry into art discourse along with a greater attention to paint handling, and it does so due to a new perception of the organ as itself textured, as 'skin tissue', another expression that should not be taken for granted.

The term 'tissue' – today generally used to describe organic matter – is, after all, itself a metaphor and one deriving from the realm of textiles. It was introduced into the language of botany and later medicine only in the middle of the seventeenth century as advances in the technology and uses of the microscope changed the ways in which the structure of organic substances was seen and put into words. The material of plants, animals and humans was now perceived as structured and metaphors enabled the naturalists to describe what they saw through the lens. The English natural philosopher Robert Hooke introduced, in his 1665 *Micrographia*, the term 'cell' into botany thus comparing

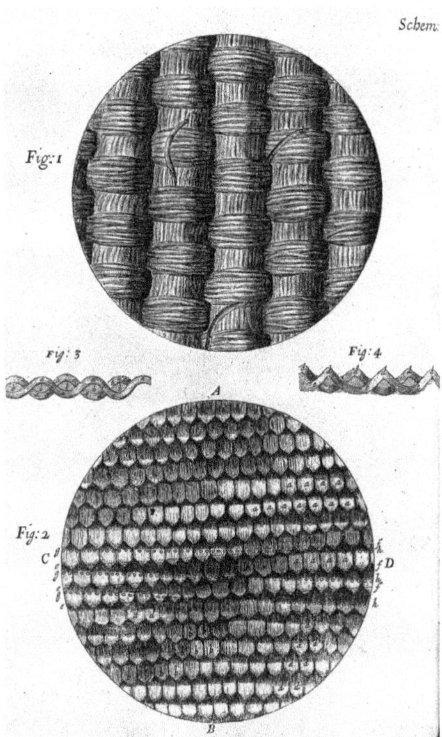

Microscopic view of silk and of watered silk, engraving from Robert Hooke, *Micrographia*, 1665, scheme 3, engraving, 29 x 19 cm. 2.8

the individual little compartments of a slice of cork he saw through a microscope to an architectural structure, a little chamber. But he also included the observation of a piece of textile ('fine Taffety-riband'), and the optical as well as linguistic comparison facilitates the scaling and understanding of organic structures seen through the microscope (Figure 2.8).[118] Physician and botanist Nehemia Grew employed the word 'texture' or 'contexture' to describe the composition of plant fibres thus comparing them to woven textiles. The French term used was 'tissure' and later 'tissu', and 'tissue' eventually also became the commonly used word in English.[119] The term 'merits attention', George Canguilhem remarks in an 1945 article on the history of cell theory:

> *Tissu* comes from *tistre*, an archaic form of the verb *tisser* ('to weave'). If the term *cell* appears charged with implicit significations of an affective and social order, the term tissue seems no less charged with extra-theoretical implications. A cell makes us think of the bee [he argues that it was associated with the honeycomb] and not of man. Weaving makes us think of man and not of the spider: woven fabric is human work par excellence.[120]

One does not have to follow Canguilhem's strategic dissociation of the humanly crafted fabric and the spider's web in order to make the point that the woof is a quintessential human (and often woman's) product, especially when looking at a language and culture in which the word for the animal (*araignée*) derives from the mythical weaver Arachne, whose dexterity in the textile craft were said to have been unrivalled among mortals. Moreover, in sixteenth- and seventeenth-century allegorical representations of the sense of touch, the relevance of tactility for artisanal skills was often symbolised by a spider and its web.[121] One of them, a ca 1544 print by George Pencz from a series dedicated to the five senses, represents 'tactus' both via a spider in a web and, in the foreground, a woman weaving (Figure 2.9). The association of tactile finesse with the spider's activity enhances the significance of weaving as emblematic for human crafts and skills. In any case, naturalists like Grew, along with using the metaphor 'texture', saw organic material as 'nature's handicraft' and associated it with the 'most elaborate Woof or Needle-Work in the World'.[122] When textile metaphors

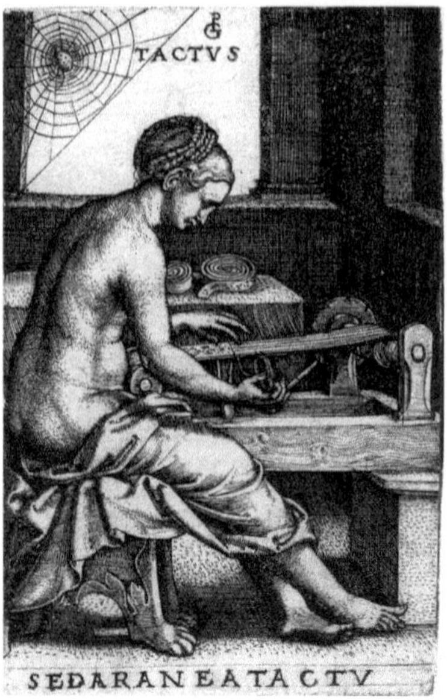

2.9 Georg Pencz, *Touch* (from a series of Five Senses), ca 1544, engraving, 7.7 x 5.1 cm.

like these were first introduced into the realm of medicine to describe the substance of the human body they seemed to have an affinity with one particular organ: skin.

It was the Italian physician Marcello Malpighi, another prolific seventeenth-century microscopist, who used the instrument to analyse the structure of the organ of touch. In his *De externo tactus organo anatomica observatio*, first published in 1665, he described one of the layers of skin as *reticulare corpus* (reticular body) or *rete mucosum* (mucous net), thus using yet another metaphor from the realm of textile fabrics.[123] The first French usage of the word *tissu* in a medical rather than botanical context was in a publication on skin so far overlooked by the etymologies of the term. It is a short note on observations by anatomist Alexis Littré based on the dissection of a black subject in the 1702 proceedings of the Académie royale des sciences which engaged closely with Malpighi and also confirmed his hypothesis about the location of the body's colouring matter in the skin (an aspect I will come back to in chapter 5). It reported that Littré 'thought he could attribute the blackness in parts to this particular *tissu* of the reticular membrane'.[124] By the mid-eighteenth century the notions *tissu* and *tissu cellulaire* were commonly used, for example in the French version of Haller's 1744 *Physiologia* or in Diderot and d'Alembert's *Encyclopédie*, published from 1751 onwards, to describe the variously textured organic material of the human body.[125]

The scrutiny given to the microscopic structure of skin since the second half of the seventeenth century excited a heightened interest in the build-up and functioning of the dermis, and impacted medical definitions of skin well into the eighteenth century. Most studies and entries to medical dictionaries dedicated to skin referred to Malpighi and generally defined the organ as an envelope whose main functions were to cover the human body and to serve as the sense of touch. They agreed that papillae (*mamelons* in French) shaped like little pyramids or cones, connected with the reticular body and, themselves made up of 'nervous filaments', served as the actual organ of touch. Among those taking up Malpighi's work in France was Joseph-Guichard Duverney, member of the Académie royale des sciences and since 1679 Professor of Anatomy at the Jardin du Roi (today Jardin des plantes) where his public dissections attracted considerable crowds.[126] He was in correspondence with Malpighi but also with his Dutch colleagues Govard Bidloo, Frederik Ruysch and Herman Boerhaave, and, himself investigating skin in his dissections, Duverney described the 'skin and its dependencies' as follows:

> The first of the general envelopes is the skin; it is made up of four different parts that are laid on top of each other, and are tied up with each other in a particular manner; there are a great number of vessels and glands that contribute to its composition […]

> The most interior part of the skin is composed of a very large number of fibres that interlace and cross in all directions, and form a particularly dense tissue that is nevertheless very flexible and spongy. […]
>
> The third part of the skin is a substance we call reticular body [Malpighi's *reticulare corpus*], because it is pierced by an infinite number of little openings and because it also seems in certain parts like a net or more or less extended stitches.[127]

Metaphors from the realm of textiles are abundant here: there are threads and fibres, interlacing to form nets, stitches and knitted loops or an overall tunic. An English *Medicinal dictionary* published between 1743 and 1745, and almost immediately translated into French, by Denis Diderot among others, suggests that similar notions of skin were widely disseminated in Europe. The lexicon defines the outermost part of skin, called epidermis or cuticle, as a non-sensitive membrane regenerating constantly and releasing sweat and oily liquids through its many pores. Both specialist and more generalist accounts of skin thus refer to it as netlike and porous. This understanding tied in with the ancient (Platonic and Galenic) legacy of comparing skin to a 'fisherman's net', a perforated bag that holds the organs while simultaneously allowing for exchange. Such a view of skin as vital for breathing and the excretion of fluids remained dominant throughout the early modern period.[128] It was crucial for medical attempts to restore or stabilise health through the regulation of bodily fluids and shared by patients describing their own body as porous.[129] Microscopy's ability to render these pores and netlike structures visible supported this understanding.

A question of more specifically anatomical and physiological concern – the issue of skin's layering – was rather complicated through microscopic insight. In the most simple terms, skin had been seen as consisting of an epidermis under which lay the 'true skin' (*veritable peau*), also named 'derma', 'cutis' or 'corium'. The *Medicinal dictionary* defines the latter as follows:

> The Skin is a Substance [translated as *tissu* in the French edition] of very large Extent, made up of several Kinds of tendinous, membranous, vascular, and nervous Fibres, the Intertexture of which is so much the more wonderful as it is difficult to unfold; for their Directions are as various as those of the Stuff of which an Hat consists.[130]

Skin was thus perceived as consisting of various layers but was also described as formed by parts rather than strata. The descriptive approach to skin apparently proved difficult because not everything visible through the microscope was discernible as a texture. It seemed interlaced in such complex ways that it resisted structuring and could only be approximated as the dense conglomerate of felt, which I presume the reference to a hat (usually made of that material) alludes to. This comparison had actually been previously made by Robert Hooke who suggested 'compar[ing] Paper and Hats with the Skin of an Animal' as a way of thinking about the shared properties of these materials.[131]

A microscopic view of the organ of touch

For early modern anatomy, focusing on the body's interior formation, skin was merely an integument as well as intermediary between inside and outside, and of little interest in itself. Vesalius, for example, took it very much for granted and explicitly stated that there was no need for it to be illustrated in his *Fabrica*.[132] Even the seventeenth-century accounts of the microscopic structure of the human skin and the functioning of the organ of touch remained largely without illustrations. An exception was Govard Bidloo's *Anatomia humani corporis* published in Amsterdam in 1685, the first anatomical atlas to consider previously invisible microscopic structures in its images, including a magnified view of the organ of touch.[133] The illustrations for the publication were entirely done after drawings by the then highly regarded Dutch artist Gérard de Lairesse,[134] a classicist often dubbed 'Poussin of the North'. Given that the text is condensed to the explanations of the tables, the engravings have been rightly assessed as the atlas's outstanding feature. Both Lairesse in his ink and wash drawings and the engravers (in all likelihood Abraham Blooteling and Peter van Gust) worked intensely with nuanced shadings thus giving the anatomised body a distinct kind of plasticity. The plates engaging with dissections of the abdomen, especially, probe the depths of the body in a new way, redefine the physical relations of inside and outside and lend skin a new materiality. In many images, the skin, slit and folded back in several layers, is thick and fleshy with the fatty layer like pelt worn inside (Figure 2.10).

More than an envelope that has to be removed in order to assess the interior, skin itself is made an issue of in the atlas, with an entire page of figures with accompanying explanations dedicated to the dermis and its appendages (Figure 2.1). The illustrations mostly derive from the dissection of a hand and represent the make up of dermis and epidermis in various details. Among them is one close-up view of the papillae and connected nerves serving jointly as the organ of feeling, and, as the legend explains, it also specifies roots of hair (E) and sweat vessels (D). The image depicts the dermal papillae as if sitting in a nest of nerves. It thus seems as if the draughtsman and the engravers experienced the same challenge as the physicians and naturalists describing the organ in presenting the elements of skin as simultaneously discrete *and* connected, as both layers *and* interlaced parts. The image is necessarily an interpretation of what was seen through the microscope and of the verbal descriptions of skin, but it insists on presenting an actual specimen as much as the text reinforces that the section of the dermis has been rendered as seen via

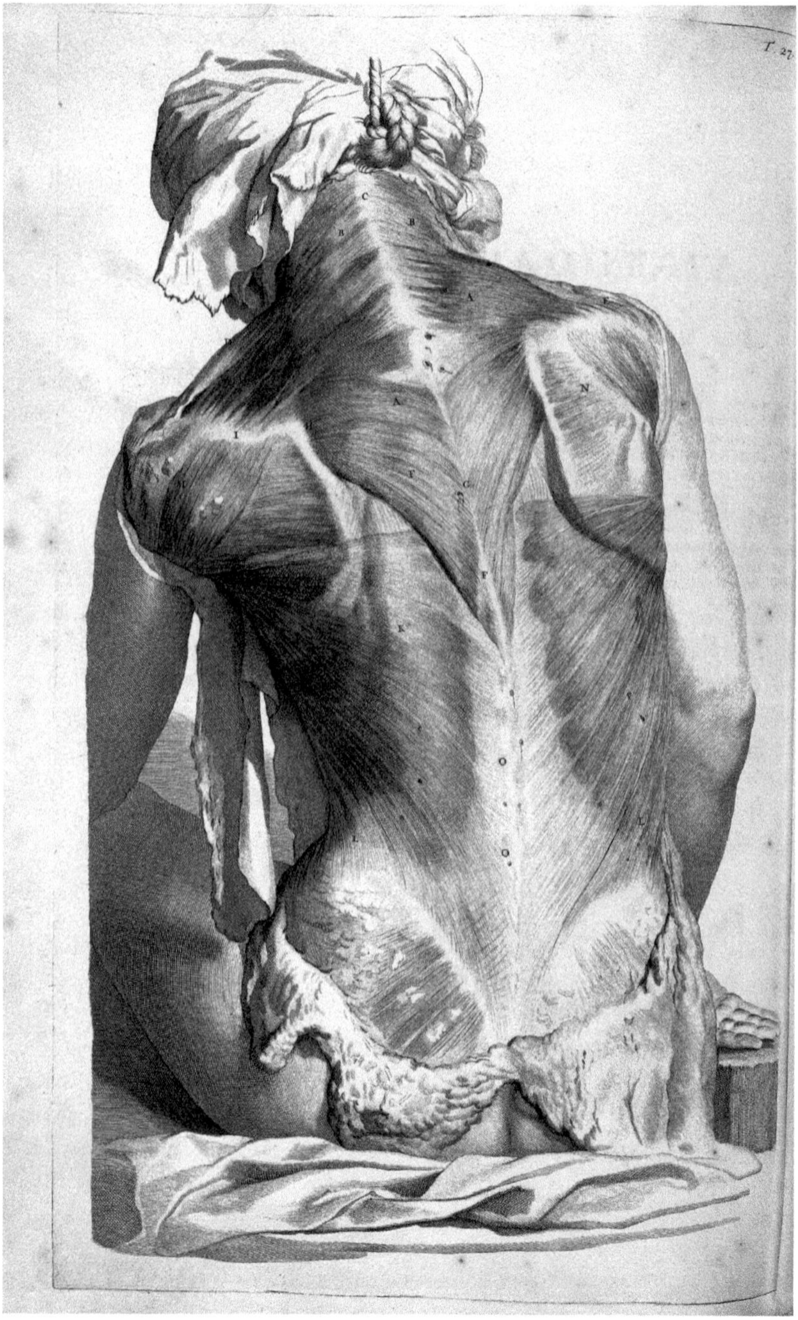

2.10 After Gérard de Lairesse, Flayed back of a woman, from Govard Bidloo, *Anatomia humani corporis*, 1685, table 27, engraving, 49 x 28 cm (platemark).

the microscope, that the 'structure, depicted through the optical instrument, is shown in figure 6'.[135] This rhetoric, which ties the image to observation, to what the artist had in front of his eyes when making his drawings, is first introduced with the treatise's extended title which announces 105 tables drawn 'from the life', *ad vivum*, or *naar het leeven* in the Dutch edition of the atlas. The notion *ad vivum* (and its Dutch companion) was well established by the time it appeared on the title page of Bidloo's atlas, and it was in the Netherlands that the term was also most systematically theorised. It is a significant term in the 1604 *Schilder-Boeck* by Karel van Mander who used it for a mode of image production in which the object is in front of the artist depicting it. Van Mander juxtaposed it to 'from the mind', referring to the capacity of artists to make new pictorial inventions thanks to their imagination.[136] This juxtaposition should not make us believe though that producing images 'from the life' does not involve imagination, and that seeing can ever be a mindless process.

So what exactly does *ad vivum* mean in the case of the little drawing of the dermis (Figures 2.11 and 2.12)? It is by no means certain whether de Lairesse himself looked through the microscope rather than following verbal instructions by Bidloo or descriptions of the organ, such as the one by Malpighi.[137] In any case, what is excluded from the illustration is precisely the instrument that allowed what is shown in the image to gain visibility in the first place. It needed to be excluded, I suggest, in order for the image to become plausible, in order for the tiny agents of human touch to become themselves tangible. To make the claim that it was drawn 'from the life', the image had to become disproportionate. The two nails with which the specimen is pinned on to the picture's ground to suggest that this is an actual piece of skin, are of an entirely different scale from the organic material. Given that the structure measures circa 6 x 8 cm in the engraving, the pins could be roughly life-size, but they are holding a tissue slice that is – if I reckon correctly from today's scaled images of this part of the dermis – circa 0.2 mm thick with minute structures seventeenth-century microscopes had allowed to render visible.[138] The elements that are meant to emphasise the veracity of the image in suggesting that we are looking at a palpable piece of organic material, are paradoxically the ones that are deliberately disproportionate thus pointing out the image's speculative character. By stressing this, I do not wish to raise doubts about the sincerity of the image, nor to chime with the accusations made by Bidloo's contemporaries, Ruysch in particular, that neither the explanations nor the illustrations were entirely drawn from the anatomist's own preparations. Ruysch took particular issue with the microscopic view in question and with the accompanying description of the cutaneous papillae. Were they pyramidal or needle-shaped cones? And what did these similes imply? In de Lairesse's image they look like neither pyramids nor needles, as the shapes are far more uneven; and the dispute only proves that the comparisons used to make sense

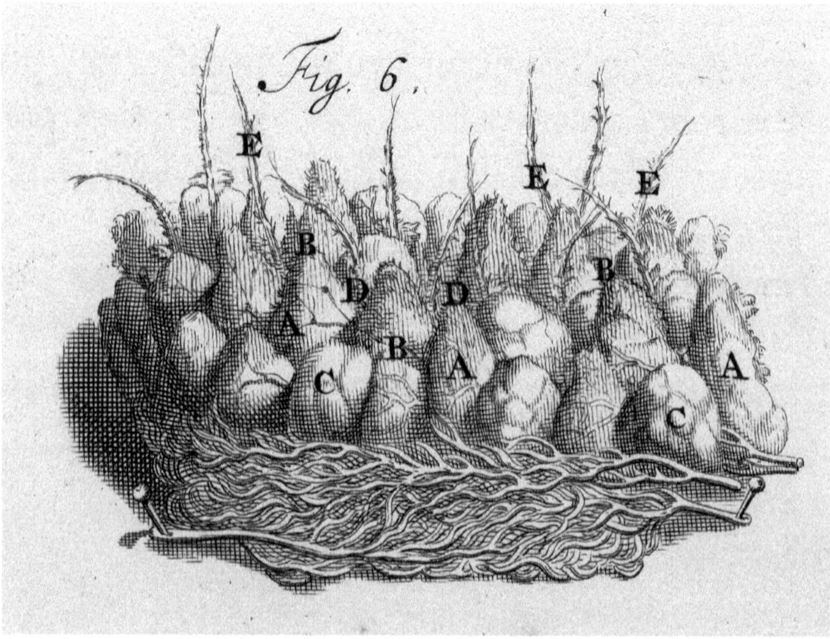

2.11 After Gérard de Lairesse, microscopic structure of skin, from Govard Bidloo, *Anatomia humani corporis*, 1685, table 4, engraving, ca 6 x 8 cm (detail).

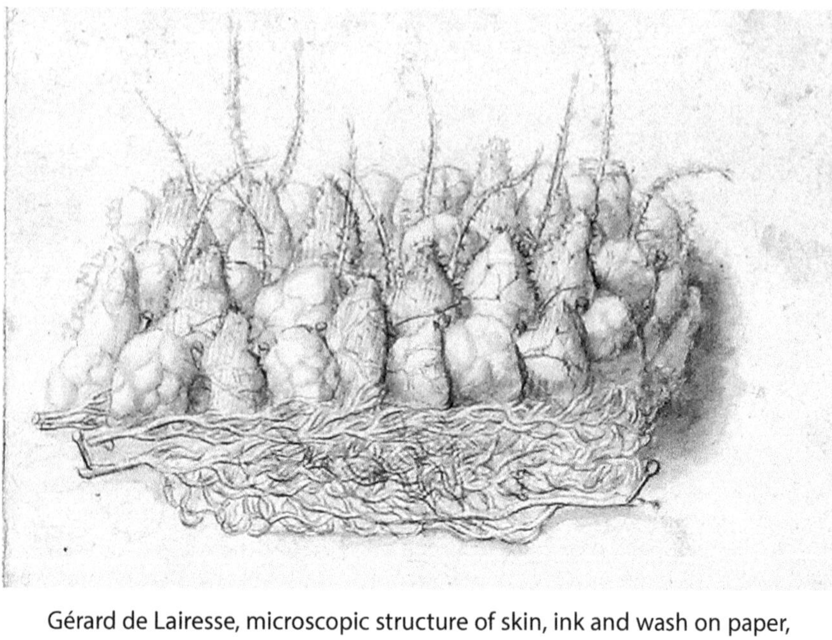

2.12 Gérard de Lairesse, microscopic structure of skin, ink and wash on paper, ca 6.2 x 8.3 cm (drawing).

of what is seen through the microscope are necessarily open to interpretation.[139] The controversy was also carried out in images (Figure 2.13). Ruysch added a more diagrammatic image of the microstructure of skin to his *Epistola* where the netlike body is a rectangle on which the pyramidal papillae are regularly distributed. In turn, Bidloo included Ruysch's image in his response, in which he reinserted de Lairesse's view with the far more irregular cones; the structure is slightly truncated though to make it more rectangular and the little pins are obliterated. This can be seen as an attempt to make the images more compatible, but also suggests that the illogical aspect of the pins started to be seen as a problem. As Margócsy has argued, the dispute between Bidloo and Ruysch, carried out in images and letters, was also about what the use of metaphors and similes implies. While Ruysch and the image he used took the comparison with pyramids as literal, for Bidloo it was rather an approximation, and de Lairesse's image accordingly shows the variability of forms.[140] In any case, the flattening microscopic views of phenomena too small to be palpable had to be re-turned into something that can be visualised spatially. The textile or architectural metaphors already discussed were indispensable not only for describing but for visibly understanding what remained difficult

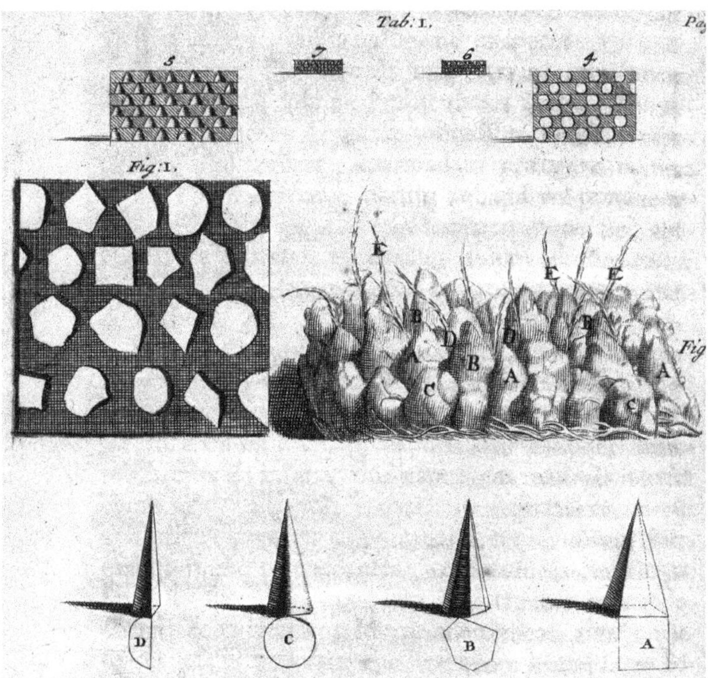

Multiple views of the papillae of the dermis, from Govard Bidloo, *Vindiciae quarundam delineationum anatomicarum*, 1697, engraving, 12.7 x 15 cm (platemark). 2.13

to discern.[141] In this sense, the nails can also be understood as the site where observation is pinned down in an image that aims to be comprehensible as a representation of a three-dimensional organic fragment. In both drawing and engraving the specimen and one of the pins cast shadows, a technique often used in *trompe l'œil* paintings, especially in *trompe l'œil* pinboards popular in seventeenth-century Dutch painting, to create the illusion that objects protrude from the picture plane.[142] The result is the image of a surface (the skin) that is turned into a thick segment of organic tissue through dissection, microscopy and image making – and seen simultaneously from the top and from the side. This oblique orientation in space has since become common in images of cross-sections of the skin.

The engraver very faithfully copied the drawing by de Lairesse, as the meshwork of nerves on which the irregular cone shaped papillae sit and the shades are duplicated accurately. And yet, the respective materials – pencil, brush and India ink in Lairesse's drawing and burin and black printer's ink in the engravings – produce a different look-and-feel as to the materiality of what is delineated. Drawn in liquid India ink the cones look mucous, engraved they seem drier. The shades are homogeneous grey zones in the drawing, but when evoked via cross hatchings in the engraving, they produce a texture of their own. In the print, the nails pierce into a gauze-like texture. This zone marked by the grid of mostly right-angled cross hatchings underlies the represented specimen and surrounds it in the lower part, expanding and darkening it due to additional diagonal lines at the left side, and can be seen as depicting a shadow cast by the magnified segment of skin. But it is not only an indication of a shadow. The woof of lines is as interlaced with the organic structure it represents as the elements of skin are interwoven among themselves. The print thus establishes a kinship between the textured nature of the representation and that of the object represented. The metaphors borrowed by the naturalists and physicians from the realm of textiles to describe the 'fabric of nature' are thus taken up here on two levels: the nerve cords are visualised like tracery, and skin's 'texture' is simultaneously traced back to the actual craft of the printer who stages the texture produced with the help of the burin. This image of the skin is thus the result of multiple mediations: something seen through the microscope, and understood and verbally described through textile metaphors, is transferred into a drawing, and later copied in a print which enhances the analogy of organic material and woven textiles. But the chain of mediations does not end here. The 1690 Dutch edition of Bidloo's atlas is credited for using the Dutch word for tissue *weefsel* – equally deriving from weaving – for the first time in an anatomical context, and it is precisely in the section on skin and relating to the image of its microscopic structure that the legend states what is drawn here 'is a tissu'.[143] Given that the phrasing is slightly different in the earlier Latin edition, it might well be that the textured engraving of the dermis encouraged the use of the word *weefzel* (Bidloo's spelling) bound to make its entry into medical language at the time anyway. The little engraving is a visually interpreted and materially re-enacted model of the texture, layering and functioning of the organ of touch. And it is as a model and re-enactment that it gains its explanatory value. The image proved successful in the sense that it remained, for some time, the only attempt to visualise the microscopic structure of the dermis. It forms the basis of many medical images of the composition of skin up to today.

The engraving's association of the skin with the means by which it is depicted coincides with the metaphorisation of living matter as texture or tissue. The medical image of the microscopic structure of skin is an early example for the encounter between organic textures and the crafted texture that reproduces them. Several decades later this relationship was explored in painting as well. Even though flesh tones or *carnations* and associated notions of the body in paint did by no means become obsolete over the course of the eighteenth century, flesh had already started to become a different matter and was increasingly dissociated from the skin.

Notes

1 Leon Battista Alberti, *On the Art of Building in Ten Books*, trans. Joseph Rykwert, Neil Leach and Robert Tavernor (Cambridge/Mass.; London: MIT Press, 1988); Alberti mentions 'skin' in particular in book 3 and in book 2, chapter 10, as well as book 6, chapters 9–11. See Marianne Koos, 'Haut als mediale Metapher in der Malerei von Caravaggio', in Daniela Bohde and Mechthild Fend (eds), *Weder Haut noch Fleisch: das Inkarnat in der Kunstgeschichte* (Berlin: Gebr. Mann, 2007), pp. 65–85 (p. 67); and more generally on the metaphoric uses of skin and the metaphor of skin for the façade or outer layer of architecture Claudia Benthien, *Skin: On the Cultural Border Between Self and the World* [1999], trans. Thomas Dunlap (New York; Chichester: Columbia University Press, 2002), p. 24.

2 Daniela Bohde, '"Le tinte delle carni": zur Begrifflichkeit von Haut und Fleisch in italienischen Kunsttraktaten des 15.–17. Jahrhunderts', in Bohde and Fend (eds), *Weder Haut noch Fleisch*, p. 43.

3 Christiane Kruse, *Wozu Menschen malen: historische Begründungen eines Bildmediums* (München: Fink, 2003).

4 Ann-Sophie Lehmann, 'Jan van Eyck und die Entdeckung der Leibfarbe', in Bohde and Fend (eds), *Weder Haut noch Fleisch*, pp. 21–40; and 'Fleshing out the body: the "colours of the naked" in workshop practice and art theory, 1400–1600', in Ann-Sophie Lehmann and Herman Roodenburg (eds), *Body and Embodiment in Netherlandish Art. Neederlands Kunsthistorisch Jaarboek* 58 (Zwolle: Wanders, 2008), pp. 86–109. See on early treatises on flesh tones also Wilhemina Lepik-Kopaczyńska, 'Das antike Inkarnat in der Überlieferung der mittelalterlichen Humanisten', in Johannes Irmscher (ed.), *Renaissance und Humanismus in Mittel- und Osteuropa* (Berlin: Akademie Verlag, 1962), pp. 76–83; on ancient painting see her *Die antike*

Malerei (Berlin: Akademie Verlag, 1963); and more recently Yvonne Schmuhl, 'Das Inkarnat in der griechischen Malerei', *RIHA Journal* 0061, 26 November 2012, www.riha-journal.org/articles/2012/2012-oct-dec/schmuhl-inkarnat.

5 Christiane Kruse, 'Fleisch werden – Fleisch malen: Malerei als "incarnazione". Mediale Verfahren des Bildwerdens in Cennino Canninis Libro dell'Arte', *Zeitschrift für Kunstgeschichte*, 63 (2000), 305–26; and a more extensive discussion of the historical rationale for painting as a medium her *Wozu Menschen malen*. On Cennini and the *incarnat* see also George Didi-Huberman, *La Peinture incarnée: suivi de Le chef-d'œuvre inconnu par Honoré de Balzac* (Paris: Les Éditions de Minuit, 1985), pp. 22–3.

6 Kruse, 'Fleisch werden – Fleisch malen', p. 322.

7 Ibid., pp. 315–18; on early Christian notions of incarnation, Georges Didi-Huberman, 'La couleur de la chair ou le paradoxe de Tertullien', *Nouvelle revue de la psychanalyse*, 35 (1987), 9–49, Special issue: *Le champ visuel*.

8 Cennino d'Andrea Cennini, *The Craftmen's Handbook: The Italian 'Il libro dell'Arte'*, trans. Daniel V. Thomspon, Jnr. [1933 Yale University Press] (New York: Dover Publications, 1960), chapter 1, p. 1.

9 Ibid.

10 Ibid., chapter 39, p. 23. See also Kruse, 'Fleisch werden – Fleisch malen', pp. 324–5; Kruse, *Wozu Menschen malen*, p. 189.

11 Pamela Smith, 'Vermilion, mercury, blood, and lizards: matter and meaning in metalworking', in Ursula Klein and Emma Spary (eds), *Materials and Expertise in Early Modern Europe: Between Market and Laboratory* (Chicago; London: University of Chicago Press, 2009), pp. 29–49 (especially pp. 42–5); Karin Leonhard, *Bildfelder: Stilleben und Naturstücke des 17. Jahrhunderts* (Berlin: Akademie Verlag, 2013), pp. 287–96.

12 Cennini, *The Craftmen's Handbook*, p. 42, and on this chapter Kruse, 'Fleisch werden – Fleisch malen', pp. 314–17.

13 Among the few sources in which a similar term, *incarnatura*, is used is the anonymous fourteenth-century treatise on miniature painting, see Franco Brunello (ed.), *De arte illuminandi e altri trattati sulla tecnica della miniatura medievale* (Vincenza: N. Pozza, 1975), see Esther Pia Wipfler, '"Color humanus": das Inkarnat in den Quellenschriften des Mittelalters', in Esther Pia Wipfler (ed.), *Kunsttechnik und Kunstgeschichte: das Inkarnat in der Malerei des Mittelalters* (München: Zentralinstitut für Kunstgeschichte, 2012), 48–65 (p. 49); Kruse, *Wozu Menschen malen*.The term interestingly reappeared from the 1920s onwards as *Inkarnat*, a technical term for flesh tones in German-language art historical writings within the context of phenomenological (and often onthologising) approaches to colour. See Bohde and Fend (eds), *Weder Haut noch Fleisch*, pp. 9–19; and Victor Stoichita, 'L'inconscient iconographique de George Wilhelm Friedrich Hegel: la rose et les raisins', in Hubert Locher and Peter Schneemann (eds), *Grammatik der Kunstgeschichte. Sprachprobleme und Regelwerk im 'Bilddiskurs': Oskar Bätschmann zum 65. Geburtstag* (Emstetten; Berlin: Edition Imorde, 2008), pp. 162–77.

14 Bohde, '"Le tinte delle carni"', p. 49.

15 Étienne [René François] Binet, *Essay des merveilles de nature et des plus nobles artifices* (Rouen: R. de Beauvais, 1621), pp. 193–4; I am following here the trans-

lation of Lebrun in Mary P. Merrifield, *Medieval and Renaissance Treatises on the Arts of Painting: Original Texts with English Translations* (Mineola/N.Y.: Dover Publications, 1999), pp. 770–3; see on the two texts also Ann Massing, 'French painting technique in the seventeenth and early eighteenth centuries and De La Fontaine's *Académie de la peinture* (Paris 1679)', in Erma Hermens (ed.), *Looking Through Paintings: A Study of Painting Techniques and Materials in Support of Art Historical Research* (Baarn: de Prom, 1998), pp. 319–90 (pp. 328–9).

16 See Bohde, '"Le tinte delle carni"', p. 46, with particular respect to Lodovico Dolce; see also Patricia L. Reilly, 'Writing out color in Renaissance art theory', *Genders*, 12 (1991), 79–99.

17 Bohde, '"Le tinte delle carni"', pp. 54–6.

18 See for a discussion of the *Bartholomew* from the Sistine Chapel, Victor Stoichita, 'Michelangelos Haut', in Hans-Georg Arburg et al. (eds), *Mehr als Schein:* Ästhetik *der Oberfläche in Film, Kunst, Literatur und Theater* (Zürich; Berlin: diaphanes, 2008), pp. 34–51; Daniela Bohde, 'Skin and the search for the interior: the representation of flaying in the art and anatomy of the cinquecento', in Florike Egmond and Robert Zwijnenberg (eds), *Bodily Extremities: Preoccupations with the Human Body in Early Modern European Culture* (Aldershot: Ashgate, 2003), pp. 10–47.

19 Bohde, 'Skin and the search for the interior'.

20 Theophilus Presbyter, *De diversis artibus*, ed. and trans. C. R. Dodwell (Oxford: Clarendon Press, 1961), p. 5: 'Color qui dicitur *membrana*, quo pinguntur facies et nuda corpora, sic componitur … Deinde tere eum et admisce ei albam cerosam et cenobrium, donec *carni similis fiat*.' Emphasis mine. The original text was probably produced in a German monastery and is assumed to date from the first half of the twelfth century; it was handed down in various twelfth- to fourteenth-century copies. See Erhard Brepohl, *Theophilus Presbyter und das mittelalterliche Kunsthandwerk: Gesamtausgabe der Schrift* De diversis artibus. 2 vols (Köln: Böhlau, 1999), pp. 30–6. Brepohl also discusses the pigments and techniques Theophilus refers to. See further, Lehmann, 'Fleshing out the body', p. 89; Kruse, *Wozu Menschen malen*, p. 179; Stoichita, 'L'inconscient iconographique', p. 168.

21 Lehmann, 'Fleshing out the body', discusses Dutch and German 1400–1600 manuscripts with recipes for 'body tint'.

22 Merrifield, *Medieval and Renaissance Treatises*, pp. 482–3.

23 Ann-Sophie Lehmann, 'Hautfarben: zur Maltechnik des Inkarnats und der Illusion des lebendigen Körpers in der europäischen Malerei der Neuzeit', in Christoph Geissmar-Brandi et al. (eds), *Gesichter der Haut* (Frankfurt a. M.: Stroemfeld/Nexus, 2002), pp. 93–128 (p. 95).

24 Lebègue's compilation is dated 1431, and it is transcribed in Merrifield, *Medievial and Renaissance Treatises*, pp. 18–321; for *carnatura*, p. 22; see also Wipfler, '"Color humanus"', pp. 54–5; Lehmann, 'Fleshing out the body', p. 88.

25 Stefan Germer, *Kunst, Macht, Diskurs: die intellektuelle Karriere des André Félibien im Frankreich von Louis XIV* (München: Fink, 1997); for the dictionary see pp. 433–4.

26 André Félibien, *Des principes de l'architecture, de la sculpture, de la peinture et des autres arts qui en dépendent* (Paris: J. B. Coignard, 1676), p. 511.

27 *Dictionnaire de l'Académie française*, 1st edn, 1694, entry 'Carnation', (accessed via

the University of Chicago: The ARTFL Project. *Dictionnaires d'autrefois* https://artfl-project.uchicago.edu/content/dictionnaires-dautrefois).

28 *Nouveau Dictionnaire de l'Académie française*, 2nd edn, 1718, entry 'Carnation'.

29 *Dictionnaire de l'Académie française*, 1st edn, 1694, entry 'Incarnat'.

30 Ibid., entry 'Incarnation'.

31 Ibid., entry 'Chair'.

32 Ibid.

33 See for example Le Brun's 1667 lecture on Raphael's *Saint Michael*, the first lecture after the reorganisation of the *conférences* initiated by Colbert, in *Les conférences de l'Académie royale de la peinture et de sculpture*, ed. Jacqueline Lichtenstein and Christian Michel; 5 vols (Paris: École nationale supérieure des Beaux-Arts, 2007–12), vol. 1, p. 114; Nicolas Mignard's 1667 lecture on the so-called *Holy Family of Francis I* then attributed to Raphael, ibid., pp. 143–4; or Nocret's 1670 lecture on Poussin's *Ecstasy of Saint-Paul*, ibid., p. 393.

34 Christian Michel, *L'Académie royale de peinture et de sculpture (1648–1793): la naissance de l'école française* (Genève: Droz, 2012), pp. 22–54. Thomas Puttfarken, *Roger de Piles' Theory of Art* (New Haven; London: Yale University Press, 1985), p. 3; and *The Discovery of Pictorial Composition: Theories of Visual Order in Painting 1400–1800* (New Haven; London: Yale University Press, 2000), p. 230; on the role of portraits of its members in the academicisation of the arts and a changing notion of the artist, Hannah Williams, *Académie Royale: A History in Portraits* (Farnham; Burlington/Vt.: Ashgate, 2015), pp. 17–75.

35 See Lichtenstein and Michel on 'La réflexion artistique des academicians', in their introduction to the first volume of the new edition (2008) of the *Conférences*, vol. 1, pp. 25–42; Michel, *Académie royale*, p. 64.

36 Germer, *Kunst, Macht, Diskurs*, pp. 370–84.

37 This has been highlighted in particular by the editors of the recent complete edition of the lectures. See the introductory essays by Gaethgens, Lichtenstein and Michel in *Conférences*, vol. 1, pp. 13–23, and pp. 25–42. Jutta Held, *Französische Kunsttheorie des 17. Jahrhunderts und der absolutistische Staat: Le Brun und die ersten acht Vorlesungen an der königlichen Akademie* (Berlin: Reimer, 2001), especially pp. 135–6, also pleads for a more complex understanding of the early lectures, arguing that there was never a doctrinaire preference for the *disegno*. See on early academic theory in France also Thomas Puttfarken 'Composition, perspective and presence: observations on early academic theory in France', in John Onians (ed.), *Sight and Insight: Essays on art and culture in honour of E. H. Gombrich at 85* (London: Phaidon Press, 1994).

38 For an overview see Jennifer Montagu, 'The quarrel of drawing and colour in the French Academy', in Victoria V. Flemming and Sebastian Schütze (eds), *Ars naturam adiuvans: Festschrift für Matthias Winner* (Mainz: Philipp von Zabern, 1996), pp. 548–56.

39 See in particular Max Imdahl, *Farbe: kunsttheoretische Reflexionen in Frankreich* (München: Fink, 1987), a study on the art theoretical discussions on colour in seventeenth- to early twentieth-century France; and to a lesser degree Puttfarken, *Roger de Piles' Theory of Art*. See for an opinionated assessment of the methodological stakes in art historical studies of French seventeenth-century art theory Jutta Held's introduction to her study of the first eight *conférences*, in Held, *Französische Kunsttheorie des 17. Jahrhunderts*, pp. 7–19.

40 *Conférences*, vol. 1, p. 123.
41 Ibid., p. 435.
42 Ibid., p. 436.
43 Puttfarken, *Roger de Piles' Theory of Art*; and *Pictorial Composition* – on de Piles see in particular pp. 263–77.
44 On de Piles's lectures at the Académie see Lichtenstein and Michel in their introduction to *Conférences*, vol. 3, pp. 15–20.
45 See Ugo Dionne, 'Félibien dialoguiste: les Entretiens sur les vies des peintres', *Dix-septième siècle*, 53:210 (2001), 49–74.
46 Roger de Piles, *Dialogue upon Colouring*, trans. Mr. Ozell (London: printed for Daniel Brown and Bernard Lintott, 1711), p. 13; *Dialogue sur le coloris* (Paris: Nicolas Langlois, 1673), p. 20. The anecdote is retold in Roger de Piles, *Cours de peinture par principes* (Paris: chez Jacques Estienne, 1708), pp. 329–30.
47 De Piles, *Dialogue upon Colouring*, p. 15; *Dialogue sur le coloris*, p. 23.
48 De Piles, *Dialogue upon Colouring*, p. 37; *Dialogue sur le coloris*, pp. 67–8.
49 Lodovico Dolce had made a similar argument for Titian in his *Dialogo della Pittura* (1557), making the mastery of the flesh tones the litmus test of a painter's ability to evoke lifelikeness. See Bohde, '"Le tinte delle carni"', pp. 45–6; and Stoichita, 'L'inconscient iconographique', p. 165.
50 De Piles, *Dialogue upon Colouring*, p. 9, *Dialogue sur le coloris*, p. 13.
51 Roger de Piles, *Conversations sur la connoissance de la peinture et sur le jugement qu'on doit faire des tableaux. Où par occassion il est parlé de Rubens* (Paris: Nicolas Langlois, 1677), p. 260: 'Le Poussin n'a veu que l'Antique & a donné dans la Pierre'.
52 Puttfarken, *Roger de Piles' Theory of Art; and Pictorial Composition.*
53 Mary D. Sheriff, *Fragonard: Art and Eroticism* (Chicago; London: University of Chicago Press, 1990), pp. 47–9; equally sceptical is Tom Holert, *Künstlerwissen: Studien zur Semantik künstlerischer Kompetenz im Frankreich des 18. und frühen 19. Jahrhunderts* (München: Fink, 1998), p. 89.
54 John Beldon Scott, 'The meaning of Perseus and Andromeda in the Farnese Gallery and on the Rubens House', *Journal of the Warburg and Courtauld Institutes*, 51 (1988), 250–60; Joanna Woodall, 'Wtewael's *Perseus and Andromeda*: looking for love in early seventeenth-century Dutch painting', in Caroline Arscott and Katie Scott (eds), *Manifestations of Venus: Art and Sexuality* (Manchester; New York: Manchester University Press, 2000), pp. 39–68 (especially pp. 48–9).
55 De Piles, *Conversations*, pp. 137–8. See on this passage also Jacqueline Lichtenstein, *The Eloquence of Color* (Berkeley: University of California Press, 1993), p. 167.
56 De Piles, *Conversations*, p. 272.
57 Ibid., p. 273.
58 See Jennifer Montagu, *The Expression of the Passions: The Origin and Influence of Charles Le Brun's Conférence sur l'expression générale et particulière* (New Haven; London: Yale University Press, 1994), on the drawings in particular pp. 126 and 144.
59 'Sentiments sur le discours de Blanchard', 9 January 1672, in: *Conférences*, vol. 1, p. 450.
60 Le Brun in *Conférences*, vol. 1, p. 276, quoted from Montagu, *The Expression of the Passions*, p. 136.
61 Ulrich Heinen, 'Haut und Knochen – Fleisch und Blut: Rubens' Affektmalerei', in Ulrich Heinen and Andreas Thielemann (eds), *Rubens Passioni: Kultur der Leiden-*

schaften im Barock (Göttingen: Vandenhoeck & Ruprecht, 2001), pp. 70–109; and on Rubens and de Piles, 'Peter Paul Rubens: Barocke Leidenschaften', in Nils Büttner and Ulrich Heinen (eds), *Rubens: Barocke Leidenschaften*, exh. cat. Herzog Anton Ulrich Museum Braunschweig (Braunschweig; München: Hirmer, 2004), pp. 28–38.

62 See on the body and the passions of the soul also Held, *Französische Kunsttheorie des 17. Jahrhunderts*, pp. 139–62.

63 De Piles, *Conversations*, p. 273.

64 De Piles, *Cours de peinture par principes*, pp. 346–8: 'L'on sait assez que la peinture n'est qu'un fard, qu'il est son essence de tromper, & que le plus grand trompeur en cet Art, est le plus grand Peintre.' De Piles had made similar remarks already in his *Dialogue sur le coloris*, p. 68.

65 Lichtenstein, *Eloquence of Color*, pp. 182–95.

66 Reilly, 'Writing out color'.

67 De Piles, *Conversations*, pp. 145–6.

68 See Bohde, '"Le tinte delle carni"', pp. 45–6; and Lichtenstein, *Eloquence of Color*, p. 167.

69 See the introductions in Sheriff, *Fragonard*, and Melissa Hyde, *Making Up the Rococo: François Boucher and his Critics* (Los Angeles: Getty Publications, 2006).

70 See Jaucourt's two entries on 'Cosmetique' in the *Encyclopédie ou dictionnaire raisonné des sciences, des arts et des metiers*, ed. Denis Diderot and Jean le Rond d'Alembert (accessed via University of Chicago: ARTFL Encyclopédie Projet (winter 2008 edn), ed. Robert Morrissey, http://encyclopedie.uchicago.edu/), vol. 4, 1754, p. 291; and the one on 'Fard', vol. 6, 1756, pp. 408–9.

71 Catherine Lanoë, *La poudre et le fard: une histoire des cosmétiques de la Renaissance aux Lumières* (Seyssel: Champ Vallon, 2008), p. 167.

72 As has been suggested by Benthien, *Skin*, p. 102.

73 Lanoë, *La poudre et le fard*, on the popular use of cosmetics in particular pp. 287–94.

74 Ibid., p. 240.

75 Hyde, *Making Up the Rococo*, pp. 94–101.

76 Ibid., pp. 107–44; Ewa Lajer-Burchardt, 'Pompadour's touch: difference in representation', *Representations*, 73 (2001), 54–88; and on the 'The Painted Face' in this double sense and nineteenth-century portraits of women Tamar Garb, *The Painted Face: Portraits of Women in France 1814–1914* (New Haven; London: Yale University Press, 2007), in particular pp. 3–9.

77 Lanoë, *La poudre et le fard*, pp. 53–7; Alex Paré, 'Peindre la chair: rendu des carnations et image du corps dans la peinture française des années 1680–1740' (MA dissertation, École du Louvre, Paris, 2009).

78 Of the few copies that have been located by Lilien I am using the one in the British Library which includes four further illustrations and their explanation. The title page does not mention a publisher, place of publication or date, but it is listed in the *Monthly Catalogue … of all Books Publish'd in London* in May 1725, see Otto M. Lilien, *Jacob Christoph Le Blon 1667–1741: Inventor of Three and Four Colour Printing* (Stuttgart: Hiersemann, 1985), in particular pp. 94–6.

79 Jacob Christoph Le Blon, *Coloritto; or the Harmony of Colouring in Painting: Reduced to Mechanical Practice, under Easy Preceps, and Infallible Rules* [London, 1725], p. 6.

80 Lilien, *Le Blon*, pp. 11–85; on Le Blon and the question of patents and copyright see Katie Scott, 'Invention and privilege in early modern France: the case of colour', in Liliane Hiliare-Pérez and Anne-Françoise Garçon (eds), *Les chemins de la nouveauté: innover, inventer au regard de l'histoire* (Paris: Éditions du CTHS, 2003), pp. 167–86; Dániel Margócsy, *Commercial Visions: Science, Trade, and Visual Culture in the Dutch Golden Age* (Chicago: University of Chicago Press, 2014), pp. 167–99.

81 Lilien, *Le Blon*, pp. 118–19; Margócsy, *Commercial Visions*, pp. 170–89.

82 John Gage, *Colour and Culture: Practice and Meaning from Antiquity to Abstraction* (London: Thames & Hudson, 1993), p. 153.

83 This has been a major argument of a 1964 article by Hans Sedlmayr on Rubens's flesh tones, 'Bemerkungen zur Fleischfarbe bei Rubens' [1964], in *Epochen und Werke: gesammelte Schriften zur Kunstgeschichte*, vol. 3 (München: Mäander, 1982), pp. 165–78. With an ontological approach to colour, Sedlmayr interprets the fact that Rubens used the three primary colours for his flesh tones as a way by which the human is allocated – by the means of colour – a central place in the cosmos as a well-ordered system. This is implicitly racist, and closely related to ideas he developed in his 1948 *Verlust der Mitte* (*Art in Crisis: The Lost Centre* [1948], trans. Brian Battershaw, with a new introduction by Roger Kimball (New Brunswick/ N.J.; London: Transaction, 2007), where he deplored loss of harmony and centre in contemporary art, as he projects into Rubens's painting the idea of a harmonious unity of the cosmos with a nacre-skinned (multi-coloured but white) human at its centre. See Bohde and Fend (eds), *Weder Haut noch Fleisch*, p. 11. More recent studies on Rubens, such as Heinen, 'Haut und Knochen', have provided a physiological reading of the colours in Rubens's flesh tones, interpreting the blues as a reference to veins etc.

84 Roger de Piles, *Les premiers* éléments *de la peinture pratique* (Paris: chez Nicolas Langlois, 1684), pp. 43–9.

85 More generally on the difference between the optical and physical mixture of colour, Leonhard, *Bildfelder*, pp. 369–9.

86 According to an eighteenth-century source; there seem to have been no further editions. See Lilien, *Le Blon*, p. 97. For the lecture see *Conférences*, vol. 4, pp. 263–72.

87 Although this book reproduces a slightly altered version of the text of *Coloritto*, it is, according to Lilien, *Le Blon* (p. 102), wrong to consider it as a reprint of Le Blon's 1725 *Coloritto* as it comes without the plates. He assumes the author was Gaultier de Montdorge, a friend of Le Blon who also wrote the entries on colour printing and mezzotint for the *Encyclopédie*; for 'Gravure en couleur' see vol. 7, 1757, pp. 899–903, where Montdorge grants Le Blon the invention of the technique.

88 Le Blon, *Coloritto*, p. 6.

89 Ibid., p. 8.

90 I elaborate on this choice of the material plaster and on Le Blon's claims for colour printing as faithful reproduction in my article 'Flesh-tones, skin-color and the eighteenth-century color print', in *Aesthetics of the Flesh*, Felix Ensslin and Charlotte Klink (eds) (Berlin: Sternberg Press, 2014), pp. 203–27.

91 Le Blon, *Coloritto*, p. 8.

92 Ibid., p. 12.

93 According to Lilien, *Le Blon* (p. 97), the original colours, with the exception of the red pigment, have faded considerably.
94 See on Pygmalion and the myth of the living image Victor Stoichita, *The Pygmalion Effect: From Ovid to Hitchcock* (Chicago; London: University of Chicago Press, 2008).
95 Le Blon, *Coloritto*, pp. iv–v.
96 Florian Rodari, *Anatomie de la couleur: l'invention de l'estampe en couleurs* (Paris: Bibliothèque nationale de France, 1996), p. 12.
97 De Piles, *Premiers* élémens *de la peinture pratique*, p. 54.
98 Ibid., p. 29.
99 He talks in two consecutive paragraphs about lively flesh and the preserved liveliness of paintings, thus linking the two aspects, see De Piles, *L'art de peinture de C.A. Du Fresnoy. Enrichie de Remarques, & augmenté d'un Dialogue sur le coloris* (Paris: Nicolas Langlois, 1668), p. 134.
100 De Piles, *Conversations*, p. 146.
101 De Piles, *Cours de peinture par principes*, p. 286.
102 Coypel in *Conférences*, vol. 4, pp. 87–8.
103 Antoine-Joseph Pernety, *Dictionnaire portatif de peinture, sculpture et gravure* (Paris: Bauche, 1757), p. 537, entry 'Touche'.
104 See on the double meaning of *la touche* as brushstroke and touch Sheriff, *Fragonard*, pp. 138–48; Lajer-Burcharth, 'Pompadour's touch', in particular p. 57. In relation to late nineteenth-century painting Anthea Callen, 'Degas's *Bathers*: hygiene and dirt – gaze and touch', in Richard Kendall and Griselda Pollock (eds), *Dealing with Degas: Representations of Women and the Politics of Vision* (New York: Universe, 1992), pp. 159–85.
105 Marc Bloch, *The Royal Touch: Sacred Monarchy and Scrofula in England and France* [1961], trans. J. E. Anderson (London: Routledge and Kegan Paul, 1973).
106 On the quest for transparency in the Enlightenment see Jean Starobinski, *Jean-Jacques Rousseau: Transparency and Obstruction* [1957], trans. Arthur Goldhammer (Chicago; London: University of Chicago Press, 1988), especially chapter 1; and for notions of the genius Sheriff, *Fragonard*, pp. 137–49.
107 Sheriff, *Fragonard*, pp. 122–7; Uwe Fleckner, '"Pourquoi une belle esquisse nous plaît-elle plus qu'un beau tableau?" Fragonard, Diderot et l'eloquence du pinceau dans quelques portraits du XVIIIe siècle', in Thomas W. Gaethgens et al. (eds), *L'art et les normes sociales au 18ième siècle* (Paris: Éditions de la Maison des sciences de l'homme, 2001), pp. 509–33.
108 Comte de Caylus, *Vies d'artistes du XVIIIe siècle. Discours sur la peinture: Salons*, ed. André Fontaine (Paris: Librairie Renard, H. Laurens, Éditeur, 1910), pp. 149–59. *Vie d'artistes* was first published in the *Mercure* in September 1756.
109 See on Cochin's attitudes towards *le faire* Christian Michel, *Charles-Nicolas Cochin et l'art des Lumières* (Rome: École française de Rome, 1993), pp. 257–78, in comparison with Caylus in particular pp. 274–6; and generally on *le faire* Sheriff, *Fragonard*, pp. 122–5; Marianne Koos, *Haut, Farbe und Medialität: Oberfläche im Werk von Jean-Étienne Liotard (1702–1789)* (Paderborn: Fink, 2014), pp. 149–91.
110 Coypel in *Conférences*, vol. 4, p. 86.
111 Louis Tocqué, 'Reflexions sur la peinture et particulièrement sur le genre du portrait' [1750], in Arnauld Doria (ed.), *Le discours de Tocqué sur le genre du portrait* (Paris:

Jean Schemit, 1930), pp. 1–40 (p. 22). See on Tocqué and more generally on the notion of the *touche* in eighteenth-century French art theory Koos, *Haut, Farbe und Medialität*, pp. 148–91; on Tocqué and the lifelikeness of portraits, Williams, *Académie Royale*, p. 139.

112 Tocqué, 'Réflections sur la peinture', p. 22.

113 On changing notions of the artist's knowledge in eighteenth-century France see Holert, *Künstlerwissen*.

114 In his 1667 lecture in *Conférences*, vol. 1, p. 163.

115 See Martial Guédron, *De chair et de marbre: imiter et exprimer le nu en France (1745–1815)* (Paris: Éditions Champion, 2003), p. 29; Holert, *Künstlerwissen*, pp. 127–91; and more specifically on the rise of art criticism in eighteenth-century France Richard Wrigley, *The Origins of French Art Criticism: From the Ancien Régime to the Restoration* (Oxford; New York: Oxford University Press, 1993).

116 Annamaria Ducci, '"Leur chair chante des Marseillaises": la main dans les écrits sur l'art en France, repères pour un parcours', in Mariacarla Gadebusch Bondio (ed.), *Die Hand: Elemente einer Medizin- und Kulturgeschichte* (Berlin: LIT, 2010), pp. 239–64.

117 Pernety, *Dictionnaire portatif*, pp. 537–8, entry 'Touche'. Pernety, who was familiar with the botanical literature of the time, referred to the *Encyclopédie* in his *Dictionnaire portatif* and might have encountered the notion *tissu* among others in the entry 'Anatomie' in the first volume of the *Encyclopédie* published in 1751.

118 Robert Hooke, *Micrographia: or some Physiological Descriptions of Minute Bodies made by Magnifying Glasses* (London: Jo. Martyn and Ja. Allestry, 1665), pp. 6–7.

119 See in particular Nehemia Grew, *The Anatomy of Plants. With an Idea of a Philosophical History of Plants* (London: W. Rawlins, for the Author, 1682), originally presented as lectures to the Royal Society. The word 'texture' is used throughout the *Anatomy of Plants*, see for example pp. 11, 108, 119, 120. The first French translation – *Anatomie des Plantes* – appeared in 1685; for usages of the term 'tissure' see for example pp. 40, 66–7. See also Ilse Jahn (ed.), *Geschichte der Biologie*, 3rd edn (Berlin: Spektrum, 2000), pp. 209–11.

120 George Canguilhem, 'Cellular Theory' [1945], in *Knowledge of Life* [1963], ed. Paola Marrati and Todd Meyers, trans. Stefanos Geroulanos and Daniela Ginsburg (Ashland/Ohio: Fordham University Press, 2008), pp. 25–56 (p. 43).

121 Benthien, *Skin*, p. 188.

122 Grew, Dedication to the *Anatomy of Plants* (no pages).

123 The tract was republished in Marcello Malpighi, *Opera Omnia. Tomis duobus comprehensa* (London: Prostant apud Robertum Scott, 1686), pp. 21–32. See Domenico Bertoloni Meli, *Mechanism, Experiment, Disease: Marcello Malpighi and Seventeenth-Century Anatomy* (Baltimore: Johns Hopkins University Press, 2011), pp. 76, 88–92.

124 Alexis Littré, ['De la structure de la peau'], in *Histoire de l'Académie Royale des Sciences*, Année MDCCII (Paris: chez Gabr. Martin, Jean-Bapt. Coignard, et les Frères Guerin, 1743), p. 31: 'M. Littré a donc crû qu'il falloit rapporter la noirceur en partie au tissu particulier de la membrane réticulaire.'

125 The *Dictionnaire culturel en langue française*, ed. Alain Rey, 4 vols (Paris: Dictionnaires le Robert, 2005), vol. 4, pp. 1,415–16, only mentions Diderot and d'Alembert's

Encyclopédie (1751), itself following Haller's *Physiologia* (1744), as source for the use of the term *tissu cellulaire*. The term is indeed widely used in the *Encyclopédie*, for example in the article on anatomy. The lemma 'tissu' itself however notes only the textile dimension of the term. The *Dictionnaire de l'Académie française* notes this signification of the word for the first time only in its sixth edition of 1832–35.

126 Andrew Cunningham, *The Anatomist Anatomis'd: An Experimental Discipline in Enlightenment Europe* (Farnham; Burlington/Vt.: Ashgate, 2010), pp. 100–3.

127 Published posthumously in Joseph-Guichard Duverney [also Du Verney], *Œuvres anatomiques* (Paris: C. A. Jombert, 1761), pp. 281–5.

128 Mieneke te Hennepe, 'Of the fisherman's net and skin pores: reframing conceptions of the skin in medicine 1572–1714', in Manfred Horstmanshoff, Helen King and Claus Zittel (eds), *Blood, Sweat and Tears: Changing Concepts of Physiology from Antiquity into Early Modern Europe* (Leiden: Brill, 2012), pp. 524–48.

129 Barbara Duden, *The Woman beneath the Skin: A Doctor's Patients in Eighteenth-century Germany* [1987], trans. Thomas Dunlap (Cambridge/Mass.: Harvard University Press, 1991).

130 *A Medicinal Dictionary, Including Physic, Surgery, Anatomy, Chymistry, and Botany, in all their Branches Relative to Medicine, by R. James*, 3 vols (London: T. Osborne, 1743–45), vol. 2, entry 'Cutis'.

131 Robert Hooke, 'A General Scheme, or Idea of the Present State of Natural Philosophy', in *The Posthumous Works of Robert Hooke* (London: Richard Weller, 1705), p. 57, quoted from Matthew Hunter, *Wicked Intelligence:, Visual Art and the Science of Experiment in Restoration London* (Chicago; London: University of Chicago Press, 2013), p. 91, who discusses Hooke's interest in the making and materiality of paper and felt in more detail.

132 Te Hennepe, 'Of the fisherman's net and skin pores', p. 528.

133 Marian Fournier, *The Fabric of Life: Microscopy in the Seventeenth Century* (Baltimore; London: Johns Hopkins University Press, 1996), pp. 138–9.

134 The complete set of drawings is held by the Bibliothèque interuniversitaire de santé (BIU Santé) in Paris; it has been digitised and can be accessed via www2.biusante.parisdescartes.fr/livanc/?do=livre&cote=ms00026. See also Paule Dumaître, *La curieuse destinée des planches anatomiques de Gérard de Lairesse, peintre en Hollande: Lairesse, Bidloo, Cowper* (Amsterdam: Rodopi, 1982); and more generally on the artist Lyckle de Vries, *Gerard de Lairesse: An Artist between Stage and Studio* (Amsterdam: Amsterdam University Press, 1999).

135 Govard Bidloo, *Anatomia humani corporis, centum & quinque tabulis, per artificiosiss. G. de Lairesse ad vivum delineatis* (Amsterdam: for the widow of Joannes van Someren, the heirs of Joannes van Dyk, Henry Boom and widow of Theodore Boom, 1685), text for table 4.

136 On the notion of *ad vivum* or *naer het leven* see Claudia Swan, '"Ad vivum", "naer het leven", "from the life": considerations on a mode of representation', *Word and Image*, 11 (1995), 353–72; Robert Felfe, '*Naer het leven:* eine sprachliche Formel zwischen bildgenerierenden Übertragungsvorgängen und ästhetischer Vermittlung', in Claudia Fritzsche, Karen Leonhard and Gregor J. M. Weber (eds), *Ad Fontes: Niederländische Kunst des siebzehnten Jahrhunderts in Quellen* (Petersberg: Michael Imhof Verlag, 2013), pp. 165–95.

137 Bertoloni Meli, *Mechanism, Experiment, Disease*, p. 300, has made a similar argument for the image of the glands of the cerebral cortex in Bidloo's atlas.

138 Marian Fournier, 'De Microscopische Anatomie in *Bidloo's Anatomia Humani Corporis* (1685)', *Tijdschrift voor de Geschiedenis der Geneeskunde, Natuurwetenschappen, Wiskunde en Tecknick*, 8:4 (1985), 187–208 (p. 204), argues that Bidloo used less powerful instruments, capable of a magnification by 20 or 30 times, than other microscopists of the time, such as Leeuwenhoek.

139 Cunningham, *The Anatomist Anatomis'd*, pp. 283–5; Margócsy, *Commerical Visions*, pp. 135–66.

140 Ibid., p. 146.

141 Matthias Bruhn, 'Beyond the icons of knowledge: artistic styles and the art history of scientific imagery', in Horst Bredekamp, Birgit Schneider and Vera Dünkel (eds), *The Technical Image: A History of Scientific Imagery* [2008] (Chicago: University of Chicago Press, 2015), pp. 36–45 (pp. 39–40).

142 On *trompe l'œil* effects produced by the use of shadows in natural history imagery see Angela Fischel, 'Sehen, Darstellen, Beschreiben: mikroskopische Beobachtung in den Kupferstichen der Micrographia', *kunsttexte.de* 1.2002, http://edoc.hu-berlin.de/kunsttexte/download/bwt/fischel.pdf.

143 *Woordenboek der Nederlandsche Taal*, accessed via the online database of the Instituut for Nederlandse Lexicologie, http://gtb.inl.nl/. Govart Bidloo, *Ontleding des menschelyken lichaams* (Amsterdam: By de weduwe van Joannes van Someren, de erfgenaamen van Joannes van Dyk, Hendrik en de weduwe van Dirk Boom, 1690), text for table 4. Using the term 'structure', Cowper's English version remains closer to Bidloo's Latin text. See on textiles, human tissue and skin in anatomical preparations by Ruysch and Albinus, Marieke Hendriksen, *Elegant Anatomy: The Eighteenth-Century Leiden Anatomical Collections* (Leiden; Boston: Brill, 2015).

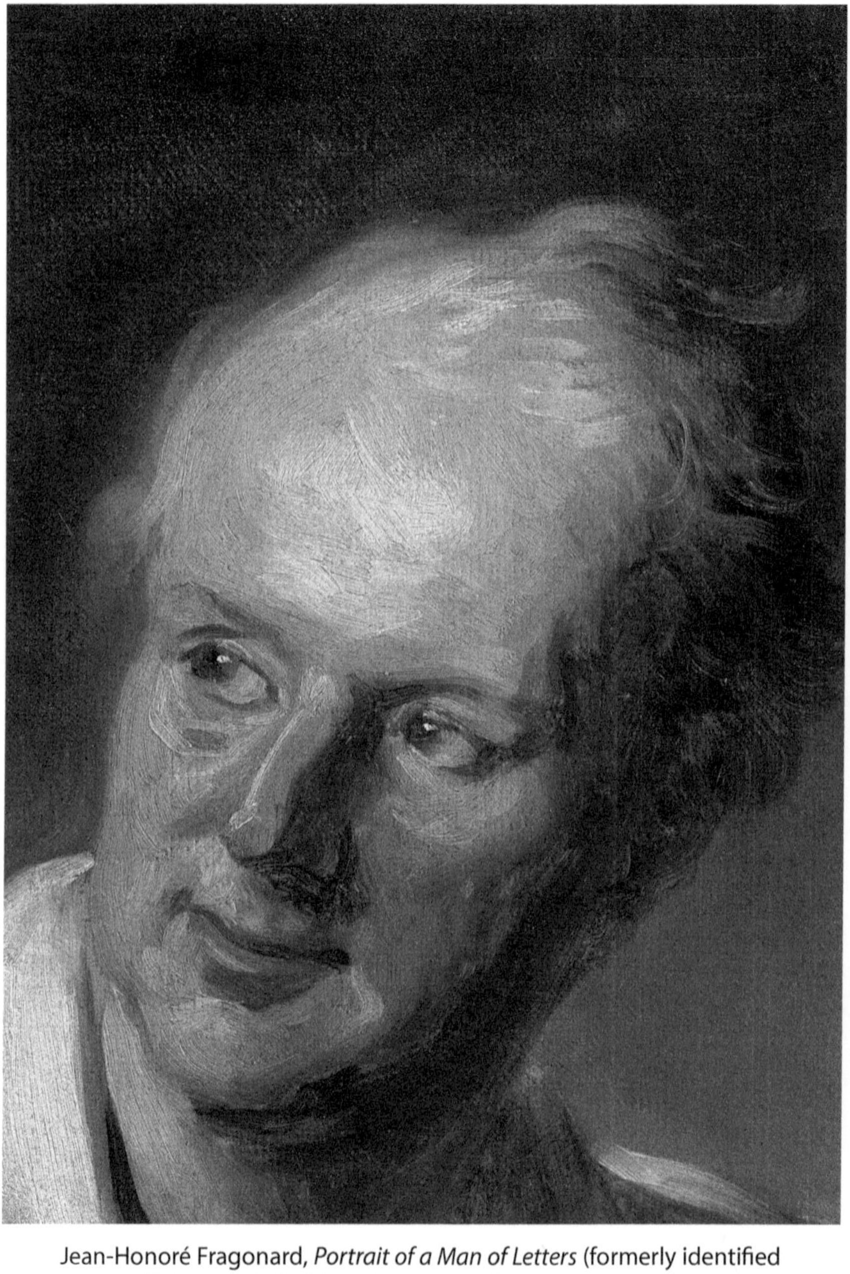

3.1 Jean-Honoré Fragonard, *Portrait of a Man of Letters* (formerly identified as Diderot; detail of head), ca 1769, oil on canvas, 81 x 65 cm.

3 Nervous canvas

The new understanding of organic substances as textured and the extensive use of textile metaphors in medical descriptions of skin, which I discussed in the last chapter, joined a special attention to the artist's hand in mid-eighteenth-century French art practice and theory. This conjuncture prompted attempts to imitate the skin's tissue with an appropriate facture produced by the brush. If metaphors can be defined as the encounter of two semantic fields, in this case medicine on the one hand, and the crafts and the arts on the other, I will, in what follows, take the medical metaphorisation of skin as a 'nervous canvas' as my guide in discussing relations between medical and artistic visions of skin in mid-eighteenth-century France. My example is the so-called *portraits de fantaisie* by Jean-Honoré Fragonard, a painter who was particularly associated with a visible *touche* and a sophisticated handling of the brush with which he drew attention to the painting's surface as crafted texture. Following on from my previous discussion of brushwork, textures and tissues, the argument will be that the simultaneous attention to the manually produced surface of the painting and to the body's surface signals a new understanding of the body in paint. Fragonard's *carnations* in the *portraits de fantaisie* are as much about flesh as they are about the materiality and vitality of skin (Figure 3.1, plate 5). I propose that there is, in mid-eighteenth-century France, a further rapprochement not only between the artist's *touche* and the sense of touch, but also between the inspired brushstrokes thought to enliven a painting and the contemporary medical understanding of skin as a vital organ and a primary site of sense activity. And it is in this context – around the notion of skin as an organ particularly gifted with sensibility – that the metaphor of skin as a 'nervous canvas' appears in the entry 'Sensibilité' in volume 17 of the *Encyclopédie* published in 1765. In my analysis of such interconnections between the fields of medicine and the arts, the philosopher and art critic Denis Diderot will function as an important mediator. Writing simultaneously on Salon exhibitions, on the significance of the sense of touch and on physiology, and fictionalising the latest medical theories in his *Rêve de d'Alembert*, Diderot thought about skin in the various arenas under consideration here. This chapter will thus look at skin, sensibility and touch in painterly practice and the art literature, and in medical as well as philosophical discourses during the period 1750–80.

Fragonard's *portraits de fantaisie* and the epidermis of nature

Fragonard skilfully adapted his *faire* to the subject matter he was treating and to the various audiences of his works.[1] In his 1765 *The High Priest Coresus Sacrificing Himself to Save Callirhoe* for example, a large format history painting that served as his reception piece for the Académie, he used a finished handling to lure the viewer into the dramatic action and dreamlike atmosphere. In contrast, in his 1763–64 *Bathers* (Figure 3.2), a relatively small easel painting representing a group of women enjoying themselves in water and reeds, he merged figures and nature with broad sweeps of the brush thus associating via the artist's lively *faire* 'nature's vitality and woman's sexuality', as Mary Sheriff has put it.[2] Such a painting would be tuned towards an audience of male connoisseurs

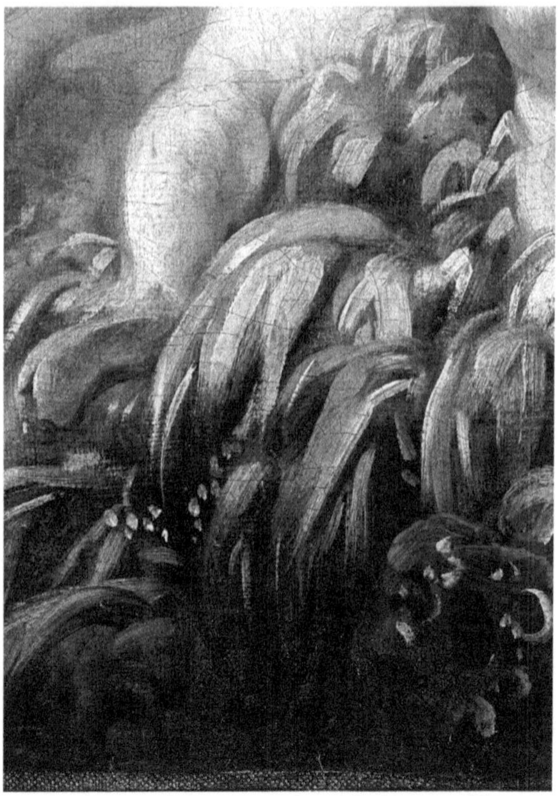

3.2 Jean-Honoré Fragonard, *Bathers*, 1763–64, oil on canvas, 64 x 80 cm (detail).

able to appreciate the artist's hand as much as the subject matter, and to enjoy the pleasure of displacement between the artist's *touche* and what it signified, in this case flesh. Finally, there is the set of circa fifteen same-sized canvases now known as *portraits* or *figures de fantaisie* painted between 1765 and 1773 in vibrant, highly visible brushstrokes. They were never shown in public during Fragonard's lifetime and remained for the most part at the artist's premises until his death in 1806.[3] The consideration of this group of paintings as *portraits de fantaisie* has recently been discussed and contested.[4] Previous assumptions about potential sitters have been challenged after the spectacular find of a set of sketches, authenticated as being by Fragonard, constituting eighteen portraits, most of them identifiable with known *portraits de fantaisie* and annotated with names believed to indicate the sitters.[5] If this assemblage of sketches encourages the inclination to see likenesses of actual people in these paintings, it also frustrates earlier identifications: the portrait which many scholars (myself included) liked to see as the image of Diderot, was now dissociated from the philosopher and linked instead with the journalist Ange-Gabriel Meusnier de Querlon.[6] The new possibility of naming the portrayed does not, however, disqualify the labelling of the paintings as *portraits de fantaisie*, a notion within the scope of eighteenth-century understandings of portraiture resonating in particular with Diderot's remarks that resemblance is not the main point of a good portrait. Whether referring to named individuals or not, these portraits have playful and imaginative aspects, as they foreground the work of the artist's hand while simultaneously staging the figures in fancy costumes and often caught in a dreamy or contemplative mood. In any case, for the argument I am making in what follows, the question of specific sitters is irrelevant, and I will therefore refer to them in the generic terms in which some of them, such as *Inspiration*, *Study* or *The Young Artist* (Figures 3.3–3.5), had already been known;[7] and I will neutrally call the portrait formerly known as that of Diderot, *Portrait of a Man of Letters* (Figure 3.1, plate 5).

Fragonard exposed his expertise in paint handling with what the eighteenth century called the 'intelligence of his art', and there is every reason to assume that he was familiar with contemporary art theoretical positions on *la touche* and *le faire*. After winning the Rome prize in 1752, Fragonard was admitted to the École royale des élèves protégés instituted shortly before as part of the attempts to reform the Académie and to re-establish a more rigorous art training. Among his teachers at the prestigious school was the artist and theorist Michel-François Dandré-Bardon whose 1765 *Traité de peinture suivi d'un essai sur la sculpture* provided a summary of earlier eighteenth-century art theoretical ideas and reiterated de Piles's views on colouring. It is distinguished through its special attention to the making of art works, and was particularly sensible to the contribution of materials and the artistic treatment of surfaces to the effects of sculptures and paintings.[8] In consequence, the

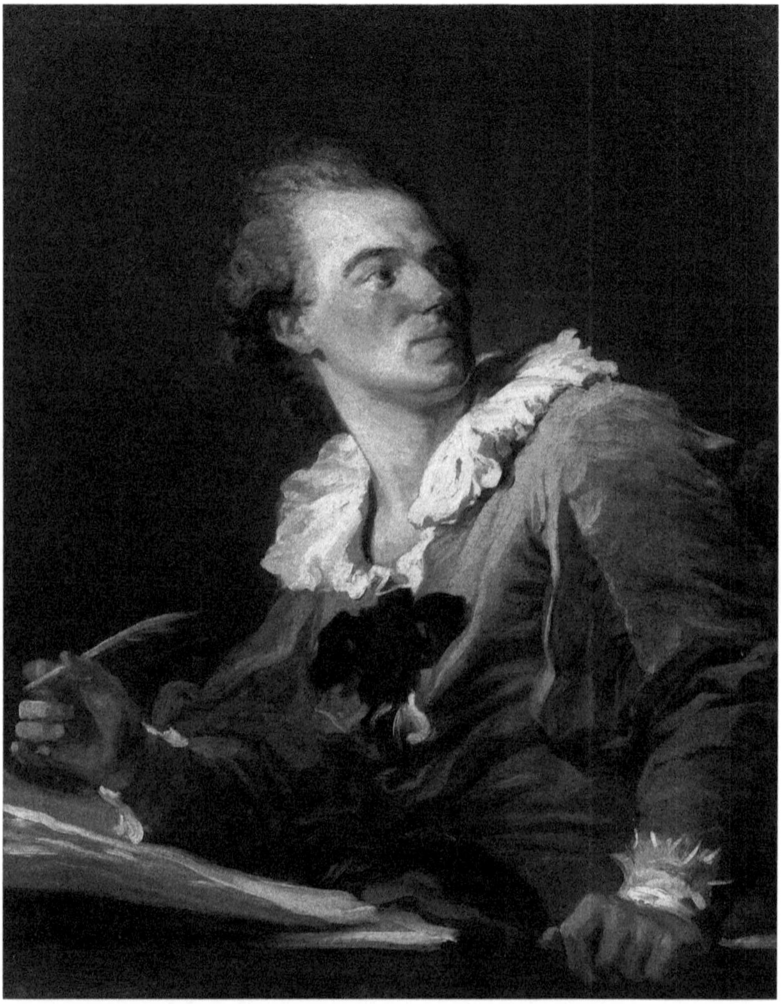

3.3 Jean-Honoré Fragonard, *Inspiration*, ca 1769, oil on canvas, 80 x 64 cm.

treatise is highly interesting in relation to skin, as it considers the rendering of flesh not only in terms of the right mixture of pigments but also with regard to the differentiating use of brushwork textures. If this was in keeping with the attention to paint handling in mid-eighteenth-century French art discourse more generally, Dandré-Bardon explored and systematised this aspect of painterly practice in unprecedented detail.

The treatise's section on colour generally highlights the fundamental significance of paint handling: 'A beautiful colouring results from a beautiful manner of painting. The most seductive and admirable manner is to paint in full colours, always adding tint on tint … and conducting the brush in

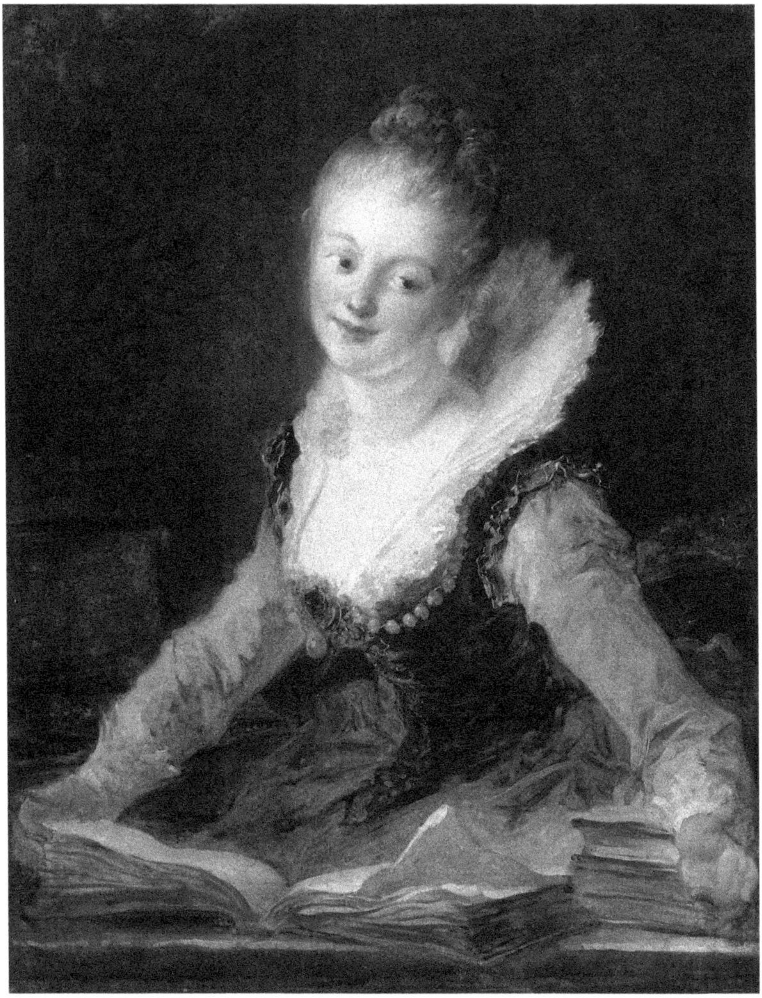

Jean-Honoré Fragonard, *Study*, ca 1769, oil on canvas, 81.5 x 65 cm. 3.4

the direction of the flesh and the muscles. This is the best way to imitate the epidermis of nature.'[9] Similar to Tocqué, Dandré-Bardon envisaged the painting of human figures as a physical engagement of the artist's touch and brush with the body. Working in layers and producing textures, the artist builds up a body in paint and mimics its structure with the brush. Like Pernety, Dandré-Bardon occasionally used the notion of skin – or in this case its outermost layer, the epidermis – to designate the crafted surface that represents the human envelope. In the following paragraph on 'the handicraft varied according to the character of figures',[10] he mostly employed the term *chair* but described minutely how the texture of this organic substance is to be rendered

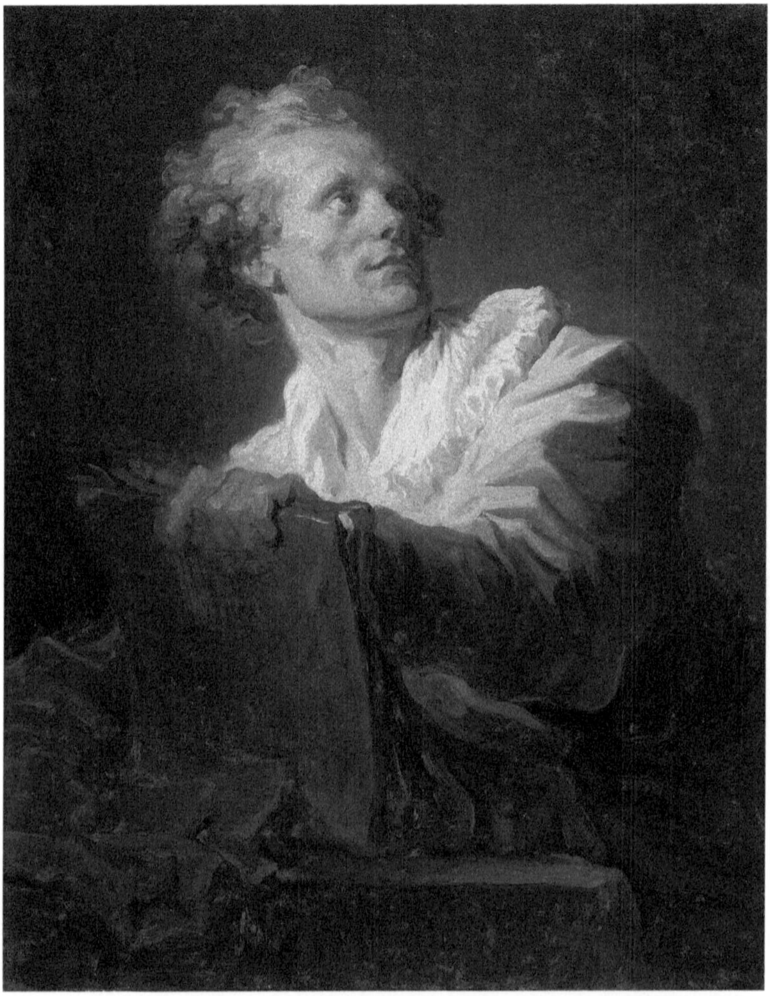

3.5 Jean-Honoré Fragonard, *The Young Artist*, ca 1769–70, oil on canvas, 81 x 65 cm.

according to the age, gender and character of a person. Starting with women he postulated: 'The flesh of women should be treated with a soft and rounded brush, and with fresh and shimmering tints [*teintes fraîches & lumineuses*].' Children, on the other hand should be given flesh tones that are

> tenderly coloured and rounded with a flimsy brush [*pinceau flou*]. Their extremities should be of a sanguine tone [*teinte sanguine*]. The diverse folds of flesh that nature has placed at the joints of their members, and the little dimples with which nature has embellished their chubby parts allow repeated, soft and sensible brushstrokes that characterise their suppleness and the grace of all their movements.[11]

Adolescents should have a *teinte plus décidée* and should, according with the greater solidity of their flesh, 'be formed with a firmer brush'. Once they reach adulthood, Dandré-Bardon continues, somewhat tautologically, men acquire a complexion in keeping with their masculinity: 'In their virile age men have a tone of male colour [*un ton de couleur male*]. It is convenient to give them fresh flesh tones, sensible half-tones and coloured shadows.' All male body parts should equally contain reddish nuances, so that 'the reflections resonate the abundance of blood circulating in all these parts'.[12] Colour is so prevalent in this characterisation of masculinity that brushwork is actually forgotten for a moment, while Dandré-Bardon took this aspect up again in his considerations of the elderly whose hands and feet are thought to be 'less sanguine'. To render persons of that age, he recommended brownish tones [*teintes basanées*], the use of a less rounded brush in order to produce a clipped touch, and for the luminous parts impasto work produced by a brush with stiffer bristles. It is with regard to the representation of elderly people that he suggested dragging the brush in the direction of the wrinkles thus giving a sense of a literal, manual mimesis in the re-production rather than a representation of furrows. The painter was expected almost to metamorphose his gestures into the physical state of the mimicked body, in rendering the 'dry skin and the emaciated muscles of the decrepit age' with a loose brush.[13] Here too, Dandré-Bardon explicitly referred to skin, but in this case in a sense in which the notion had been already employed by Italian and French art theorists describing the human envelope in rather negative terms in cases where it does not seem to form a unity with a fleshy body.

The variation of flesh tones had, of course, been a means of differentiating men and women, or persons of various ages since antiquity,[14] and it was common practice in early modern painting. The practice was explicitly spelled out in an artist's manual by Antoine Le Blond de la Tour, published in 1669, almost a century before Dandré-Bardon's *Traité*. Le Blond gave minute directions for the rendering of diverse flesh tones, generally stating that there were barely two people with the same complexion, but focusing in particular on the differences between the flesh tones of men and women:

> If you want to make a woman's beautiful flesh tone [*une belle carnation de femme*], you have to choose a fresh, beautiful and white woman, and one who is well, since health is the true source of good colour … When I say that one should choose a woman who is beautiful, fresh & white, to make a good colouring, I do not mean to speak of those tones of plaster [*teintes de plâtre*] that gleam only by their grand whiteness, … but I wish to speak of a rose complexion [*teint rose*] that has something softer, more vivid and animated to it which also pleases the senses more strongly. The complexions of men should be stronger and more charged than that of women; because men are more

> robust and vigorous than women their expressions should express it more strongly. I don't say this of those who are yellowish and brown, as they seem to tend more towards the sick, but of the healthy man whose colour is normally reddish and full of a certain vivacity.[15]

In consonance with early modern notions of complexions, Le Blond drew implicitly on the theory of humours for which well-being was a result of the right balance of bodily fluids. Humoral theory in the tradition of the Ancient Greek physician Hippocrates assumed that the main four humours – black bile, yellow bile, phlegm and blood – were in differentiating proportions in men and women, and characterised men as being more sanguine thus featuring a more reddish complexion. It is hence on the basis of this theory that Le Blond posited a difference between men's and women's complexions, recommending the representation of the flesh tones accordingly. If Dandré-Bardon operated less explicitly with notions of health, he still resorted to humoral theory when claiming the sanguine and active character of men and he equally built on a well-established tradition when arguing for the use of flesh tones for the distinction of persons of different gender and age. There is however one aspect that is totally absent in the seventeenth-century treatise: while it explains in much detail which pigments are to be used for rendering flesh tones, paint handling is not addressed at all. Le Blond briefly considered that painters have different manners of painting, that is to say they choose different procedures for sketching and executing a painting, but (like with other seventeenth-century manuals) notions of *le faire* or *la touche* are entirely absent. For Le Blond, the rendering of the flesh tones is an issue of the right mixture of colours, not of the appropriate handling of the brush. In contrast, Dandré-Bardon paid close attention to the physical mimesis of the brush-work. Painting the different appearances of male and female, of young and old bodies had become an issue of mimicking the various textures of skin and its underlying structures.

Fragonard, I propose, had techniques like those noted by his former teacher in mind and at hand when painting the *portraits de fantaisie*. He employed an exceptional variation of tints as well as manifold painterly textures to render the skin. The portrait of an old man, today at the Art Institute in Chicago, for example, is dominated by brownish colours applied with a large brush (Figure 3.6). The complexion features a rusty red at the hand, checks and nose, while the side of the forehead turned towards the viewer is painted in brighter colours applied in impasto. The *Portrait of a Man* representing a younger man (associated with Fragonard's patron and friend the Abbé de Saint-Non) is generally much more colourful (Plate 6).[16] On a slightly violet brown ground painted in thin *frottis*, the figure is modelled mostly with broad brushstrokes in thickly applied paint. The garment is made of lively colours, dominated by Prussian blue, combined with the acidic Naples yellow and a warm orange. The

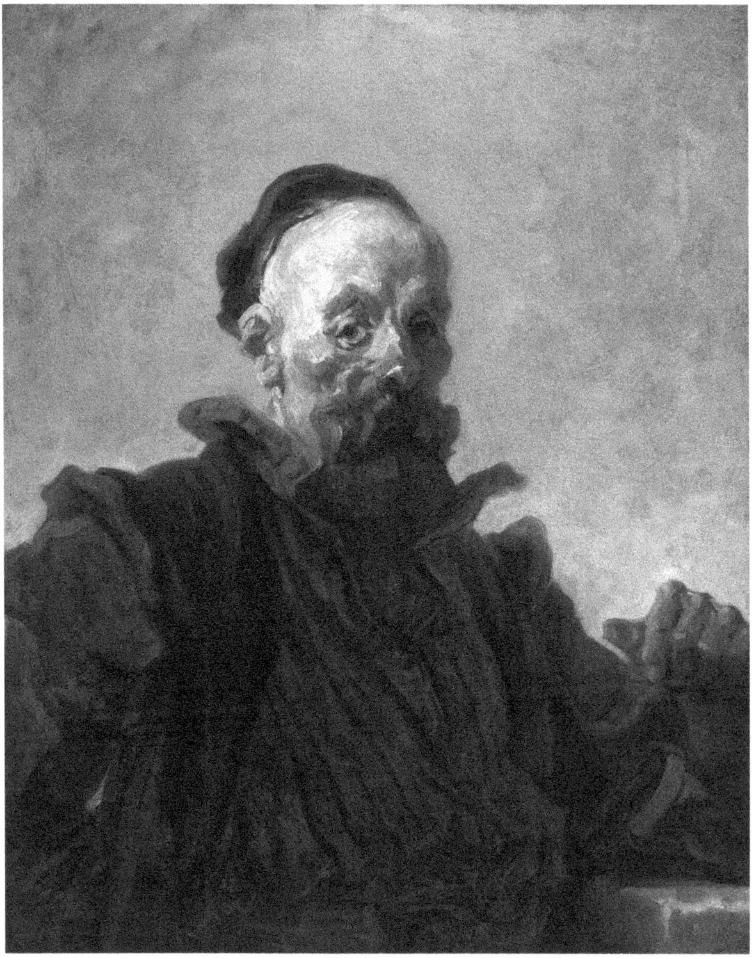

Jean-Honoré Fragonard, *Portrait of a Man in Spanish Costume*, ca 1768–70, oil on canvas, 80.3 x 64.7 cm. 3.6

collar painted in white impasto highlights by means of contrast the variegated complexion that is far brighter than that of the old man. The basic flesh tint is yellowish while the upper layer is formed by an irregular network of patches of blue, thin touches of rose and more thickly applied strokes of white paint.[17]

The painting called *Inspiration* (or *The Writer*, figure 3.3), staging a young man who pauses in his writing, turning around and directing his eyes towards an undefined distance located outside the picture frame, as if indeed caught in a moment of inspiration, is dominated by warmer ochre tones while blue is almost entirely absent. The ample sleeves of the yellowish costume feature deep slashes opening up a ruby interior the colour of which matches the reddened cheeks of the meditating young man. The reddish tones on the yellowish basic tint of the face and neck stage the moment of inspiration not as a passive reception of ideas but as a sanguine, manly mental activity.

The female figures among the *portraits de fantaisie* are rendered in a manner distinct from all the male ones, however varied the latter may be. There is a striking differentiation between the paint handling of the clothes and that of the female flesh tones. While the dresses are executed with the same lively brush as the costumes of the male figures, the paint handling of the faces is much more finished. The skin of the young woman in *Study* is fairly light overall, ranging from almost white at the décolleté via a slightly yellowish tint in the face to rose hues marking the cheeks (Figure 3.4). Traces of the brush are barely visible, making the surface homogeneous; a dryer application of paint in the areas where skin is depicted seems powdery as if to indicate the use of this type of make-up.

In another female figure (previously held to be a portrait of the dancer Marie-Madeleine Guimard), with a playing card in her right hand and a number of sketches at her left, Fragonard treated the skin in yet another manner (Plate 7).[18] Almost no yellow is employed for the flesh tones that are of a light rose with more reddish zones around the eyes, the cheeks and at the tip of the nose. From a distance, the painted surface representing the face looks finished and as if the paint had been finely blurred. Coming closer, however, impasto areas become visible, in particular the dot of white paint that simultaneously represents light on the nose and does itself reflect light. In other areas, furrows left by a flat brush are discernible and model the face (Figure 3.7, detail). They are a remaining indexical sign of the movement made by the artist's hand, but rather than being traces of a speedy process, seemingly distributed at random, they indicate in this case that the impasto paint has been applied with precision. The relief left by the brush looks, especially around the left eye, like the memory of a caressing gesture. At the same time, Fragonard conducted the brush here in the direction of the muscles, imitating, as Dandré-Bardon had suggested, 'the epidermis of nature'. The ridges around the eye indeed bear an astonishing resemblance to the lines that indicate the orbicular muscle in the illustrations for a renowned contemporary anatomical atlas: the 1747 *Tabulae sceleti et musculorum corporis humani* by the German-born and Leiden-based anatomist Bernhard Siegfried Albinus with engravings by Jan Wandelaar (Figure 3.8). The muscles of the eye socket of the full figure écorché (flayed man) demonstrating the exterior muscles, and those in the detail of the 'orbicularis' in a separate illustration, are engraved with parallel lines that cover the lid and surround the eye. Wandelaar's engravings for Albinus were at the time highly praised for their accuracy, in the article 'Anatomie' of the *Encyclopédie* authored by Denis Diderot and Pierre Tarin, for example. Moreover, the écorché figure by Wandelaar was used for the anatomical illustrations in the

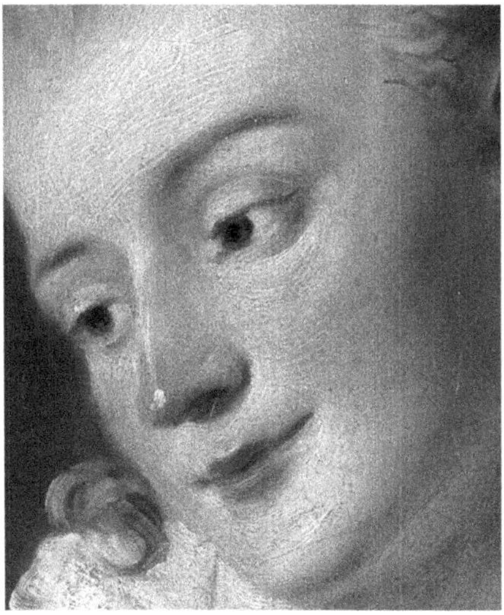
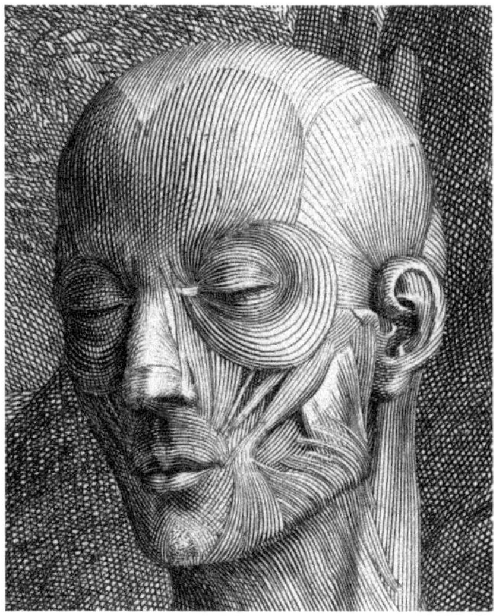

[*left*] Jean-Honoré Fragonard, *Portrait of a Woman* (formerly identified as Marie-Madeleine Guimard), ca 1769–70 (detail). 3.7–8
[*right*] Jan Wandelaar, Muscles of the head, from: Bernhard Siegfried Albinus, *Tabulae sceleti et musculorum corporis humani*, 1747, detail of table 1.

first volume of plates of the *Encyclopédie* published in 1762.[19] Reproducing the eye socket in this particular way, Fragonard seems to demonstrate that 'feeling in the brush that grubs for the muscles', evoked some years earlier by Tocqué,[20] as he simulates the distribution of the muscle strands with the flow of his hand in a process of anatomical mimesis.

If Fragonard used his brush and touch to mimic the muscular structure under the skin at this particular site, he did not do so consistently. He employed his facture in a flexible and playful manner throughout his work and in the *portraits de fantaisie* in particular. In most of the male portraits brushstrokes forming the face lead a life independent of any underlying muscular texture. The *touche* is here as least as much an indexical sign of the artist's activity as a means to represent an object. Such a distinction between the two ways in which the artist's touch could signify was theorised in the eighteenth century. In the article 'Touche' of his influential *Dictionnaire des beaux arts* (1788–91) Claude-Henri Watelet, largely following the mid-eighteenth-century consensus on the significance of the artist's hand and extensively quoting from Dandré-Bardon, distinguished between *touche* as *signe imitatif* and as *signe communicatif*. He conceived of the former as being in the service of imitation, as 'drawn from nature', while the latter transports an artist's personality and enthusiasm by communicating, 'how the artist has seen and felt while making the imitation'.[21] These two modes of signification could even be recognised in the colouring of a painting and of the flesh tones. According to a theory received from Lomazzo by Félibien, taken up by Pernety in his *Dictionnaire portatif de peinture*, and repeated into the nineteenth century, the temperament of a painter had an impact on his choice of colours; while the melancholic artist favours yellow and greenish colours, the phlegmatic employs pale ones, and the sanguine is inclined to animate the flesh tones thanks to his predilection for red.[22]

Eighteenth-century theorists such as Diderot understood however that the *signe communicatif* would always remain a paradoxical concept. Just as much as an actor conveys a passion convincingly, not because he actually experiences it but because he has learned to professionally simulate its expression, a painter needs a trained hand to transmit the signs of his enthusiasm.[23] Fragonard dealt with this paradox and used it productively in his *portraits de fantaisie*. Especially in the images featuring artists, writers or philosophers the two aspects of *la touche* enhance each other. Shown musing rather than drawing, reading or writing, the subjects are caught in moments of enthusiasm, so that the object and the mode of rendition are equally inspired. This correspondence of inspired artists or thinkers represented by an artist striving to display

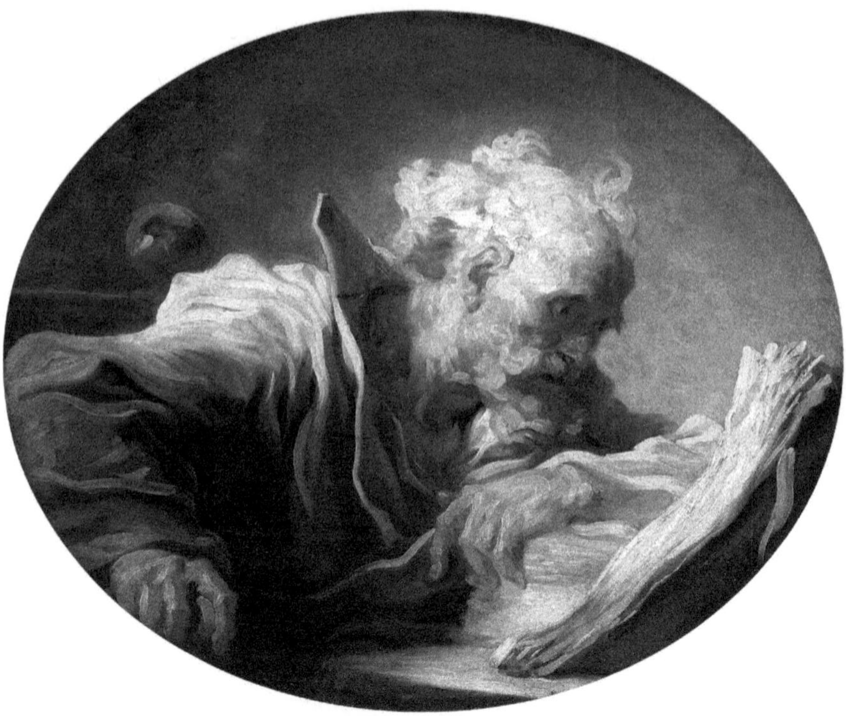

3.9 Jean-Honoré Fragonard, *A Philosopher* (*St Jerome Reading*), ca 1764, oil on canvas, 72.2 x 79 cm.

his own inspiration, lends the images, as Sheriff has argued, a self-referential aspect. All of them employ conventional as well as natural signs (in Watelet's sense), since they represent the figures in the traditional iconography of inspiration, with the eyes directed into an undefined distance, and simultaneously aim to transmit Fragonard's 'fire' via the lively brushstrokes.[24] Above all in the *Portrait of a Man of Letters* or in a painting known as *A Philosopher* (similar to the other *portraits de fantaisie*, but of oval format), the visible brushstrokes can refer to both the enthusiasm of the painter and the active mind of the portrayed (Figure 3.9). Whether representing a figure directing acute attention to the book or a person in more dreamy contemplation, the agitated brushstrokes turn thinking into a physical activity and a state of sensory and mental alertness. They capture a process (thinking, reading, painting) at a moment in time, and store this in the brushstrokes as remaining visible traces of the artist's momentary gestures. The paintings thus engage with the possibilities of portraits in capturing fleeting emotions and dealing with the changeability of the flesh and of facial expressions discussed in the contemporary art literature, such as Diderot's Salon criticism.

Diderot and portraiture

Diderot discussed portraiture at various occasions in his critiques of the Salon exhibitions, which circulated in Grimm's *Correspondance littéraire*.[25] One of these occasions was the exhibition at the 1767 Salon of a portrait of himself done by Michel Van Loo (Figure 3.10). The painting captures Diderot working at a desk, but apparently interrupted either by something outside the space of action of the painting or by a thought. The eyes do not fix on anything, as if directed into a void. Unlike Fragonard, Van Loo largely effaced the traces of his brush, and modelled the face via the use of colour by employing, on top of a yellowish basic tone, grey-blue for the shadows, and red for the cheeks and chin. In view of the striking similarities with, as well as significant departures from, Van Loo's painting, Fragonard's *portrait de fantaisie*, which used to be considered a portrait of Diderot (Figure 3.1, plate 5), has been discussed by a number of scholars as a meta-portrait of Van Loo's.[26] In view of the changes Fragonard made, it seems as though the painter had taken into account the philosopher's critique of his likeness. Whether specifically a meta-portrait of Diderot, that is, a painted comment on Van Loo's earlier portrait of Diderot and the sitter's responses to it, or more generally a different proposition for a philosopher's portrait, this particular *portrait de fantaisie* engages by pictorial means with several problems the philosopher and art critic was concerned with.

Although Van Loo was a friend, Diderot expressed in his *Salon of 1767* that he was not happy with this image of himself. He stated that it had 'a fairly good likeness' but was nevertheless lacking truth.[27] In fact, as Diderot had pointed

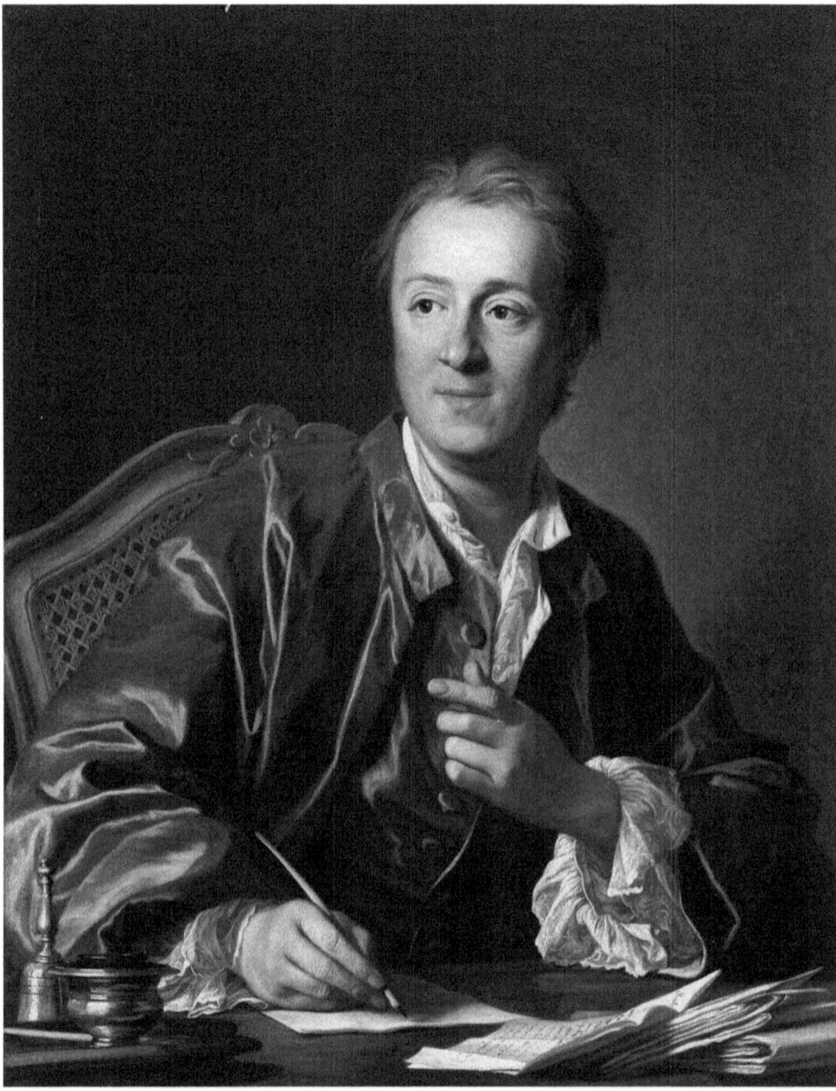

3.10 Michel Van Loo, *Denis Diderot*, 1767, oil on canvas, 81 x 65 cm.

out in more general remarks on portraiture prompted by a 1763 self-portrait by Michel Van Loo (which he quite liked) resemblance is not necessarily what makes a good portrait. It is, Diderot observed, a quality the *gens du monde* value, as they are familiar with the sitters, while he himself esteemed portraits for their composition and their rendering. Artists themselves argued that what we appreciate about Van Dyck's portraits is not resemblance but the way they are painted, as it is the brush that 'immortalizes the work of art'.[28]

Diderot generally valued a paint handling that refers to the work process, and praised the aesthetics of the sketch. Regarding Greuze's sketch for the *Well-Loved Mother* exhibited at the Salon of 1765 he stated:

> Sketches frequently have a fire that the finished paintings lack; they're the moment of the artist's zeal, his pure verve, undiluted by any carefully considered preparation, they're the painter's soul freely transferred to canvas. The poet's pen, the skilled draftsman's pencil seem to frolic and amuse themselves. Rapid sketches characterise everything with a few strokes. The more ambiguity there is in artistic expression, the more comfortable the imagination.[29]

In line with other eighteenth-century art theorists such as Coypel (discussed in the previous chapter), Diderot associated fire and enthusiasm, understanding the sketchy strokes of a pencil or brush as immediate traces of an artist's inspired ardour. Allying himself with the professionals in his esteem for a visible *touche*, Diderot, at this point, downplayed the mimetic function of the artist's brushwork. For his own portrait, however, Diderot sought 'truth', that is he wished the image to match his personality and to some extent his looks. He probably envisaged some reciprocal 'fire' and along with it a mutual immortalisation via a touch that both refers back to the artist and to the sitter, by plausibly rendering the facial expression of an inspired subject. In his humorously phrased critique of Van Loo's portrait, he was indeed concerned with his posthumous image, since he wondered what his grandchildren might think of the portrait and commented upon his likeness first in the third person and later in the more personal first person:

> Very lively. It has his kindness, along with his vivacity. But too young, his head too small. Pretty like a woman, leering, smiling, dainty, pursing his mouth to make himself look captivating … My pretty philosopher you will always serve me as precious testimony to the friendship of an artist, an excellent artist, and a more excellent man. But what will my grandchildren say, when they compare my sad works to this smiling, affected, effeminate old flirt? My children I warn you that this is not me.[30]

Diderot's main problem with Van Loo's portrait was that he could not identify with the facial expression the artist had given him. The appearance of a human being, affected by external and internal stimuli, changed constantly, and the 'sensitive philosopher' (this is how Diderot referred to himself) may have a hundred different physiognomies a day – 'sad, pensive, tender, violent, passionate or enthusiastic',[31] but never looked the way Van Loo depicted him. While criticising Van Loo's view of him, Diderot drew his own self-portrait in words. Anticipating his posterity he declared that he had 'penetrating eyes, rather large features, a head quite similar in character to that of an ancient orator'. He wished not only to be captured in a characteristic moment, rendered as an inspired person with a distracted glance 'focused on the distance', but also to be inscribed into the iconography of great men, and especially that of the philosopher featuring 'a large forehead'. What is more, Diderot pretended that he was particularly hard to portray: 'I have a facial mask that fools artists, either because too many features blend together or because the impressions of my soul succeed one another very quickly and register themselves on my face, such that the painter's eye does not perceive me to be the same from one moment to the next.'[32]

Describing the versatility of his countenance, he turned the face into a screen that transmits internal occurrences to the outer world as it reflects the thoughts and feelings of a person. Although establishing a meaningful rapport between inside and outside, this approach is decidedly non-physiognomic as it rejects any stable relations between a person's appearance and their character. It accords in this respect with Diderot's 1765 entry 'Physionomie' for the *Encyclopédie*. Dismissive already by its very shortness, it defines physiognomy as the 'expression of the character and also of the temperament' and bluntly states that one should not judge a person on their physiognomy.[33] It is likely that the disregard for this 'imaginary science' – as another heading of the *Encyclopédie* labels it – was at least partly due to the fact that French physiognomy was at the time mostly associated with occultism.[34] The more contemporary work on physiognomy by Pernety (also the author of the previously mentioned *Dictionnaire portatif de peinture*), published from 1769 onwards while the author was working in Berlin as conservator for the library of Frederick the Great, was, in some respects, concerned with similar questions to those of Diderot in his art criticism. Diderot would have certainly had issues with Dom Pernety's moralism which came with his belief in facial analysis as a tool of judgement as well as with his valuation of physiognomy as a basis of human communication and hence community. Still, both were interested in the physical manifestations of human emotions, or more generally speaking in the relations between the interior and the exterior. Inside and outside relations and reading the body's surface were also a major concern for Swiss pastor Johann Caspar Lavater, whose influential writings on physiognomy would appear from 1775 onwards. In contrast to the latter's focus on the skull as a stable and essential sign of a person's character, Pernety was much more concerned with the passions of the soul and their traces on the face. He explained the more stable appearance with the fact that people with a particular character or prevalent mood would repeat certain expressions that consequently inscribe themselves more permanently on a person's face. Skin is the predominant site where these physical traces of the soul are left, as passions become visible when 'the muscles of the forehead and of the entire face extended under the skin tighten and loosen following the motions that the spirits and nerves imprint on them. These muscle contractions build the furrows and lines in the skin that become more visible the more the contraction is repeated.'[35]

Interestingly, Pernety compared the art of the physiognomist with that of the connoisseur, as he claimed that the same observational techniques were needed to read a face and to judge a work of art. In fact, he frequently drew an analogy between the face and a picture (*tableau*), both being an image or a mirror 'that presents the passions to our eyes'.[36] As already discussed in the previous chapter, the idea that emotions 'paint' themselves on a face was quite common.[37] Diderot used similar metaphors in a passage of his *Notes on Painting*, an appendix to his *Salon of 1765*, in which he described the difficulties of portrait painting and of the attempts to freeze the countenance of a person whose facial expression might change constantly:

> But what drives a great colorist to distraction is flesh's mutability [*vicissitude de la chair*], how it can become more vivacious or moribund in the blink of an eye. This is because while the artist's gaze is focused on the canvas and he's doing his best to trap me with his brush, I move on, and when he looks up again he no longer finds me as I was. Because I think of the Abbé le Blanc and am overcome by boredom … Because I picture Grimm or my Sophie, and my heart beats fast, tenderness and serenity becoming visible on my features; joy is released through the pores of the skin [*par les pores de la peau*], my heart dilates, my small sanguinary reservoirs are set vibrating and the barely perceptible colour of the fluid thus activated augments the bloom and life of my flesh [*l'incarnat et la vie*] … What torment for them, then, is the human visage, this canvas that becomes excited, animated, flushed, or pale, that expands or contracts in tandem with the infinite multitude of alternatives sustained by this light, fleet expiration we call the soul?[38]

Diderot used three different notions here to refer to the body, its surface and their painterly representation: *chair*, *incarnat* and *peau*. Speaking of 'flesh's mutability' (*vicissitude de la chair*) so hard to grasp for the artist, he referred back to the traditional art theoretical terminology of *chair* and *carnations*, and indirectly to the idea that it is the lifelike rendering of the flesh that is the primary way to animate art works. Further on, he associated colour and life, by conflating sanguine as a pigment and as actual blood on the one hand and 'flesh and life' (*l'incarnat et la vie*) on the other. At this point he thus chose a term that etymologically still carried the reference to the Christian mystery of incarnation but had, in its abbreviated form, become a word for the red colour of flesh in the French art literature of the seventeenth and eighteenth century. Diderot transformed these mystifying ideas about the animation of art works by grounding them in the physicality of the living body. He uses the word *peau*, giving a materialist account of the transmission of the emotions via coloured fluids that migrate 'through the pores of the skin'. The face thus seems like an image that is painted from within as colours push through 'this canvas that becomes excited'. Initially a pars pro toto for the painting, the word 'canvas' transforms into a metaphor for the human face. Diderot thus closely connected the woven tissue that serves as a support for paintings and the facial skin as an organic tissue that colours or de-colours according to a subject's fleeting emotions and thoughts. Both the support of a painting, the woven fabric of the canvas, and its crafted surface, the texture of brushstrokes produced by the painter, could thus be associated with skin as a surface and/or tissue itself. The association of skin and canvas has however further connotative layers resonating in Diderot's and other eighteenth-century writings. I will discuss them discretely and in more detail in what follows: firstly, the understanding of skin and canvas as expressive media that serve the communication of affectations or more generally speaking as supports that carry signs; secondly, the medical notion of skin as a 'nervous canvas', as an envelope that is imbued with life and sensibility, and keeps the human being in touch with the exterior world.

Sensible skin as nervous canvas

The eighteenth-century association of skin and canvas builds on a long material history of skin as a medium. A different area where skin was seen as a surface on which signs become visible was the exercise of medical diagnosis. In particular the eighteenth-century medical practice explicitly labelled 'semiotic medicine' regarded skin as a privileged site for medical deciphering.[39] 'Médecine Séméiotique' is one of the special aspects under which skin is treated in the *Encyclopédie*. The article, authored by Jean-Jacques Ménuret de Chambaud, focuses on skin as a site and instrument of medical analysis for a wide range of diseases.[40] With characteristic Enlightenment rhetoric the author claimed right at the outset: 'The state of skin should elucidate us about their [the diseases'] nature, their course and their termination; any phenomenon can be a sign under the attentive eyes of an adept observer.'[41] Fully in keeping with a holistic approach to the body (to which I will come back later) he assumed an 'admirable harmony among all parts of the human body',[42] the skin's activity counterbalancing that of the internal organs. Skin is thus seen as an organ that has an important stabilising function and that has hence to be affected whenever there is a physical imbalance. He carefully considered the many effects diseases may have on the condition of the outermost organ. Using similar criteria, most medical practitioners at the time would have resorted to skin – its colour, moisture or dryness – as one of the first sites of diagnosis.

Later on, the emerging field of dermatology – particularly dedicated to the diseases of skin – expanded and specialised the visual scrutiny and reading of the body's surface. While there had been specialised treatises on skin diseases since the sixteenth century, when skin started to become an object of anatomical and medical interest, it was only around 1800 that dermatology became an independent branch within medicine. This development, which was linked in France to the establishment of specialised clinics, most famously the Saint Louis hospital in Paris, went along with the publication of richly illustrated atlases that helped to establish dermatology as a discipline engaged with surface inspection. The first French volume of this kind was Jean-Louis-Marie Alibert's 1806 *Description des maladies de la peau observées à l'hôpital Saint Louis*.[43] Concerned with lesions that present themselves on the body's exterior, dermatology developed techniques of observation that looked at skin as a carrier of symptoms and turned it into a signifying surface.

If skin became an important medium for pathological enquiry, it was at least as prominent for the eighteenth-century understanding of the functioning of the vital and healthy body. The human's envelope and organ of touch became indeed closely associated with *the* paradigmatic Enlightenment quality: sensibility. Not only a psychological capacity for refined emotion and compassion, sensibility was also understood as physical perceptiveness and as such considered a dominant if not *the* dominant force of life. For those areas of eighteenth-century medicine considered in what follows, skin became the exquisite organic outpost of sensibility. The physicality of sensibility was far from a specialist concern of medics and Diderot's *Notes on Painting* demonstrate how closely art and physiological discourse were connected at the time.[44] His passage on flesh's mutability is quite a complex account of both the problems of portraiture and issues concerning the human body's vitality. The importance Diderot generally allocated to the physical aspects of human existence clearly transpires from this passage. Subscribing to the central role that the newly emerging sciences of man awarded the human body, Diderot argued that nothing could be explained without it.[45] Although still operating with the notion of the 'soul', he described its emanations as purely physical. No longer a metaphysical entity but embedded in the materiality of the body,[46] the organ 'called soul' makes fluids pulsate through the body in order to surface on the skin. Diderot's understanding of the body in the *Notes on Painting*, his emphasis on its vitality and the materiality of its emotional utterances can be aligned with an important current in Enlightenment medicine: vitalism. One of the eighteenth century's attempts to comprehend the specificity of living organisms, vitalism assumed that the functions of a living organism rely on a specific vital force, a spark or energy, that could not sufficiently be explained by the laws of physics. Particularly prominent in France, vitalist medicine departed from the Cartesian dualism of body and soul and developed a dynamic conception of matter in which every single element of a living body was considered as animated.[47] Vitalism has often been contrasted with another approach of eighteenth-century medicine and philosophy, 'Mechanism', since vitalists understood the human being as an organism rather than a mechanical apparatus, and life was defined by sensitivity rather than movement.[48] Most vitalists still supposed the existence of an immaterial soul and associated the vital force with it; publicly stating otherwise would have certainly resulted in a confrontation with the authorities of the Ancien Régime.[49] However, the vitalists did not really need the concept of a soul to explain the nature of life and their focus on the vital functions of the organs opened up the debate about the existence of a soul and disclosed the possibility of its non-existence.[50] Despite employing the word 'soul', Diderot, who has often been called a 'materialist vitalist',[51] characterised even emotional processes in material terms in the passage on the difficulties of portraiture from his *Notes on Painting*. In his *Rêve de d'Alembert*, a text that remained unpublished during his lifetime, Diderot reached a particularly materialist point of view of life and living organism (that I will discuss later on). He engaged with and contributed to vitalist positions throughout his adult life, and was acquainted with many vitalist physicians, such as Théophile Bordeu who was a close friend. Vitalist approaches to the body were also prominent in the original edition of the *Encyclopédie* published from 1751 onwards.[52] Moreover, Diderot engaged with the writings by Swiss physiologist Albrecht von Haller, another scholar concerned with the specificity of living organisms and whose work was widely received and critically discussed in France.[53] Despite disagreements between Haller and Bordeu, Diderot read Haller's physiological writings closely, compiling comprehensive notes of his reading.[54]

In France, vitalism was especially prominent among the members of the so-called medical school of Montpellier; besides Bordeu, there was Ménuret de Chambaud and Paul-Joseph Barthez. The vitalists of the École de Montpellier shared a holistic approach to the human body, one of the reasons why they were opposed to Haller's experimental method. They combined observation of physical phenomena with philosophical reasoning about the nature of life and the body, and were thus also referred to as *médecins-philosophes*. Among their main concerns was the interplay of body and soul or physical and moral aspects of human life, and many of their writings explicitly addressed this issue: from La Caze's *Idées de l'homme physique et morale* (1755) via the later revolutionary Jean-Paul Marat's *De l'homme, ou Des principes et des loix de l'influence de l'*âme *sur le corps et du corps sur l'*âme (1775–76) to Pierre-Jean-George Cabanis' *Rapports du physique et du moral de l'homme* (1802). Sensibility was a key concept in these integrating accounts, as it was considered both a physical property and a psychological quality; and it was, as Anne Vila has put it, the 'grand-scale effort to study the multi-faceted effects of sensibility in all of its various human types that made eighteenth-century medicine an overtly "philosophical" endeavour'.[55]

Due to its philosophical, non-specialist perspective, medical theory also became a major issue of Enlightenment debates. Medical discourse was at the heart of contemporary concerns with the constitution of the human, the materiality of the body and the definition of life. Michel Foucault has consequently argued, both in *The Birth of the Clinic* and *The Order of Things*, that medicine played a defining role in the emerging Sciences of Man and their account of the human. And one might add, as Claudia Honegger claims, that it was precisely the holistic, anti-Cartesian attempt to integrate body and soul, the physical and the social, so prominent in French medicine, that had a major impact on the scientisation of gender difference.[56] During the short period between 1750 and 1770 in focus here, when the first volumes of the *Encyclopédie* appeared, Diderot wrote his Salon criticism and Fragonard painted his *portraits de fantaisie*, this debate was still in flux, and medical discourse was questioning the constitution of the human and its body as much as it was redefining it. And I assume that it must have been – wittingly or not – a matter of concern for anyone who tried to understand or represent the body in its liveliness, physicians and philosophers as much as artists and art theorists. This is all the more likely as, due to the particular approach of the French *médecins philosophes* and their attempt to integrate medical and philosophical explanations of life and the functioning of the human, these discussions far exceeded the domain of medical specialists.[57] Among the most important sites for such debates were social gatherings, like the famous salon of Anne-Cathérine de Ligniville d'Autricourt, Madame Helvétius, hosted from 1751 onwards with her husband the philosopher Claude-Adrien Helvétius in their mansion in Paris, and later, after his death in 1771, at her retreat at Auteuil. Friends and regulars of her salon were the overlapping groups of the *Encyclopédistes* and the *médecins philosophes*, but also artists such as the sculptor Jean-Antoine Houdon, and during the Revolution and the Directory scientists and *idéologues* such as Antoine Lavoisier or Cabanis.[58]

Neither Haller nor the French *médecins philosophes* ever devoted a special study to skin, but the external organ became crucial for their understanding of life and the body, as it was closely linked to their notion of sensibility. This new attention to skin was one of the consequences of the rise of the nervous system and of sensibility as determining forces of life within medical theories. In her study *Body Criticism*, Barbara Stafford has described the new significance of the sub-epidermal region: 'the volatile nervous system – governed by an impressionable *sensibilité* responsive to environmental effluvia – created a new medium or "atmospheric" third world of fleeting emotions and fluid instincts coursing beneath the skin'.[59] The sub-cutaneous zone (a notion that is itself an eighteenth-century neologism) worked like a vivid whole body antenna whose perceptions are transported by nerves. These nerves are themselves imagined as operating with fluids as their medium. The new focus on the nerves did not imply a supersession of humoral theories in the tradition of Hippocrates and Galen. The theory of the humours remained an important aspect of vitalist medicine and was crucial for its anti-mechanistic, holistic approach that went along with a trust in the body's self-regulatory potential. Healthy skin, however much filled with nerves and sensibility, was still regarded as a moist and oily organ releasing sweat and other saps, and as a membrane whose complexions were an indication of the humours circulating in the body.[60]

The conceptual transition from the seventeenth-century *homme machine* to the eighteenth-century *homme sensible* had an important impact on the understanding of skin.[61] For Diderot skin is a complex, vivid organ in itself playing an active role in sensual perception, as his notes on touch in his 'Élemens de physiologie' suggest: 'If the impression is made on the skin, the sensation is that of touch. No part of the skin is not sensible … The skin is a dense tissue composed of a large number of cells that are very close to each other and whose fibres are interlaced … It is extensible, contractile and porous.' Diderot thus described the general features of the sense organ very much in the manner the anatomists discussed in the previous chapter had done since the late seventeenth century, but emphasising the sensibility and receptiveness of the organ. He continued his account with the papillae that are situated underneath the epidermis and are formed by vessels and nerves tied together by the cellular tissue: 'Pressed on the object of touch those papillae receive the impression on their nervous part which transmits it to the trunk of the nerve. I conceive a feeling of touch so exquisite that it could make up for all the other four senses.'[62]

Diderot argued as a sensualist here, defining human existence not through the act of thinking but through sense perception. He connected the materiality of the skin with the perceptual finesse that makes it a particularly apt and alert sensual organ full of nervous activity. Touching for Diderot is not only a way of gaining knowledge about the shape and extent of an object; the act of touching is a pleasurable experience in itself. He thus blurred the distinction between skin as the organ that makes the hand a precise manual tool and touch as a sense associated with pleasure and voluptuousness. Although there were occasional voices in French eighteenth-century medical or philosophical discourse that dismissed touch as a 'coarse sense',[63] the interest was predominantly not in a moralising hierarchisation of the senses, and hence dismissal of touch, but, especially from a sensationalist perspective, in the understanding of sense perception and its potential for the acquisition of various forms of knowledge of the world.[64] For Diderot, touching, in its emotional and physical sense of 'feeling', was more a way of enjoying oneself as a being that is connected with the world through the senses, than a means of taking pleasure in the objects touched.

For a physiologist like Haller, skin was equally important, but he associated its sensibility with pain instead of pleasure. In his famous lecture on the sensible and irritable parts of the human body (delivered at Göttingen in 1752 and disseminated at the time mainly via Tissot's French translation published in 1755) he considered the dermis as particularly sensible.[65] The results Haller presented in this lecture were based on a series of physiological experiments with the help of which Haller tried to comprehend the properties that constitute life. In these experiments he exposed individual body parts of living animals to stimuli such as touching, cutting, burning or aggressive substances like vitriol. Haller then registered the animal's behaviour and distinguished two main reactions enabling him to deduce whether a body part was irritable or sensible. At the outset of his paper he gave the following definition:

> I call that part of the human body irritable, which becomes shorter upon being touched; very irritable if it contracts upon a slight touch … I call that a sensible part of the human body, which upon being touched transmits the impression of it to the soul; and in brutes, in whom the existence of a soul is not so clear, I call those parts sensible, the irritation of which occasions evident signs of pain and disquiet in the animal.[66]

Haller classified the heart, the intestines and muscles in general as irritable, and body parts endowed with nerves as sensible. Among them, skin holds a prominent place, not only as one of the most sensible somatic zones but more importantly as the organ with which he started each set of experiments serving at the same time as a heuristic tool. Haller first stated that neither the epidermis nor Malpighi's reticular membrane have any feeling but that the skin lying underneath is

> sensible, and indeed more so than any other part of the body; for in whatever manner you irritate it, the animal makes a noise, struggles, and gives all the marks of pain that it is capable of. This great sensibility of the skin has determined me to take it as a fixed standard of that property; and I reckon as insensible, or at least only in a small degree, those parts which may be irritated without disturbing the animal, while it discovers signs of pain if the neighbouring skin is irritated.[67]

Haller thus not only described the skin as extremely sensible but also turned it into the very gauge of sensibility. Not surprisingly then, the famous article 'Sensibilité' of the *Encyclopédie* (published in 1765) also talks about skin and refers in detail, albeit critically, to Haller. The author was the Montpellier physician Henri Fouquet, since his youth closely tied to Bordeu. Taking up arguments by the latter and by other French vitalists, he questioned Haller's distinction between irritability and sensibility. Right at the outset of his article Fouquet defined sensibility as the 'faculty to sense, … the basis and the conserving agent of life, liveliness par excellence',[68] hence declaring it the one and only principle of life. Moreover, Fouquet doubted not only the results of Haller's trials but his experimental method as such. The isolation of individual body parts already distorts the picture, as it does not take the interrelatedness of parts within an organism into account. Fouquet highlighted the 'consensus of the skin with the internal parts',[69] indirectly questioning any harming of the skin and opening of the body in experiments that are supposed to illuminate the functioning of the living body. The arguments against vivisection are logical rather than ethical: how valid are results from experiments inflicting pain on animals? Fouquet's arguments were in line with the general concerns French vitalists raised against such experiments. Arguing that experiments disregard the unity of the body, they favoured non-invasive methods for examining it.[70]

Despite these differences, Haller and Fouquet agreed upon considering skin a particularly sensible organ. Stressing again the embracing role of skin for the interplay of organs Fouquet postulated: 'The skin, this nervous canvas [*toile nerveuse*] forming a general organ the activity of which counterbalances that of the internal organs, is also eminently imbued with that instinct [sensibility].'[71] Labelling skin a canvas, the physician employed a metaphor similarly to Diderot who had named the 'human visage' in his *Notes on Painting* a 'canvas that becomes excited', thus imagining facial skin as a screen on which emotions paint themselves. At the same time, the physician as well as the art critic likened the tissue of skin to the crafted tissue of the very fabric that painters use as a support for their images.

Touching the self

The new notion of the human being as an organism dominated by nerves and vested with a sensitive membrane, also brought up the issue of the borderlines of the body and the unity of the self. These questions were most urgently raised in Diderot's *Rêve de d'Alembert*, a text debating contemporary medical theories and their wider implications from a philosophical and radically materialist perspective. Diderot produced the first version of this piece (that remained unpublished at the time) in 1769.[72] The text takes the form of fictional dialogues between non-fictional persons, the first (*A Conversation between d'Alembert and Diderot*) between the two editors of the *Encyclopédie*, the second (*D'Alembert's Dream*) between the physician Théophile Bordeu and Julie de L'Espinasse, an intimate friend of d'Alembert and host of a famous Parisian salon frequented by the *Encyclopédistes*. In the first dialogue Diderot and d'Alembert discuss the question whether all matter is sensible. Interestingly, the issue is introduced by using a thought-experiment from the realm of the arts, thereby associating the problem of potential animateness of matter with that of artistic animation and creation. By raising the question about the difference between 'man and statue, flesh and marble',[73] the text takes up art theoretical topoi that opposed, with respect to painting, a stiff and a lifelike rendering of the body, and alludes, with regards to sculpture, to the

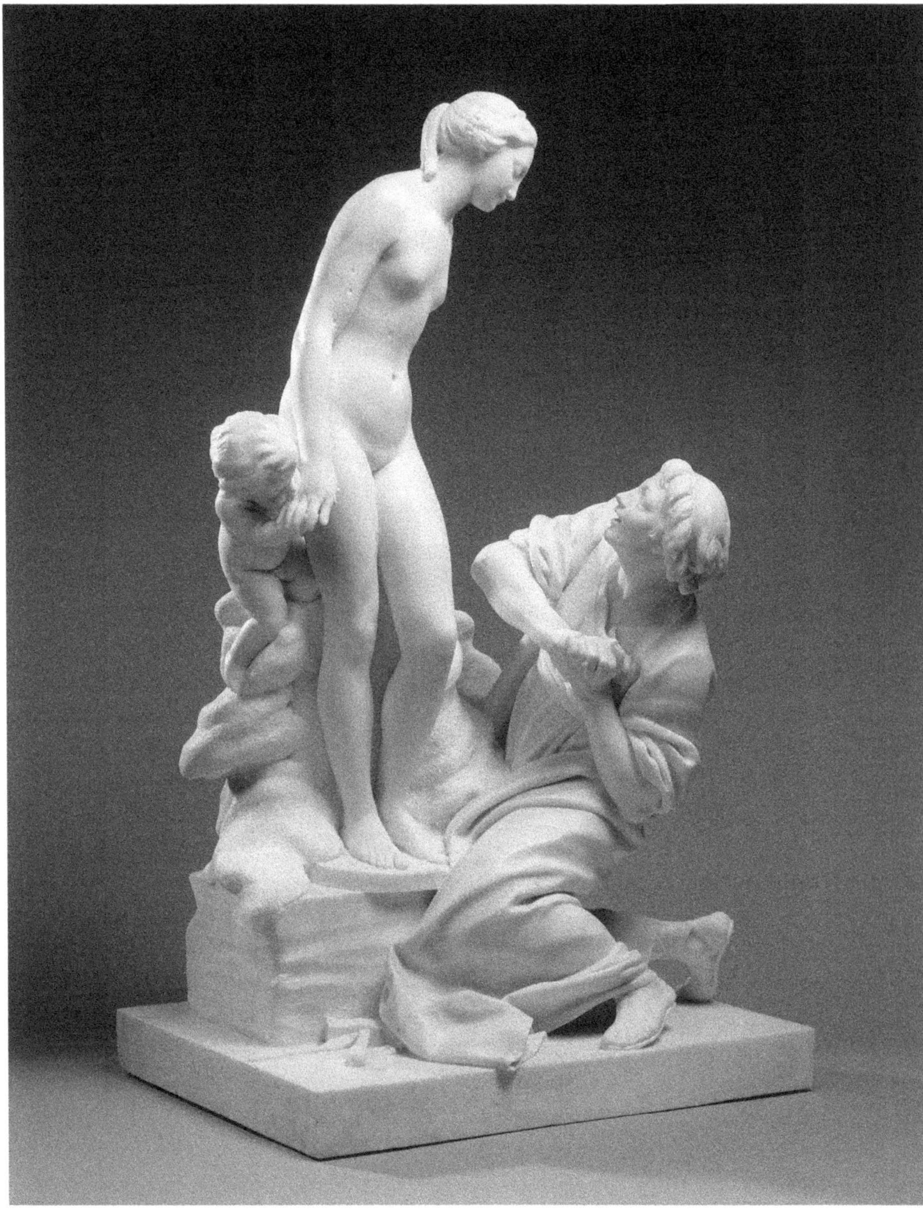

Etienne-Maurice Falconet, *Pygmalion and Galatea*, 1761, marble, 83.5 cm. **3.11**

challenge a sculptor faces when striving to make stone look like flesh. They evoke 'Falconet's masterpiece' without further naming the sculpture they have in mind. But given the context of the experiments in philosophy using the model of the animated sculpture then so popular, it has been assumed that they refer to *Pygmalion and Galatea* (Figure 3.11), not only one of Falconet's most acclaimed pieces, but also an art work that deals itself with a myth of artistic creation and, indeed, animation.[74]

Ovid's tale of the sculptor Pygmalion, whose desire for an ideal woman and wish to animate his ivory statuette became fulfilled with the help of Venus, was equally fashionable in the visual arts and in the literature of the time. In most eighteenth-century versions Pygmalion's sculpture is made of marble (rather than ivory) and hence matches its maker in size. Moreover, many of them eliminate the goddess, thus transferring the divine power of animation solely to the artist. Some of them include a little Cupid, suggesting that the powers of love contributed alongside the artist's inspiration to the marble's animation.[75] At the same time, the formerly anonymous creature is now given a name – Galatea, the name of a nymph, thus insinuating that the artist's creation derives from the realm of nature. For painters, such as Lagrenée in his 1777 version of *Pygmalion*, the topic was an ideal opportunity for staging a rivalry between sculpture and painting in demonstrating painters' ability to imitate marble as well as flesh. By representing the animation of the statue as a process of colouring, they used their expertise in the rendering of flesh tones to visually argue that painting is much more apt than sculpture for making an imitation of flesh or skin lifelike. On the other hand, the particular challenge for a treatment of the theme in a sculpture (and it was rarely done in this medium in the eighteenth century) was that, unlike the painter, the sculptor could not resort to colour to visualise the process of animation, but had to do it in the same material Pygmalion had used. In other words, sculptors had to imitate with one material – then usually white marble – both marble representing flesh, and living flesh as such. In addition, a sculptor could be more immediately aligned with Pygmalion himself. Falconet's sculptural version of the topic, shown at the Salon of 1763 as *Marble Group Representing Pygmalion at the Feet of his Statue, at the Moment when she Comes to Life*, was immediately interpreted as taking up this challenge, and Diderot himself discussed it in this sense in his critique of the exhibition. For Diderot, Falconet solved this problem through the admirable *faire* with which he distinguished between different kinds of flesh: 'This is one matter, one from which the statuary has drawn three different kinds of flesh. That of the statue is not that of the child [the Cupid], nor are these the flesh of Pygmalion.'[76] The critic particularly lauded the figure of Galatea for its *morbidesse*, exclaiming: 'What softness of flesh! No, this is not marble.'[77] And praising the lifelikeness of the figure of Pygmalion which, in this case, is based on his pose and the convincing expression of the sculptor's emotions, Diderot allocated Falconet the powers of godlike creation: 'O Falconet! … Emulator of the gods, if the gods have animated the statue, you have renewed the miracle by animating the sculptor.'[78]

In the *Conversation*, however, Diderot envisaged a far more down-to-earth way of animating inorganic matter. Still assuming a difference between a 'block of marble and the flesh tissue', he let d'Alembert state, 'the chisel of the most cunning sculptor does not create even an epidermis.'[79] In deploying the latter term, Diderot simultaneously invoked a part of the body that serves as a passage between inert matter and sensitive flesh,[80] and used a technical term for the surface of a sculpture. The notion of the 'epidermis of sculpture' referred in the French and Italian art literature from the seventeenth century onwards to the traces of an artist's chisel as well as to the bodily surface represented with them.[81] Eighteenth-century art literature entangled chisel work and the epidermis in the case of sculpture, facture and skin tissue in the case of painting, and often insinuated a mystical transformation of paint or marble into flesh when praising the lifelikeness of an art work. In contrast, the conversation between d'Alembert and Diderot provided a materialist version of the conversion of stone into life. They imagine pulverising Falconet's sculpture, mixing it with humus to compost it, and sowing seeds in it. When the resulting vegetables are finally harvested and eaten by an animal or human, stone is literally transferred into flesh.[82] This is, I suggest, an explosive materialist critique of myths of godlike artistic creation re-mobilised in many interpretations of the tale of Pygmalion and his animated statue. Diderot's account of the transformation of stone into flesh raised also the issue of what animates a human being, a topic that is further discussed in a second conversation, *D'Alembert's Dream*.

The setting is that Bordeu is called in, as d'Alembert is ill. The first thing the doctor does is touch the patient. Just as in Bordeu's actual medical case observations the fictionalised physician takes the patient's pulse and feels his skin, in order to conclude: 'The pulse is good: a little weak … the skin damp, the breathing easy.'[83] In what follows, Mademoiselle de l'Espinasse reports the dream, that is the utterances that the mathematician, troubled by his earlier conversation with Diderot, makes during his restless sleep during the night. D'Alembert's snippet monologue envisages an experimental type of thinking, unfiltered by the constraints of convention and perceived wisdom. Taking up his brainstorming, the physician proves it to be sensible and matching the latest medical propositions. While Bordeu and L'Espinasse discuss the feverish speculations, they are occasionally interrupted by d'Alembert who still speaks in his sleep. They wonder among other things, what would be the consequences of assuming that every single part of a being, every molecule or fibre, consisted of living matter. And d'Alembert mumbles in his sleep that at the beginning of human life there is 'at first nothing, then a living point' which is then joined by others, so that they finally build a being. But, he then asks himself, are these assembled animated points more 'than a tissue of little feeling beings'?[84] How does a potentially indefinite structure become a unity conscious of itself? Speculating about the relationship between individual animated elements and a whole organism the interlocutors resort to a metaphor (also employed by Bordeu in his study on glands) by comparing the human being to a swarm of bees, consisting of a multitude of little animated organisms, making up a collective form, like a bunch of grapes. Eventually they state, 'this cluster is a being, an individual'.[85] But whether this being is really something indivisible is far less clear than it seems. The swarm has no skin that contains the mass of individual bees: they might scatter at any moment. There is, in fact, throughout the whole text an anxiety about the subject falling apart.[86] Just as the swarm of bees can always change shape, a human being's feeling of its extent in space may alter dramatically. The fictive Bordeu recounts for example the case of a woman who periodically had the impression of being small as a needle and who felt a terrible anxiety of getting lost, before returning to a more realistic perception of her actual size. In this context, Mademoiselle L'Espinasse also reports that d'Alembert, when he asked these questions, 'felt himself all over'. I suggest that touch, besides its sexual connotation, enters the dialogue here as a sense that establishes unity and that reassures an uncertain subject.

Touch was generally re-evaluated during the eighteenth century both as a precise perceptual tool and as a sense that grants awareness of the self. Often ranked as the lowest in the hierarchy of the senses, as it depended on direct contact with the perceived object and was associated with physical pleasures, it was newly valorised as crucial for spatial perception.[87] Late seventeenth- and eighteenth-century sensualist philosophy, generally assuming that there are no innate ideas and that no knowledge can be acquired without the senses, paid particular attention to touch. The significance of touch for the experience of space and of the shape of objects was mainly discussed around the famous Molyneux question. The problem, first formulated in 1688 by William Molyneux in a letter to John Locke, was whether a person born blind would, upon gaining sight, be able to visually recognise a globe and a sphere without touching them. Roughly speaking, for empiricist or sensualist philosophers such as John Locke, or the Anglo-Irish philosopher and bishop George Berkeley and in France especially Étienne Bonnot de Condillac, the answer was no, as they believed that the eye alone was not capable of forming an idea of space, that is of the three-dimensional shape, position and distance of objects.[88] And it was Condillac, who, rejecting the assumption of any innate ideas, most radically stated that the eyes could only perceive light and colour, thus emphasising the significance of the sense of touch.

Diderot, who engaged with the debate in his 1749 *Letter on the Blind for the Use of Those who See*, stood somewhat between the two positions and complicated the issue by introducing, among others, the notion of experience. He suggested that the formerly blind person would be able to recognise the geometric forms with their eyes alone, but not at first sight, that is only after a period of exercising the newly gained sense organ.[89] However, he also disputed the idea of any innate ideas of space and shape and even claimed that the world and morals of a blind person were different from those of the seeing. Moreover, he not only pointed out that no human could live without the sense of touch, while the sight is dispensable, but also elaborated on the sophistication the sense of touch of blind people can reach. Taking the blind Cambridge mathematician Nicolas Sauderson as his example, he described how the skin had replaced Sauderson's eyes:

> Sauderson, then, saw by the means of his skin, and this integument of his was so keenly sensitive that with a little practice he could certainly have recognised the features of a friend traced upon his hand, and would have exclaimed as the result of successive sensations caused by the pencil: 'That is so-and-so'. Thus the blind have likewise a painting, in which their own skin serves as the canvas.[90]

Like in his later *Notes on Painting* Diderot understood skin as a canvas, in this case one on to which a portrait can be traced. However, it is an image perceived by touch not by sight. The metaphor had yet another connotation: the skin-canvas is here not the expressive medium (the face that transmits emotions), but a highly sensible perceptive organ, accurate enough to recognise a person from a contour drawn on its extended surface.

Étienne Bonnot de Condillac, in his *Treatise on the Sensations* of 1754, gave an even more elaborate account of the sense of touch. In this influential text, the philosopher constructed a thought-experiment in imagining a statue that becomes animated – just like Pymalion's sculpture. However, this nameless statue of indeterminate gender is not vitalised in a single miraculous moment, but step by step as it is bestowed with individual senses.[91] Condillac thus systematically explored which faculties and what specific knowledge of itself and the surrounding world the statue would have when given individual senses or various combinations of them. Touch is acknowledged as the 'only sense that judges external objects on its own',[92] and the only perceptual tool able to judge the distance, size and shape of objects at all. More importantly, it is the sense via which the statue learns to know its own body and thus apprehends itself, due to the double sensation which this sense alone provides: when the organ touches an object it feels both itself and the external item touched and 'in placing the hand on itself, the statue will only discover that it has a body when it distinguishes the different parts of that body and when it recognizes itself in each part to be the same sentient being'.[93] According to Condillac, it is thus via the double sensation generated by touching that we are able to experience we have a body and to become an individual by differentiating our own body from external objects. As a consequence, it is the sense of touch that enables a human being to say 'Me'.[94] This moment of self-recognition is dramatised in Jean-Jacques Rousseau's short play *Pygmalion* (1762), which brings the idea of the animated statue back to the realm of the arts. The first step Rousseau's Galatea takes is discovering herself. She exclaims 'Me' when she first touches herself, when she senses with the skin of her hand her own warm and living skin, finding herself by learning to distinguish between marble and flesh.[95] However, in the next moment she touches Pygmalion and believes his flesh to be 'me again'. Flesh is the distinguishing matter of life here, but does not again allow the double sensation of touch which is the basis of tactile self-recognition.

This moment of uneasy self-recognition is curiously echoed in Diderot's account of his visual encounter with his own portrait in the *Salon of 1767*, which opens 'Moi'. The recognition of the self does not quite work vis-à-vis the unloved likeness of Van Loo's painting, but is established via the portrait in writing that is set against it.

Painting in touch with thinking

Coming back to Fragonard and the way skin and touch feature in the portrait of a man of letters (Figure 3.1, plate 5), I propose that the sophistication with which artists employed hand and brush while painting skin could add to the complexity of the verbal discourses. Fragonard made his *portraits de fantaisie* as multilayered as the organ of skin, both in the literal and figurative sense. On the technical level, the paintings visibly demonstrate their build-up. Fragonard tended to work with two coloured preparatory layers, the first of which was usually red, the second in variations of grey, adapted in the case of the *portraits* to the overall colour effect of the individual painting. Here and there the grey underpainting remains uncovered. Occasionally even the canvas shows through, as in one spot of this portrait, at the lower part representing the desk on which the arm rests. It looks as if the artist purposefully made the tissue structure of the canvas visible here.[96] As for the upper layers, they often expose the brushwork as an interlacement of strokes.

If many of Fragonard's paintings are made of palpable brushstrokes, forming a vibrant and animated surface, such handling is particularly prominent in this portrait. The painting is generally dominated by a palette of warm tones, ochre of various shades and a fair amount of yellow, including the bright Naples yellow. The flesh tones are also dominated by various shades of yellow, emphasising brightness rather than the mature age the receding hair might indicate. Within these overall lively flesh tones, the rendering of the head stands out, as the man's facial skin is given a scintillating and mobile character. White is applied quite thickly, so that refractions on the impasto add to the vivid appearance. Bright colours are concentrated in particular on the brow and some final strokes in white impasto reflect the light. This marked brightness makes the forehead one of the centres of the painting, and both the size of the brow and the highlights inscribe the portrait into the very iconography of the philosopher Diderot had evoked in his verbal self-portrait. No matter who might be represented here, it is sensible to refer to this musing man as a philosopher, and one 'enlightened' in all senses of the term. The painting can be seen as an attempt to capture the act of thinking with a knowing and inspired brush. It is quite visibly the artist's touch that renders the sitter's skin lively and evokes the enthusiasm of his mind. The painter's activity thus performs complicity between the artist and the philosopher, suggesting an alliance of painting and thinking. By doing so, Fragonard not only inscribed himself along with the philosopher into the enlightened ideal of the *homme de génie*, a category comprising at the time poets, philosophers, painters and musicians,[97] but also established a further bond by turning the philosopher into a subject who touches. Fragonard painted him as an alert person with an active tactility, as he made the sense an issue by transforming the hands that would more typically write and gesticulate into hands that touch. In fact, the artist made no particular effort to indicate printed letters on the painted book: the man is sitting in front of a blank page, touching instead of reading a book. With his eyes directed elsewhere, he feels the paper like the blind man who reads with his skin, fingering one page of the book, as if he was sensing the materiality of the paper. The book thus comes into play as a material object rather than a carrier of information. Such emphasis on the physicality of the book recalls the fact that books were themselves often made of skin: in the eighteenth century they would still be mostly bound in leather made from animal hides. While the philosopher feels the paper with his right hand, the other arm moves towards the body, in a gesture that is not necessarily to be read as one of arguing. It looks as if the hand were about to be laid on the collar or possibly directed towards the uncovered neck. In fact, if we abstract from the spatial illusion, the paint that represents the hand does touch the paint that represents the neck thus provoking a sense of the double sensation occurring when a body touches itself. This encounter of the skin with itself also evokes the story of Pygmalion and Galatea and it might be a touch needed for self-affirmation. After all, the painted man, both caught in thought and distracted, consists of a bundle of individual brushstrokes that are – like the swarm of bees in *D'Alembert's Dream* – not contained within a clear outline. Even if this irregular tissue forms a recognisable entity, the vibrant strokes might provoke the anxiety of scattering, and the touch would be a way of testing the materiality of the body and the coherence of the self. On the other side, there is also Fragonard who affirmed himself as an artist by leaving behind traces of his touch.

The painter's brush produces a fictive intersubjectivity that is literally based on contact. Making visible a thinking and touching subject via a skin rendered with brio, the painting turns the body's surface into a nervous organ imbued with sensibility. The activity of the nerves, inextricably linked with alert perceptiveness, is staged at the site of the painting and of the painted. Painter and painted thus materialise on the canvas as vital, touching and sensitive men. In mid-eighteenth-century France, sensibility and nervous activity, understood as *the* vital forces, could still be considered manly qualities. Only a little later, the nerves were increasingly associated with their uncontrolled abundance to which women were allegedly more prone.[98] Voltaire proudly considered himself as *sensible*,[99] much as Diderot called himself 'philosophe sensible' in the written self-portrait with which he contrasted Van Loo's painted portrait. Sensible could mean at the time, reasonable and feeling, and having a perceptual alertness that formed the emotional and physiological hinge between the self and the surrounding world. This is how Fragonard envisages his subject as a 'philosophe sensible', producing a 'nervous canvas' in a double sense: in fabricating the thick multilayered and vibrant surface that is the painting and in representing the skin as an envelope imbued with sensibility.

The new understanding of skin, taken forward from the second half of the seventeenth century, left its mark in the art literature and in art practice. Skin came into focus alongside flesh and was perceived as a complex, textured and highly sensible organ. In turn, medical and philosophical discourses relied heavily on metaphors and examples from the visual arts. Medical texts, using verbal images such as tissue or canvas, associated organic materials like flesh with humanly crafted stuff, and by describing skin as 'canvas' likened the human envelope to an image. In many of Diderot's texts these discourses are entirely intermingled, fusing art theoretical and physiological concerns. Moreover, the appreciation of the painterly *touche* in the eighteenth century was hardly independent of the re-evaluation of the sense of touch during the same period. Skin as the organ of touch became an exquisite perceptual tool, able even to recognise portraits. The painter's *touche* would accordingly be not only a medium of enthusiasm but also an instrument of precision lending artists the tactile skills particularly needed to appropriately render this same delicate organ of the skin. There is inspired manual expertise and pleasure in the nervous impasto of the *portraits de fantaisie*, and the painted human envelope is for a moment both skin and flesh, surface and materiality.

Notes

1 Mary D. Sheriff, *Fragonard: Art and Eroticism* (Chicago; London: University of Chicago Press, 1990), here in particular pp. 117–18.
2 Ibid., p. 116.
3 Pierre Rosenberg (ed.), *Fragonard*, exh. cat., Paris, Grand Palais; New York, Metropolitan Museum (Paris: Réunion des musées nationaux, 1987), pp. 255–93. Rosenberg assembled seventeen paintings under the grouping, others such as

Carol Blumenfeld, *Une facétie de Fragonard: les révélations d'un dessin retrouvé* (Montreuil: Gourcuff Gradenigo, 2013), p. 9, have restricted the number to a core group of fourteen same-sized canvases.

4 See on the notion of the *portrait* or *figure de fantaisie* Melissa Percival, *Fragonard and the Fantasy Figure: Painting the Imagination* (Farnham; Burlington/Vt.: Ashgate, 2012), in particular pp. 17–47.

5 On the consequences of the find for the interpretation of the group see Blumenfeld, *Une facétie de Fragonard.*

6 Ibid., p. 40.

7 See on the problem of associating the *portraits de fantaisie* with individual sitters Sheriff, *Fragonard*, pp. 162–5. Despite the recent discussion I still agree with her assessment, already made in Mary D. Sheriff, 'Invention, resemblance, Fragonard's *Portraits de Fantaisie*', *Art Bulletin*, 49 (1987), 77–87 (p. 78), that the works in question 'cannot be characterised as face paintings'.

8 Klaus Herding, *Pierre Puget: das bildnerische Werk* (Berlin: Gebr. Mann, 1970), pp. 18–19.

9 Michel-François Dandré-Bardon, *Traité de peinture suivi d'un essai sur la sculpture* (Paris: Saillant, 1765), p. 185.

10 Ibid., p. 185.

11 Ibid., pp. 186–7.

12 Ibid., p. 187.

13 Ibid., pp. 187–8.

14 Yvonne Schmuhl, 'Das Inkarnat in der griechischenMalerei', *RIHA Journal* 0061, 26 November 2012, www.riha-journal.org/articles/2012/2012-oct-dec/schmuhl-inkarnat.

15 Antoine Le Blond de La Tour, *Lettre du Sieur Le Blond de La Tour,* à *un de ses amis, contenant quelques instructions touchant la Peinture* (Bordeaux: P. Du Coq, 1669), pp. 48–9. See on the treatise and generally on flesh tones in French late seventeenth- and early-eighteenth-century painting also the MA dissertation by Alex Paré, 'Peindre la chair: rendu des carnations et image du corps dans la peinture française des années 1680–1740' (École du Louvre, Paris, 2009), pp. 34–5. I would like to thank Elisabeth Martin for making this dissertation accessible to me.

16 Blumenfeld, *Une facétie de Fragonard*, p. 32.

17 For Fragonard's painterly technique see Ségolène Bergeon et al., 'Dossier Fragonard', *Science et technologie de la conservation et de la restauration des oeuvres d'art et du patrimoine*, no. 1 (April 1988), pp. 8–40.

18 The association with La Guimard was already questioned by Sheriff, *Fragonard*, p. 169; for the recent reallocation see Blumenfeld, *Une facétie de Fragonard*, p. 22.

19 *Encyclopédie ou dictionnaire raisonné des sciences, des arts et des metiers*, ed. Denis Diderot and Jean le Rond d'Alembert (accessed via University of Chicago: ARTFL Encyclopédie Projet (winter 2008 edn), ed. Robert Morrissey, http://encyclopedie.uchicago.edu/), vol. 1, 1751, p. 415, and for the illustration: *Receuil de planches*, vol. 1, 1762, part 3, p. 3, planche 4: 'L'écorché vû de face d'après Albinus'.

20 Louis Tocqué, 'Reflexions sur la peinture et particulièrement sur le genre du portrait'[1750], in Arnauld Doria (ed.), *Le discours de Tocqué sur le genre du portrait* (Paris: Jean Schemit, 1930), p. 22. See chapter 2, p. 42.

21 The actual title of the first edition is *Encyclopédié méthodique. Beaux-Arts*, ed.

Claude-Henri Watelet and Pierre-Charles Levesque, 2 vols (Paris: Panckoucke, 1788–91), vol. 2, 1791, p. 409. See more extensively on this issue Sheriff, *Fragonard*, pp. 146–8.

22 Antoine-Joseph Pernety, *Dictionnaire portatif de peinture, sculpture et gravure* (Paris: Bauche, 1757), entry 'Coloris', p. 69; see also Martial Guédron, *Peaux d'âmes: l'interprétation physiognomonique des œuvres d'art* (Paris: Éditions Kimé, 2001), p. 41.

23 Diderot discussed this in his 1773 *Paradoxe sur le comédien*, see Sheriff, *Fragonard*, p. 146.

24 Sheriff, *Fragonard*, pp. 153–62.

25 *Correspondance littéraire, philosophique et critique*, ed. Friedrich Melchior Baron von Grimm et al. Revised from the original by Maurice Tourneux, 16 vols (Paris: Garnier Frères 1877–82). Even though the *Correspondance littéraire* circulated only in the form of handwritten letters in a number of copies, as a newsletter from Paris sent to various German courts and eventually that of Catherine the Great and other European monarchs, its content was relatively public with the advantage of not being subject to censorship, as it circulated and was read aloud in the Parisian salons and even at the Court in Versailles. See on the *Correspondance littéraires* of the Enlightenment, Dena Goodman, *The Republic of Letters: A Cultural History of the Enlightenment* (Ithaca; London: Cornell University Press, 1994), pp. 136–82.

26 Sheriff, *Fragonard*, has argued that while several of the *portraits de fantaisie* can be seen as indirectly engaging with the eighteenth-century debate over the portrait, the so-called portrait of Diderot is directly involved in that discussion as it 'operates between two other portraits', and is thus a 'meta-portrait' of Van Loo's portrait and of Diderot's own self-portrait in words in his *Salon of 1767*. See for the older debate on the portrait Isabelle Combin and Pierre Rosenberg, 'Quatre nouveau Fragonard au Louvre', *La revue du Louvre*, 24 (1975), pp. 183–92, here in particular 186–8; and for a more recent discussion which takes up Sheriff's point Percival, *Fragonard and the Fantasy Figure*, pp. 126–31.

27 *Diderot on Art*, trans. John Goodman, introd. Thomas Crow, 2 vols (New Haven; London: Yale University Press, 1995), vol. 2, p. 19.

28 Diderot, *Salon de 1763*, in *Œuvres complètes*, ed. Herbert Dieckmann and Jean Varloot, 33 vols (Paris: Herrmann, 1975–), vol. 13, pp. 352–4: 'Le mérite de ressembler est passager; c'est celui du pinceau qui émerveille dans le moment, et qui éternise l'ouvrage.'

29 Diderot, *Diderot on Art*, vol. 1, p. 104. See on this passage also Uwe Fleckner, '"Pourquoi une belle esquisse nous plaît-elle plus qu'un beau tableau?" Fragonard, Diderot et l'éloquence du pinceau dans quelques portraits du XVIIIe siècle', in Thomas W. Gaethgens et al. (eds), *L'art et les normes sociales au 18ième siècle* (Paris: Éditions de la Maison des sciences de l'homme, 2001), pp. 509–33 (pp. 525–6).

30 Diderot, *Diderot on Art*, vol. 2, pp. 19–20.

31 Ibid., p. 20.

32 Ibid.

33 Diderot 'Physionomie', in *Encyclopédie*, vol. 12, 1765, p. 538. A second, equally short and dismissive article 'Physionomie (Scienc. Imagin.)' was authored by Louis Jaucourt.

34 See Guédron, *Peaux d'âmes*, p. 40. More extensively on physiognomy in France Melissa Percival, *The Appearance of Character: Physiognomy and Facial Expression in Eighteenth-Century France* (Leeds: Modern Humanities Research Association, 1999); and Melissa Percival and Graeme Tytler (eds), *Physiognomy in Profile: Lavater's Impact on European Culture* (Newark/Del.: University of Delaware Press, 2005).

35 Antoine-Joseph Pernety, *Discours sur la physionomie, et les avantages des connoissances physionomiques* (Berlin: Georges Jacques Decker, 1769), pp. 52–3.

36 Ibid., p. 52. See on the historical relationship between art historical practices and physiognomy also Guédron, *Peau d'âmes*, pp. 27–45; and more generally on the relationship between art history and physiognomy Daniela Bohde, *Kunstgeschichte als physiognomische Wissenschaft: Kritik einer Denkfigur der 1920er bis 1940er Jahre* (Berlin: Akademie Verlag, 2012); and Frederic Schwartz, *Blindspots: Critical Theory and the History of Art in Twentieth-Century Germany* (New Haven; London: Yale University Press, 2005), in particular pp. 177–210.

37 See for example Barthez's entry 'Face' in vol. 6, 1755, of the *Encyclopédie*, p. 355: 'M. de Buffon, dans le second tome de son histoire naturelle, a exprimé parfaitement les traits caractéristiques qui *peignent* les passions fortes par le changement de la physionomie.' Emphasis mine.

38 Diderot, *Diderot on Art*, vol. 1, p. 201. I am slightly altering John Goodman's translation here, as it omits the word 'skin'. See on this passage also Claudia Benthien, *Skin: On the Cultural Border Between Self and the World* [1999], trans. Thomas Dunlap (New York; Chichester: Columbia University Press, 2002), pp. 87–8.

39 On semiotical medicine see Volker Hess, *Von der semiotischen zur diagnostischen Medizin: die Entstehung der klinischen Methoden zwischen 1750 und 1850* (Husum: Matthiesen, 1993); and Roland Barthes, 'Semiology and Medicine', in *The Semiotic Challenge* [1985], trans. Richard Howard (Berkeley: University of California Press, 1994), pp. 202–13.

40 Ménuret also contributed a comprehensive article on skin diseases. See on Ménuret's articles regarding skin, Roselyne Rey, *Naissance et développement du vitalisme en France de la deuxième moitié du XVIIIème siècle à la fin du Premier Empire* (Oxford: Voltaire Fondation, 2000), pp. 166–7.

41 *Encyclopédie*, vol. 12, 1765, entry 'Peau (Médec. Séméiotiq.)', p. 219.

42 Ibid.

43 See on the history of dermatology with a particular focus on nineteenth-century visualisations of skin and skin diseases: Mieneke te Hennepe, *Depicting Skin: Visual Culture in Nineteenth-Century Medicine* (Wageningen: Ponsen & Looijen, 2007); Mechthild Fend, 'Portraying skin disease: Robert Carswell's dermatological watercolours', in Kevin Siena and Jonathan Reinarz (eds), *A Medical History of Skin* (London: Pickering and Chatto, 2013), pp. 147–64.

44 Tomas Macsotay has thus referred to it as 'medico-physiological' art criticism – see his article 'Suffering bodies, sensible artists: vitalist medicine and the visualizing of corporeal life in Diderot', in Manfred Horstmanshoff, Helen King and Claus Zittel (eds), *Blood, Sweat and Tears: Changing Concepts of Physiology from Antiquity into Early Modern Europe* (Leiden: Brill, 2012), pp. 267–91.

45 See for a general account Angelica Goodden, *Diderot and the Body* (Oxford:

Legenda, 2001), here in particular p. 1. On the emergence of the *sciences humaines*, Michel Foucault, *The Order of Things: An Archaeology of the Human Sciences* [1966], trans. A. M. Sheridan Smith (London: Tavistock, 1970).

46 Ann Thomson, 'Mechanistic materialism vs vitalistic materialism', *La lettre de la Maison française d'Oxford*, 14 (2001), 21–36.

47 For a comprehensive study see Rey, *Naissance et développement du vitalisme*.

48 Sergio Moravia, 'From *homme machine* to *homme sensible*: changing eighteenth-century models of man's image', *Journal of the History of Ideas*, 39 (1978), 45–60 (p. 55).

49 Laurence Brockliss and Colin Jones, *The Medical World of Early Modern France* (Oxford: Clarendon Press, 1997), p. 430, argue that 'neither Bordeu nor Barthez were materialists'.

50 See Philipp Sarasin, *Reizbare Maschinen: eine Geschichte des Körpers 1765–1914* (Frankfurt a. M.: Suhrkamp, 2001), a study on the history of the body as 'irritable machine' spanning the period from the Enlightenment to 1914, here p. 59; and Dominique Boury, 'Bordeu et Barthez: le malentendu "vitaliste"', *La Lettre de la Maison française d'Oxford*, 14 (2001), 71–84. Scholars such as Goodden, *Diderot and the Body*, have highlighted that most vitalists still assumed an immaterial soul, while Diderot reached a more radical materialist position in his late works. See also Charles T. Wolfe and Motoichi Terada, 'The animal economy as object and program in Montpellier vitalism', *Science in Context*, 21 (2008), 537–79 (pp. 544–5).

51 For example Sarasin, *Reizbare Maschinen*, pp. 57–62; Charles T. Wolfe, 'The allure of the flesh and the vitality of materialism: aporias of embodiment', in Felix Ensslin and Charlotte Klink (eds), *Aesthetics of the Flesh* (Berlin: Sternberg Press, 2014), pp. 83–106; see for a discussion of the notion 'vitalist materialism', Thomson, 'Mechanistic materialism vs vitalistic materialism'.

52 See Rey, *Naissance et développement du vitalisme*, in particular pp. 403–13, with a list of articles in the *Encyclopédie* attributed to vitalist physicians. The Montpellier physician Ménuret de Chambaud was the most prolific of the vitalists, contributing almost one hundred articles on medical topics and representing vitalist medicine, along with Fouquet, in the *Encyclopédie* most effectively and coherently (see Rey, pp. 57–122).

53 For Haller's reception in France see Hubert Steinke, 'Haller's concept of irritability and sensibility and its reception in France', in *La lettre de la Maison française d'Oxford*, 14 (2001), 37–69; and Hubert Steinke, *Irritating Experiments: Haller's Concept and the European Controversy on Irritability and Sensibility, 1750–90* (Amsterdam: Rodopi, 2005).

54 Haller's earlier writings on physiology had been translated by Pierre Tarin and Toussaint Bordenave as *Élémens de physiologie ou Traité de la structure et des usages des différentes parties du corps humain* (Paris: chez Prault fils, 1769). Between 1757 and 1766 Haller published his *Elementa physiologiæ corporis humani* (Lugduni Batavorum: Apud Cornel Haak) in eight volumes. It is unclear whether Diderot's own 'Éléments de physiologie' were ever meant for publication; they have been handed down in the form of two substantially different manuscripts. See the introduction to Diderot's 'Éléments de physiologie' by Jean Mayer, in: Diderot, *Œuvres*, vol. 17, pp. 263–90.

55 Anne C. Vila, *Enlightenment and Pathology: Sensibility in the Literature and Medicine of Eighteenth-century France* (Baltimore; London: Johns Hopkins University Press, 1998), p. 44.
56 Claudia Honegger, *Die Ordnung der Geschlechter: die Wissenschaften vom Menschen und das Weib, 1750–1850* (Frankfurt a. M.; New York: Campus, 1991).
57 Steinke, *Irritating Experiments*, p. 231.
58 On Madame Helvetius's salon and the *médecins philosophes* see Honegger, *Die Ordnung der Geschlechter*, pp. 137–8; and more generally Antoine Guillois, *Le Salon de Madame Hélvetius: Cabanis et les idéologues* (Paris: Callmann Lévy 1894); Jean-Paul Lagrave (ed.), *Madame Helvétius et la Société d'Auteuil* (Oxford: Voltaire Foundation, 1999). See more generally on the significance of the salons for the French republic of letters Goodman, *Republic of Letters*, and more recently Antoine Lilti, 'Sociabilité et mondanité: les hommes de lettres dans les salons parisiens au XVIIIe siècle', *French Historical Studies*, 28 (2005), 415–45.
59 Barbara Maria Stafford, *Body Criticism: Imaging the Unseen in Enlightenment Art and Medecine* (Cambridge/Mass.; London: MIT Press, 1991), p. 38.
60 The emphasis on liquids and internal ointments is particularly strong in Christianus Gottlieb Ludwig, respondente F. Grützmacher, 'De humore cutem inungente pro loco', [Leipzig 1748], in Albrecht von Haller (ed.), *Disputationum anatomicarum selectarum*, vol. 7, pars 2 (Göttingen: Vandenhoek, 1751), pp. 33–64, but is also evident in the entries on skin in eighteenth-century medical dictionaries. The significance of humoral theory for eighteenth-century medicine has been highlighted among others by Sarasin, *Reizbare Maschinen*, on neo-hippocratism in particular pp. 33–51.
61 Moravia, 'From *homme machine* to *homme sensible*'.
62 Diderot, 'Élemens', in *Œuvres*, vol. 17, pp. 447–8.
63 See for example Le Cat's 1740 *Traité des sens* (Rouen [*s.n.*], 1740), p. 3: 'Le Toucher est le sens le plus grossier.' At the same time, Le Cat considers touch as the safest sense and 'le dernier retranchement de l'incrédulité'.
64 For a recent overview see Anne C. Vila (ed.), *A Cultural History of the Senses in the Age of Enlightenment* (London: Bloomsbury Academic, 2014), especially Vila's introduction; on the eighteenth-century valorisation of the sense of touch Ulrike Zeuch, *Umkehr der Sinneshierachie: Herder und die Aufwertung des Tastsinns seit der frühen Neuzeit* (Tübingen: Niemeyer, 2000).
65 Albrecht von Haller, *Dissertation sur les parties irritables et sensibles des animaux*, trans. Samuel-Auguste-David Tissot (Lausanne: Marc-Michel Bousquet, 1755); *A Dissertation on the Sensible and Irritable Parts of Animals*, with a preface by M. Tissot (London: J. Nourse, 1755). See on the significance of the French translation Moravia, 'From *homme machine* to *homme sensible*', p. 53. The English translation from which I quote appeared in London 1755.
66 Haller, *A Dissertation on the Sensible and Irritable Parts*, p. 4. See for a more detailed analysis Steinke, 'Haller's concept of irritability and sensibility'.
67 Haller, *A Dissertation on the Sensible and Irritable Parts*, p. 7.
68 Fouquet, article 'Sensibilité', in *Encyclopédie*, vol. 15, 1765, entry 'Sensibilité, Sentiment (Médecine)', p. 38.
69 Ibid., p. 51. The *Encyclopédie* did of course not represent only one scholarly doctrine on this matter. Haller himself contributed the article 'Irritabilité' (1777)

to the Supplement of the *Encyclopédie*, where he conceded that irritability might depend on sensibility. See Steinke, 'Haller's concept of irritability and sensibility', pp. 48–9.

70 See Steinke, 'Haller's concept of irritability and sensibility', p. 60.

71 Fouquet, 'Sensibilité', in *Encyclopédie*, vol. 15, p. 48: 'La peau, cette toile nerveuse qui forme un organe général, & dont l'action contrebalance celle des organes intérieurs, la peau est encore éminemment douée de cet instinct.'

72 They are usually referred to together as *Le rêve de d'Alembert*. See for the history of the text the introduction and comment by Jean Varloot and the annotations by Georges Dulac in: Diderot, *Œuvres*, vol. 17, pp. 25–66, and 67–85. I am quoting here the English edition in *Dialogues by Denis Diderot*, trans. and introd. Francis Birrell (London: Routledge, 1927).

73 'A Conversation between d'Alembert and Diderot', in: Diderot, *Dialogues by Diderot*, p. 23.

74 See the notes to the text in Diderot, *Œuvres*, vol. 16, p. 93, reference no. 12; and more importantly Inka Mülder-Bach, *Im Zeichen Pygmalions: das Modell der Statue und die Entdeckung der 'Darstellung' im 18. Jahrhundert* (München: Fink, 1998), a study on eighteenth-century thought-experiments around Pygmalion's statue; as well as J. L.Carr, 'Pygmalion and the philosophes: the animated statue in eighteenth-century France', *Journal of the Warburg and Courtauld Institutes*, 23 (1960), 239–55.

75 See on this aspect in particular Mary D. Sheriff, *Moved by Love: Inspired Artists and Deviant Women in Eighteenth-Century France* (Chicago; London: University of Chicago Press, 2004); Victor Stoichita, *The Pygmalion Effect: From Ovid to Hitchcock* (Chicago; London: University of Chicago Press, 2008), on the eighteenth century and 'the nervous statue', pp. 111–60.

76 Diderot, 'Salon de 1763', in *Œuvres*, vol. 13, p. 410. See on Diderot's comment on Falconet's *Pygmalion*, Stoichita, *The Pygmalion Effect*, pp. 111–48.

77 Diderot, 'Salon de 1763', in *Œuvres*, vol. 13, p. 409.

78 Ibid., p. 410.

79 Diderot, 'Conversation', *Dialogues by Diderot*, p. 24.

80 See the notes on *Le rêve de d'Alembert* in Diderot, *Œuvres*, vol. 17, p. 92, reference no. 11.

81 The issue came first into focus with regard to the cleaning and conservation of ancient sculptures and of modern statues exposed to the weather in the gardens of Versailles when it was deplored that the works had lost their 'epidermis' or 'patina'. See in more detail on the skin of sculptures Hans Körner, '"Die Epidermis der Statue": Oberflächen der Skulptur vom späten 17. bis zum frühen 19. Jahrhundert', in Daniela Bohde and Mechthild Fend (eds), *Weder Haut noch Fleisch: das Inkarnat in der Kunstgeschichte* (Berlin: Gebr. Mann, 2007), pp. 105–32.

82 Diderot, 'Entretien', in *Œuvres*, vol. 17, p. 95.

83 Diderot, *Dialogues by Diderot*, p. 41. See for this kind of diagnosis the case descriptions in Théophile Bordeu, *Recherches sur le pouls, par rapport aux crises* (Paris: De Bure l'aîné, 1756).

84 Diderot, *Dialogues by Diderot*, p. 43.

85 Ibid., p. 45. See also Théophile Bordeu, *Recherches anatomiques sur la position des*

glandes et sur leur action (Paris: chez G. F. Quillau, 1751), § CXXV; and Boury, 'Bordeu and Barthez', p. 72.

86 See for a similar reading of this text also Sarasin, *Reizbare Maschinen*, pp. 85–6.

87 See Benthien, *Skin*, pp. 185–202; and more extensively on the reassessment of the sense in the eighteenth century Marjolein Degenaar, *Molyneux's Problem: Three Centuries of Discussion on the Perception of Forms* (Dordrecht; Boston; London: Kluwer Academic, 1996).

88 See for an overview still John W. Davis, 'The Molyneux problem', *Journal of the History of Ideas*, 21 (1960), 392–408; and in more detail: Degenaar, *Molyneux's Problem*.

89 Degenaar, *Molyneux's Problem*, pp. 73–8.

90 'Letter on the Blind for the Use of Those who See', in Denis Diderot, *Thoughts on the Interpretation of Nature and Other Philosophical Works*, introd. and annotated by David Adams (Manchester: Clinamen Press, 1999), p. 171. See on this passage by Diderot also Jacques Derrida, *Memoirs of the Blind: The Self-portrait and Other Ruins* [1991], trans. Pascale-Anne Brault and Michael Naas (Chicago: University of Chicago Press, 1993), pp. 100–1; and *On Touching, Jean-Luc Nancy* [2000], trans. Christine Irizarry (Stanford/Cal.: Stanford University Press, 2005).

91 This is with regard mainly to the French original, as Condillac takes on the one hand universal man ('homme') as the test figure for his thought-experiment, referring to him as 'il', and on the other 'la statue', a noun of female gender in French to which he refers as 'elle' – thus evoking more explicitly Pygmalion's sculpture Galatea.

92 'On Touch, or the only sense that judges external objects' is the title of Part Two of Étienne Bonnot de Condillac, 'A treatise on the sensations', in *Philosophical Writings of Étienne Bonnot, Abbé de Condillac*, trans. Franklin Philip with the collaboration of Harlan Lane (Hillsdale: N.J.: Lawrence Erlbaum, 1982), pp. 1–415 (pp. 225–63).

93 Condillac, 'A treatise on the sensations', p. 233. See on this aspect of Condillac's *Traité des Sensations* also Daniel Heller-Roazen, *The Inner Touch: Archaeology of a Sensation* (New York: Zone Books, 2007), p. 224.

94 Condillac, 'A treatise on the sensations', p. 231. See also Ewa Lajer-Burcharth, 'Pompadour's touch: difference in representation', *Representations*, 73 (2001), 54–88 (p. 56).

95 Jean Starobinski, *Jean-Jacques Rousseau: Transparency and Obstruction* [1957], trans. Arthur Goldhammer (Chicago; London: University of Chicago Press, 1988), pp. 70–2, interprets this as narcissist reunion of the artist with his own creation. For Paul de Man, *Allegories of Reading: Figural Language in Rousseau, Nietzsche, Rilke and Proust* (New Haven; London: Yale University Press, 1979), p. 181, Galatea is the figure of 'the Self as such'. See also Lajer-Burcharth, 'Pompadour's Touch', pp. 54–6.

96 Bergeon et al., 'Dossier Fragonard', p. 29, on Fragonard's preparatory layers, and p. 33, for the detail of the painting showing the canvas.

97 Claudia Denk, *Artiste, Citoyen & Philosophe: der Künstler und sein Bildnis im Zeitalter der französischen Aufklärung* (München: Fink, 1998), pp. 37–8.

98 See on the gendering of sensibility Vila, *Enlightenment and Pathology*, in particular

p. 3; Sarasin, *Reizbare Maschinen*, pp. 89–94; Honegger, *Die Ordnung der Geschlechter*, in particular p. 13; Ludmilla Jordanova, *Sexual Visions: Images of Gender in Sciences and Medicine between the Eighteenth and Twentieth Centuries* (New York; London: Harvester Wheatsheaf, 1989), pp. 27–8.

99 Vila, *Enlightenment and Pathology*, p. 3.

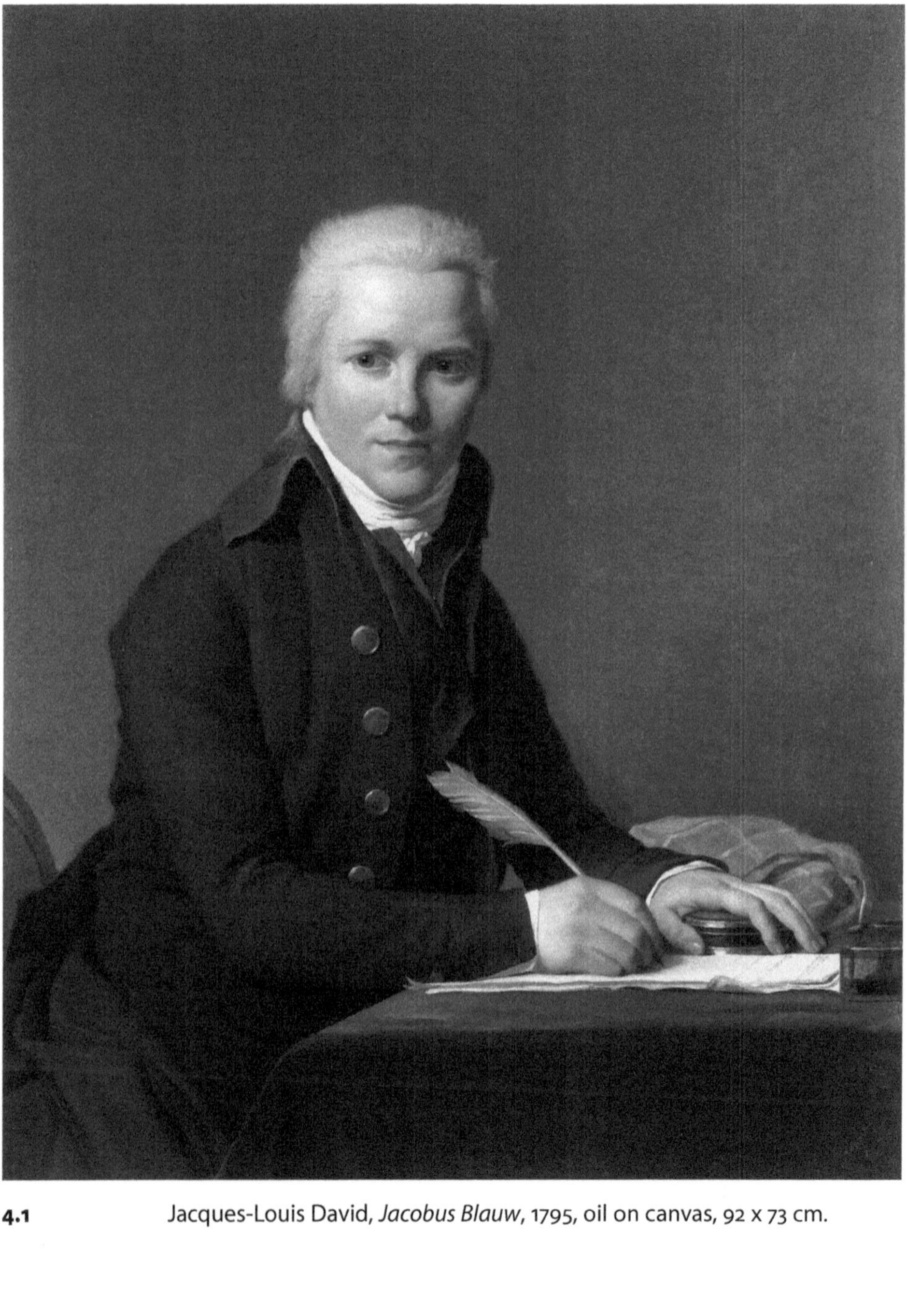

4.1 Jacques-Louis David, *Jacobus Blauw*, 1795, oil on canvas, 92 x 73 cm.

4 Sensitive limit

The appreciation of visible brushstrokes and the textures produced by them gradually faded over the course of the second half of the eighteenth century along with the rise of neoclassical aesthetics. Among the most distinctive features of neoclassicism were an emphasis on the contour and a preference for more finished surfaces. These features might be considered as purely formal attributes of artistic style, but they are equally elements crucial for the pictorial formation and understanding of the human body, its surface and borderlines. The culture of neoclassicism, extending well beyond the realm of art and art discourse, was generally characterised by a heightened concern with the shaping of the body and the safeguarding of its boundaries. The emerging bourgeoisie engaged in techniques of self-regulation and self-control, 'technologies of the self' as Foucault has called them,[1] including physical exercise, dietary regimes and procedures of hygiene, as much as routines of psychological self-inspection. Skin as the body's physical demarcation, was increasingly perceived not merely as an envelope and organ, but as the boundary of the self. Skin was thus psychologised and tied to modern notions of subjectivity and identity. Jan Goldstein suggests that older notions of selfhood were transformed during the revolutionary period into naturalised and authentic 'holistic selves', and George Vigarello notes that the term *soi* 'opens up an entirely new way of speaking about the individual'.[2] This self knows of the world through sense perception and simultaneously organises the network of sensations. It is rooted in the body and held together by the skin.

Medical discourse contributed considerably to the integrated view of the self, and the *médecins philosophes* or *idéologues* of the revolutionary and post-revolutionary period remained particularly concerned with the ties between *physique* and *morale*. Skin came under new medical scrutiny at the time and was now explicitly defined as the body's limit. However, its physiological function could, from a medical point of view, hardly be restricted to that of a demarcation or even protective barrier. From this perspective the human dermis was simultaneously border and organ, an envelope operating as the sense of touch and safeguarding the exchange between the body and its environment. In the immediate post-revolutionary period, this – to some degree paradoxical – notion of skin was elaborated in particular detail in Xavier Bichat's *Anatomie générale* (1801). Developing the vitalist understanding of the organ, discussed in the previous chapter, Bichat regarded the human envelope as a lively sense organ as well as a boundary and called it a 'limite sensitive'.

This chapter will engage with the transformations in notions of flesh and skin occurring around the period of the French Revolution, and is concerned with the interchange between medical and artistic conceptions of skin and flesh at the time. It will begin with a discussion of the period's art literature and argue that there was, in conjunction with the neoclassical privileging of the contour, an increased attention to skin in parallel to flesh and flesh tones as objects of artistic imitation. Bichat's notion of skin as *limite sensitive* will be analysed in the subsequent section, and finally will serve as a leading metaphor with which to look at the rendering of skin and the body's surface in a set of Jacques-Louis David's portraits dating from the immediate post-revolutionary period, especially his 1795 portrait of Jacobus Blauw (Figure 4.1).

Skin and contour in the *Dictionnaire des beaux-arts* and neoclassical art theory

The contour, when circumscribing a human figure in a drawing or painting, can be seen not only as indicating this figure's shape, but also as an abstracted visual sign of the skin in its function as the body's envelope and borderline. Given the neoclassical affection for lines and outlines, it is not surprising that the term 'skin' gains significance in the art literature of the period. A particularly good indicator for the gradual changes in the understanding of the body in representation is the *Dictionnaire des beaux-arts*. This important and well-known compendium both summed up eighteenth-century art theory and disseminated neoclassical aesthetics in France. The dictionary, begun by Claude-Henri Watelet (1718–86) and continued after his death by Pierre-Charles Lévesque (1736–1812), was first published in two volumes in 1788 and 1791 as part of the *Encyclopédie méthodique* and re-edited in 1792; it was thus the last of the many art dictionaries produced during the Ancien Régime and the first to be published during the French Revolution.[3] Watelet, its initial editor, was a wealthy tax collector, and an amateur painter, etcher, art collector and writer on the arts whose poem *L'art de peindre* (1760) earned him honorary membership in the Académie. Also a founding member of the Société royale de médecine, he always argued for the integration of arts and sciences, emphasising the significance of knowledge for artists, stressing in particular the benefits of anatomical training.[4] He was a regular at Mme Geoffrin's salon, flourishing between 1749 and 1776, where he mingled with the likes of Voltaire and the *Encyclopédistes* and could well have taken part in the kinds of debates around the qualities of living matter or the relation of body and mind, discussed in the previous chapter.[5] Lévesque, almost twenty years younger, was also linked with the *philosophes*, and went, on Diderot's recommendation, to St. Petersburg to teach literature, and to work and publish extensively on the history of Russia. In St. Petersburg he also befriended the sculptor Falconet, who stayed in the city between 1766 and 1778 on the invitation of Catherine the Great,[6] and whose views subsequently featured prominently in the *Beaux-arts* section of the *Encyclopédie méthodique*. Beyond that, Lévesque's contributions generally expanded Watelet's more franco-centric view, introducing a wider range of European art theoretical positions, referring for example to Gérard de Lairesse's *Groot Schilderboek* and the writings of Joshua Reynolds, but most importantly to Johann Joachim Winckelmann and the latter's friend, the painter Anton Raphael Mengs.[7] In contrast to Watelet, Lévesque took an explicitly classicist position, and his extensive dictionary article 'Sculpture' relied – in the sections on antiquity – heavily on Winckelmann, on his mode of historicising successive styles of ancient art and on his privileging of the 'beautiful' style characterised by simple forms circumscribed by flowing, continuous outlines.[8]

There are necessarily areas of disagreement between Watelet and Lévesque, and as a co-authored work taking up a variety of previous sources, the dictionary could not possibly be a homogeneous body of art theory. But it is precisely by focusing on these inconsistencies that a sense of a debate and of the shifting art theoretical notions of the body emerges. Lévesque questioned, for example, the overemphasis on the *faire*, the painterly facture of a work which had been so crucial to earlier eighteenth-century art theory and practice. Watelet, who provided the most important entries regarding the imitation of flesh and skin for the *Encyclopédie méthodique*, remained more committed to the *faire* and to authors like Dandré-Bardon. But he also slightly shifted the terms, and the dictionary thus continued the tendency, already apparent in mid-eighteenth-century art literature, to make skin an increasingly important aspect in discussions of the artistic imitation of the human body's surface.

Across the dictionary *peau* is a term quite frequently used, as it comes with a variety of significations, due partly to the multiple meaning of the word in French language, including both skin and leather. It may, in the *Encyclopédie méthodique*, refer to an object of representation, either a human's skin or, more rarely, an animal hide to be represented in drawing, painting or sculpture, but it is equally employed for skin as a material, such as leather sponges used to disperse pigments on paper,[9] or little bags made of leather or pig intestine for storing paint.[10] Skin is thus a term that is not per se associated with the human body, nor with a living entity, and can easily qualify as a raw material. It is only in relation to notions of flesh that it clearly connotes the living human body.

The representation of skin and flesh is predominantly treated in four articles of the *Encyclopédie méthodique* which all focus on painting: 'Carnation', 'Chairs' and 'Coloris', authored by Watelet, as well as the entry 'Couleur' contributed by Lévesque. On two occasions Watelet praised the encyclopaedic serendipity that united all four entries touching on flesh tones under the letter 'C', declaring in the entry 'Chairs': 'This word and the ways to employ it, have, as one will see, sensible relations with what we call *carnation*, *coloris* and *couleurs*, which fortunately find themselves close together in the collection of articles that the letter C demands.'[11] While giving it a positive twist, he indirectly addressed the conundrum of the dictionary as a medium for the exposition of knowledge: it divides knowledge into terms listed in arbitrary alphabetical order and it makes little allowance for comprehensive treatises.[12] Insisting on the systematic connection between the terms *chair*, *carnation*, *coloris* and *couleur*, and tying the three articles together, Watelet reinforced the long-lasting kinship of colour and flesh. And yet, skin makes its entry here.

A short and concise definition is given under the first heading 'Carnation':

> The word *carnation* designates, in the language of art as much as in general language, the appearance that the colour of the skin [*la couleur de la peau*] and primarily that of the face offers us in nature.
>
> The word *carnation* also signifies the imitation that painters make of this appearance when painting the human figure. Finally, it refers to the manner artists employ in order to imitate the colour of the skin and in particular that of the complexions [*la couleur de la peau & sur-tout du teint*]. It is hence in this general sense that one says that Dutch women tend to have a beautiful flesh tone [*carnation*]. Which means that they have beautiful white skin and complexions [*la peau & le teint blanc*], just as coloured as necessary.[13]

With this explanation, which is repeated almost verbatim two decades later in another *Dictionnaire des beaux-arts*,[14] Watelet took up the traditional meaning of the term *carnation* while also transforming it slightly, but significantly: on the one hand, *carnation* continues to be the key term and refers, as it used to, simultaneously to the human body and the imitation made of it. On the other, 'skin' is now employed to relate to the human body's outer appearance. Watelet chose – as far as I can see for the first time in this context – the expression *la couleur de la peau* as a synonym for *carnation*. Interestingly, the term 'skin colour' comes in the same breath as the praise of white skin.[15] As I will discuss in more detail in the chapter on skin colour, a reassessment of the human body's appearance as a surface phenomenon, the partial shift from flesh tones and complexion to skin colour, happens in conjunction with the development of racial anthropology and the privileging of whiteness during the second half of the eighteenth century.[16]

While the notions of skin, colour and complexion still co-existed during that period, there is in the *Encyclopédie méthodique* a gradual shift in focus from the substance of the body to its outer appearance. The colour of a human being was thus increasingly understood as a property of an external organ (the skin) rather than of the entire flesh tinted by humours. The article 'Chairs' confirms this. It explains that painting flesh is not only the most significant subject in the imitation of the 'living and animated' human being in history painting, and, even more so in portraiture, but also the most difficult one. This intricacy results from the multitude of hues that even the flesh of a single person can feature due to the complex ways in which the human body's matter reflects light:

> Flesh is also one the most difficult objects to render, because it is susceptible to an infinity of gradations, delicacy of tones, and of transitions that demand both intense study of nature and great lightness of brush handling ... Speaking here of the particular nature of flesh, I refer mainly to the manner in which light reflects on a substance. An observing artist who is eager to please examines the effect that the different incidences of light produce on the face of a woman, on her arms, on her hands, on her neck and bosom, in particular if she is white [*si elle est blanche*]; and if her skin is fine, transparent and slightly coloured by the blood covered by the delicate tissue of the epidermis.[17]

Though mentioning the necessity of an ease in the handling of the brush and employing the expression 'tissue of the epidermis', two aspects which resonate with the writings of Pernety and Dandré-Bardon discussed in the previous chapter, Watelet was much less preoccupied than these authors with the texture produced by the brush in order to mimic the fabric of skin and flesh. The emphasis is on the ways in which skin reflects light and on the transparency of the human's outermost organ.[18] More concerned with layering than with the artist's touch, he proposed an observational mode that results in rendering the subcutaneous substance visible as a thin organic layer through which internal physiological processes (blood circulating) interact with the external workings of light. The painter is expected to mimic not so much the fabric of various materials but the ways in which they react to light:

> The firm, supple and porous consistency that nature, the spring of age and health, bestows on a young beauty, modifies the light, which is not reflected by the tissue of the skin in the same way as by hard and rough substances …
>
> The soft and elastic flesh allows the penetration of its imperceptible pores by part of the light up to the first layer of the skin. Reflected and thrown back from there, the light conveys to the soul, via the eyes that fix it, the idea of life and sensations of voluptuousness. Observe furthermore, how the imperceptible curves of the flesh and its transparency that makes the veins noticeable, spread on the half-tones … slightly bluish nuances, which lead through soft gradations to the most radiant tones of the skin. The variations of flesh [*chairs*] are countless. It takes the most delicate and attentive eyes to discern them and a highly special talent to render them.[19]

Watelet thus promoted a painterly attention that is sensible to the physiology of the living skin as well as to the multiple effects of light on the body's surface and to the variation of flesh tones. By doing so he was himself attentive to the countless shades of skin, without being concerned with classifying the ways of imitating the skin of members of different age groups. For Watelet, there was *one* ideal skin and skin tone, and it was gendered, eroticised and geographically local: the white, radiant skin of young European women, especially those of Dutch or Flemish origins.[20]

Lévesque's entry 'Couleur' is less judgemental in this respect. After considering the influence of different environments, such as seasons or times of the day, on the appearance of objects, it urges the painter to attend to the nuances different objects require. Without being specific about any particular colour (though cautioning against the use of too-brown tones), Lévesque suggests that 'flesh, in particular delicate flesh, should be of a soft and tender tone'.[21] Moreover, any individual figure has more than one single flesh tone. 'Different tones [*teintes*] should colour the parts exposed to the sun … or affected by excessive perspiration. Certain parts are covered with a finer skin, others with a thicker one; the fat [*graisse*] is not distributed with the same abundance, the blood does not everywhere show with the same intensity: all these variations … must be observed by the artist.'[22]

Both Watelet and Lévesque highlighted close observation as a crucial component of an artist's activity, one which corresponds with a minute way of painting. They tended to favour relatively finished brushwork when it came to the imitation of flesh or skin, emphasising the smoothness of the body's surface and the subtleness of gradations that should be rendered with a finesse rivalling that of skin itself. Although Dandré-Bardon was extensively quoted by both of them, his detailed advice on the variations of paint handling was not taken up. They nevertheless conceded that too much attention to detail is as detrimental as the 'torturing' of the paint into a too-finished effect. Despite their reservations regarding overly visible brushwork, associated with liveliness and enthusiasm in much of the earlier eighteenth-century art literature, both Watelet and Lévesque maintained the importance of animating the painting and the painted body. Lévesque stressed that paint itself is dead while only the painter's art animates the colours: 'With a few colours which have no charm in themselves, he will create the flesh of Venus.'[23] And the painting as such should be given 'life' when the artist takes it up 'with a fresh eye', applying some final 'light touches'.[24] Quoting from Dandré-Bardon in this section of his article, Lévesque closely associated this process of animation, via the workings of the painter's touch, with the representation of flesh, evoking myths of Pygmalionesque creation of actual flesh. In a similar vein, *chair* is mentioned right at the outset of Watelet's article 'Touche', making it the principal subject matter to be 'touched with sentiment'.[25]

Despite the frequent occurrence of the word 'skin' in the entries on colour, flesh and flesh tones, the entry 'Peau' itself suggests a more restrictive use of the term. It was authored by the painter Jean-Baptiste Robin, responsible for a comparatively small number of articles of the *Encyclopédie méthodique*. In contrast to Watelet and Lévesque, he insisted that the word 'skin' should only be employed when speaking of drawing and sculpture: 'With respect to the usage of the word skin one has to distinguish between the art of colouring and the art of drawing, because it is only applied when referring to this latter aspect of painting. One uses the word flesh [*chair*] when speaking of anything regarding the painting of the flesh and of the human figure.'[26] Robin thus followed the traditional art parlance that associated flesh, paint and colour, while describing as epidermis or skin the worked surface of a sculpture (especially when made with a chisel in stone) and the human body's exterior of which the imitation is made in these media.[27] He underpinned this traditional approach with neoclassical ideals of the body and its representation. Looking at the ways the Gods are represented in ancient sculpture and contrasting these to then contemporary practices he stated: 'Small wrinkles, fugitive movements of the skin, all the accidental or individual unevenness, weaken the expression of the muscles, the only organs of movement in the human body.'[28] Lévesque, in his entry 'Details', similarly cautioned the history painter to 'neglect minor wrinkles, and the lines of the skin that cross the large wrinkles in old people.'[29]

These warnings are generally directed against the art of the seventeenth and eighteenth centuries, and sculptors such as Bernini or Pierre Puget, classified as 'modern' in distinction from the ancients. But again, this view was not consistently shared throughout the *Dictionnaire*. The article 'Sculpture' refers extensively to Winckelmann in the sections of ancient art for which Lévesque was responsible, while opening a different perspective in the part of modern sculpture, authored by the sculptor Falconet, and initially written for Diderot and d'Alembert's *Encyclopédie*. [30] Falconet praised Puget and voiced discontent with the ways ancient sculptors 'treated flesh', making the point that the ancients were 'so little concerned with the details that often they neglected the wrinkles and movements of the skin in the places where it stretches or folds over according to the action of the limbs.'[31] In an argument much discussed in the eighteenth century and fiercely rejected by Mengs, among others, Falconet proposed that modern sculpture had exceeded ancient art in this respect.[32] He granted sculpture the same capacity to animate the represented flesh as painting, and singled out Puget for the mastery with which the 'sentiment of the folds of the skin, the softness of the flesh [*mollesse de la chair*] and the fluidity of blood' are so well observed that one sees 'the blood circulating in the veins of the *Milo* of Versailles'.[33]

In contrast, the section on ancient sculpture sums up Winckelmann and reiterates his critique of seventeenth-century sculpture and in particular that of Bernini. In a comment very similar to Robin's later remarks in his article 'Peau', Winckelmann had critiqued the exaggerated detail in the rendering of the human body in modern sculpture in his *Reflections on the Painting and Sculpture of the Greeks*, first published in German in 1755: 'Modern works are likewise distinguished from the antient [sic] by parts; a crowd of small touches and dimples too sensibly drawn. In antient works you find these distributed with sparing sagacity, and, as relative to a completer and more perfect Nature, offered but as hints.'[34]

Winckelmann developed this view in his famous *History of Ancient Art* where he praised the pure forms of Greek art. The post-classical 'beautiful style', especially, was singled out as characterised by fluently drawn, graceful outlines.[35] This account of the representation of the body was less concerned with the imitation of physical appearance than with the circumscription of bodily forms. The contour became a visual sign of the skin in its function as a borderline and shell rather than as a layered, vital organ. It was understood by Winckelmann, and his followers in France, that Greek art was an idealising practice, and that the artist, as exemplified in the story of Zeuxis, who was said to have chosen the best parts from the five most beautiful women of Croton to compose an ideal image of Helena, abstracted from individual features. Yet, there was no clear line between the imagination of actual Greek bodies and their representation in art. Lévesque held that the basis of Greek sculpture was 'la belle nature',[36] and Winckelmann had more wishfully blurred the distinction between artistic idealisation and the shaping of the actual body through physical exercise, diet and eugenic practices.[37] Looking in particular at Sparta, his *Reflexions* set out to describe such physical activities, and assume that Greek artists always had beautiful models at hand, when they studied in the gymnasia and other sites of sports activity. Winckelmann even suggested that the statues were a true, if mediated, record of actual Greek athletes when he imagined the artist Phidias drawing from the contours the bodies of wrestlers had left in the sand of a gymnasium.[38]

When Winckelmann described beautiful statues as if they were beautiful bodies, his reconstruction of ancient sculpture was driven by a desire to re-animate the past. The followers of Winckelmann in France, especially, turned neoclassical aesthetics into the quest for an ideal human set against the allegedly decadent bodies of their time. The culture of neoclassicism was explicitly anti-aristocratic and its ideal of a beautiful body has been considered as the aesthetic equivalent of the bourgeois *homo clausus*.[39] The notion of the *homo clausus* ('confined human') was initially introduced by the sociologist Norbert Elias in his 1939 *The Civilizing Process*, a study that analyses the formation of the modern subject as a history of increasing physical control and self-restraint. Historians of the body have variously taken up this notion and associated it with Michael Bakthin's *Rabelais and His World*, where the literary scholar famously argued that the grotesque body dominating medieval and early modern popular culture was eventually superseded by a more contained body defined by a clear demarcation between self and the world.[40] With a similar sympathy for a more porous pre-modern body, Barbara Duden has elaborated in her study of the womens' patient records of a German doctor that an understanding of a body in permanent flux and with permeable boundaries still prevailed in the early eighteenth century. Pushing the emergence of the modern body even further, Dorinda Outram suggests in *The Body and the French Revolution* that the *homo clausus* only fully took shape during the French Revolution in a culture of politicised classicism in which ancient heroes became models of stoic self-control.[41]

Pursuing these arguments through my reading of art historical and medical texts, the aim is not to construct the formation of an increasingly contained and controlled body as a continuous, linear process. Rather, I suggest that the neoclassical notion of a free subjectivity residing in a body confined in clear-cut borderlines was a powerful model of anti-aristocratic critique as well as a narcissistic projection of a bourgeois self. Associated practices of sports, dieting, dressing and in particular an increasing national and individual concern with hygiene, contributed to shaping actual bodies.[42] Other bodies and models of the body always co-existed. The fully concealed human body remains an impossibility, as it would be incapable of interacting with the exterior world – and the physiologists of the late eighteenth and early nineteenth centuries were well aware of this crux. From a medical point of view skin was by necessity porous; all the more reason then to be concerned with the regulation of its exchanges. Within the field of the visual arts too, the grotesque body and the grimace, a distorting anti-physiognomical provocation, held its fascination despite, or maybe because of, the prevalence of a neoclassical aesthetic.[43] But even as such, the ideal of the body contained in undulating lines does not come without its internal antagonisms and discontents. Both firm and fluent, these lines always threaten the body with dissolution.[44]

Similar contradictions were also inherent in the artistic production of idealised bodies within the context of academic art training: the skeleton and the physical interior of the body always lurked behind the surface. While ancient artists were believed to have lived in an age of anatomical innocence, ignorant of the the messy work with the cadaver, neoclassical art discourse in late eighteenth-century France insisted on the necessity of anatomical knowledge for the artistic formation of ideal bodies. Ancient artists were imagined to have had fit and beautiful naked bodies always at their disposal, so that the correct rendering of the human physique came to them naturally. The modern artist however, with no such models at hand – and the degenerate physique of the models in art academies was subject to particular ridicule and critique – had to study anatomy in search for the ideal physique.

This situation contributed to the rise of artistic anatomy during the last decades of the Ancien Régime. Efforts to reform art training at the Académie royale under the aegis of the Comte d'Angiviller, since 1774 the Directeur général des Bâtiments du Roi, aimed at a return to the heyday of France's seventeenth-century classicism and a revival of history painting. This was in keeping with the attempts to re-establish discipline in the study of anatomy and the life model. Jean-Joseph Sue and his eponymous son, the teachers of anatomy at the Académie, and, after the abolition of the royal institution during the French Revolution, at the newly formed École de dessin (later École des beaux-arts), had established in the 1770s a regular and more rigorous training in the subject. In May 1795, under the short-lived Thermidor government that preceded the establishment of the Directory later that year, an anatomy theatre was installed for the first time in the art institution itself, and for the next couple of decades art students (women and men alike, as the lectures were public) would have studied anatomy, partly through dissection or assisting at dissections. The theatre itself was situated in the basement of the Louvre, close to the gallery of ancient sculptures, thus blending, as Sue (the younger) put it, 'the corpse, the living human, and examples of the most beautiful shape, as they can be found in antiquity'.[45]

Finding the ideal – healthy, athletic and beautiful – body in antiquity, the anatomist took a decisively neoclassical view. This is more elaborately expressed in his 1788 artistic anatomy, the *Élémens d'anatomie, à l'usage des peintres, des sculpteurs et des amateurs*. Building on Winckelmann's argument according to which regular exercise contributed to the beautiful formation of the body, Sue assumed that Greek artists had the privilege of always having sight of well-formed natural bodies not degenerated by civilisation. His praise of Greek physical perfection is paired with a rejection of the 'luxury and softness that has weakened all European nations to such an extent that natural beauty can only be found among the class of the working man'. And this was precisely the problem. While this remark chimes with the then-prevalent critique of a decadent aristocratic culture – to which Jean-Jacques Rousseau lent one prominent voice – at stake, even though not named, is the social group which articulated this critique. Sue pointed out that physical perfection could not be a mere side effect of physical labour but required conscious work on the body. The ideal bourgeois body – and the New Man of the French Revolution – was by no means natural but consciously shaped according to the gendered neoclassical ideals; formed by the 'moderate' exercise Sue suggested. Especially in women exercise should be in 'proportion with the delicacy of their constitution'. In contrast, women working outdoors in the countryside, might get a tan [*teint bruni*], a nervy body and pronounced muscles, which would be detrimental to their grace and beauty. The 'well-built woman' is an ancient model seen through neoclassical eyes, as the description of 'rounded limbs' and 'white and delicate skin' merges into the language of art when the text speaks of her 'pleasant contours'.[46]

Many physicians of the revolutionary period, and not only those teaching artists, were classicists in their own right. They shared models of the body that were informed by the aesthetics of neoclassicism and a general esteem for ancient culture. 'No matter what subject you treat', postulated the physiologist and physician Cabanis in his 1802 *Rapports du physique et du morale de l'homme*, 'it is always the ancient Greeks you have to quote.'[47] Hippocrates, Galen and the ancient theory of temperaments were studied afresh and gained new popularity as they provided a holistic vision of the body and a model of self-regulation particularly attractive to vitalist medicine.[48]

Neoclassical art theory and medical discourses, adhering to similar cultural ideals, placed particular emphasis on the body's surface and outer demarcation. It was especially in debates around sculpture, and the revival of ancient art as a universal model and along with it the imagination of an ideal Greek body, that the aesthetics of simplified outlines were aligned with a fit body, shaped by moderate exercise and contained in a unifying skin. The parallel discussions of painting and painterly practices had a slightly different outlook, mobilising different aspects of skin. While the gradual shifting from flesh to skin, already observed in mid-eighteenth-century art literature, continued, attention was paid less to textures and more to layering, transparency and the action of light. Colour remained associated with life, and along with issues of colour and colouring, the vital functions of skin came into focus. Skin was seen as a site of life and was simultaneously a demarcation and a transparent screen – artistically rendered via subtle layering of paint – through which vital processes became visible. This double function of skin as a borderline and vital organ is also at the heart of one of the period's most elaborate discussions of the organ: Bichat's chapter on the dermoidal system in his 1801 *Anatomie générale*. Defining skin as a *limite sensitive* was not the only paradox involved here, as the knowledge of life functions of the human organs derived from excessive study of the corpse.

Vital skin and questions of life and death

Anatomical and physiological discourse of the time described skin and its functions in a new way; it not only went into more detail with respect to the composition of the organ, but also researched its vital functions while simultaneously emphasising its function as a boundary. In the work of Xavier Bichat, despite his short life (1771–1802) one of most prolific and influential physicians of the immediate post-revolutionary period, the skin both demarcates the body and ensures its communication with the exterior world. As an organ which is both the limit of the body and part of it as it adheres to the tissues inside, it becomes, for Bichat, a crucial model for the understanding of the organic structure and organisation of the body.

Bichat belonged to a younger generation of vitalists who were, like the representatives of the École de Montpellier and many of the *médecins-philosophes* discussed in the previous chapter, concerned with the understanding of the vital forces of life.[49] Born in Lyon as the son of a practising physician who had studied at the medical faculty in Montpellier with the vitalist Paul-Joseph Barthez, the young Bichat was introduced to the ideas of the École de Montpellier early on. Eventually moving to Paris, he complemented his training in anatomy and surgery by studying with Pierre-Joseph Desault, then Chief Surgeon at the Hôtel-Dieux, Paris's largest hospital.[50] Bichat arrived in the capital in June 1794, and thus at the height of the Terror. Death was everywhere in a clinician's life at this period: mortality rates were high in hospitals, dissections for purposes of research and training were undertaken in considerable number, while the guillotine was almost ceaselessly in operation. The guillotine, as is well known, was more than just an instrument of capital punishment. It provoked both fascination and disgust, and provided a great public spectacle in the years after its initial operation in April 1792. Proposed by Joseph-Ignace Guillotin, a physician and deputy of the Third Estate in 1789, as an allegedly humane machine that killed reliably, quickly and in an egalitarian manner,[51] the instrument not only incited political and legal debate, but also philosophical and medical speculations about the nature of life and death and more precisely the process of dying. These questions were prompted not least by processes transmitted through the skin and observable on the face in the moments after execution.

Anatomists, besides being citizens who could witness the killing machine working on a daily basis, had a particular relationship with the guillotine, as it provided cadavers that could be accessed immediately after execution.[52] Anatomical, surgical and physiological research during this period in France relied on dissections in unprecedented numbers. According to one of his students, Bichat opened more than six hundred dead bodies in his last year alone.[53] Not surprisingly then, Bichat defined life against the backdrop of death, and famously opened his *Recherches physiologiques sur la vie et la mort* with the definition of life as 'the totality of those functions which resist death'.[54] For Foucault, who analysed the structural transformations in French medical theory between 1770 and 1820 in his influential early study *La naissance de la clinique* (1963), morbidity was at the heart of the development of modern, clinical medicine and its understanding of the workings of the body, and Bichat is a crucial protagonist in his account.[55]

Bichat was not the only physician for whom the guillotine prompted questions about the nature of, and the boundaries between, life and death. From a medical perspective it was a machine not only for killing but also for experimentation which enabled what was only then explicitly understood as 'physiological research'.[56] Designed to kill in an instant, it was paradoxically used to make observations about dying and about the time span during which certain vital processes continued after decapitation. The question, initially raised by the German physician Samuel Thomas Sömmering, was whether the decapitated head immediately loses consciousness.[57] Sue (the younger) also embarked on experiments related to the guillotine, raising research questions very similar to those that occupied Bichat. Between 1795 and 1797 he executed physiological experiments, according to his own account in front of large audiences in anatomical theatres, which were summarised in lectures for the Institut national de France in the summer of 1797. He experimented with animals, which were decapitated in order to study the time span during which movements still continued in different parts of the body.[58] With a similar focus, he presented his observations on guillotined humans, concluding from continuing movements and facial expressions visible on the severed heads, that pain is still experienced up to four minutes after decapitation. Clearly defying the idea of a clean and painless death, the guillotine was abhorred by Sue. In the same context, he got very excited about the sensibility of skin in a moment of physical crisis: 'What remarkable changes do we see in the skin when the disease becomes cutaneous? How many nuances in colour it goes through? What sensibility we notice? … What difference in its form and texture?'[59] Given that this fascination with the vital qualities of skin when in a state of crisis occurs in the midst of his reflections on the guillotine, it is hard not to think of the popular accounts of heads that grimaced or blushed after decapitation. The best known of these narratives is the one relating to Charlotte Corday, guillotined for the assassination of Jean-Paul Marat in July 1793. Her face was said to have blushed after the executioner had slapped her severed head. The account was recorded by a medical observer, who also accepted the psychologised reading of the physical reaction as 'indignation', thus doubly condemning the decapitation of the woman.[60] This episode also demonstrates that an essential part of the procedure of decapitation was its visibility, which turned the head into a juridical trophy and demonstration. The guillotined head was exposed to the crowd waiting to see emotions paint themselves on the face. Daniel Arasse has thus called the guillotine a 'portrait machine' and hence argued that the guillotine constitutes a cut in the history of portraiture: the genre's focus on the head does not feel quite the same after that post-guillotine moment; nor will the inspection of the vital processes of skin.[61]

Bichat: a body full of membranes

Bichat's first book, the *Traité des membranes* published in 1799, was, as the title suggests, entirely dedicated to these thin layers of tissue. From his vitalist perspective, Bichat was interested in the ways in which membranes cover organs, partake in their functions and connect with other parts, and a particular focus were the mucous membranes that line the orifices thus marking the mediating zones between the body's interior and exterior, establishing the communication between the two. For Foucault, Bichat's main contribution to clinical medicine was the way he rethought the corporeal space:

> The major discovery of the *Traité des membranes*, later systematized in the *Anatomie générale*, is a principle of deciphering corporeal space that is at once intra-organic, inter-organic, and transorganic. The anatomical element … is now no more than a secondary form of a primary space, which, by a process of winding round, superposition, and thickening, constitutes it. This fundamental space is entirely defined by the thinness of the tissue.[62]

Bichat looked at the interior body as a space crossed and organised by planes of tissue, and it is his focus on surfaces even within the body that makes him in Foucault's account a clinician, a physician embedded within the visual and institutional culture of the modern clinic.[63] Understood as bordering tissues, membranes are all considered after the model of the human body's external organ, the skin, as tissue sheets that circumscribe the organs and connect to them:

> We should regard the mucous membranes as barriers [*comme limites, des barrières*], which, placed between our organs and the substances which are foreign to them, should guard them against the fatal impression of these substances, and consequently contribute within to the same functions which the skin performs on the exterior, with regard to bodies which surround that of the animal, and which incessantly tend to act upon it.[64]

Bichat took this up in his 1801 *Anatomie générale*, now talking of the cellular system rather than of mucous membranes. He maintained that the cellular system 'forms an envelope or outward limit to the organs' while entering 'freely into the structure of each' organ.[65] It is a surface that crosses the threshold of the structure it segregates. The *Anatomie générale* addressed in a more systematic and elaborate way the question, what makes and demarcates the body parts? The publication departed from previous anatomical tracts in so far as it was less a description of the topography and structure of the bones, muscles and organs than an account of the tissues that form and wrap the body parts. In this vitalist anatomy, tissues are seen as media for the exchange processes between parts of the body. They are membranes that enable nourishment and secretion thus keeping the organism alive, and simultaneously demarcations that guarantee the differentiation between body parts and their distinct functionality. Bichat believed that a set of distinct tissues constituted the basic elements of the human body, comparable to the thirty-three elements of chemistry that

Lavoisier had distinguished in his *Traité élémentaire de chimie* of 1789.[66] This theory of elementary tissues was, later in the nineteenth century, replaced by cellular theory, which considered the cell as the basic unit of living beings, but it still earned Bichat the reputation of being the founder of histology (the discipline concerned with the microscopic structure of organic tissues). Bichat singled out twenty-one types of tissues – or 'systems' and the tissues proper to them; among the elements distinguished were cellular, nervous, vascular and muscular systems and finally those of the dermis, epidermis and the hair.

Unlike physicians and naturalists like Malpighi and Grew, who had first described the structures of organic material with textile metaphors, as nets, textures or woofs, Bichat rejected the use of microscopes and believed in the naked eye as a unmediated means of observation.[67] He was equally antagonistic to medical images, and none of his works including the *Anatomie générale* have illustrations. As he argued, they would keep medical students and professionals from performing dissections, in his view the prime route to medical knowledge.[68] In lieu of illustrations Bichat provided extensive verbal descriptions of the characteristics of each of the twenty-one systems and their associated tissues. More than a hundred pages of his *Anatomie générale* are dedicated to the *système dermoïde* alone. As had been common in most medical accounts of the skin since the seventeenth century, Bichat divided the dermis into three layered components: the corium, its main part that determines the depth of the skin; the papillae responsible for the sense of touch, and the reticular body. The latter forms the connection between dermis and epidermis, and was also considered by Bichat as the seat of the colouring matter responsible for the tone of the skin. Like any other system, the skin is for Bichat internally connected to other organs, but what singles it out is the fact that it is 'free on one side'.

Bichat discerned different tissues, but acknowledged that no system is ever fully distinct from others, as they are criss-crossed by nerves and vessels that establish the communications of liquids or sense impressions through the body. This conglomerate of systems exchanges fluids and transmits information gained from sense perception. No less than for Diderot and his materialist account of the human in *D'Alembert's Dream*, which saw the organism divided into sensible units, or for Bichat's contemporary Cabanis, the disquieting question remained: what guarantees the unity of the self, and what governs the co-operation of physical elements?[69] Rather than resorting to the self, Bichat used two major concepts to tackle the issue: communication and organisation. If organisation is a leading metaphor in Bichat's account of the human body,[70] the notion of communication is crucial for his account of skin.

Right at the outset of his chapter on the *système dermoïde*, skin is defined as follows:

> All animals are invested with a membrane more or less dense, generally proportionate in thickness to the volume of the body. This is intended both to protect the subjacent parts, to expel a considerable portion of the residue of nutrition and digestion, as well as to connect the animal with exterior forms. To man it is a sensitive limit, placed on the boundaries of his soul, with which limit these forms incessantly come in contact, to establish the connections of his animal life, and thus bind his existence with that of all that surrounds him. This envelopment is the dermis, or the skin; and the parts of which it is composed we will term the dermoidal system.[71]

More specifically than any physician before, Bichat highlighted the function of the dermis as a hinge between the body's internal processes and its environment, turning it into what we call an interface today. By naming skin a 'sensitive limit' Bichat stressed both the boundary character and the sensibility of the organ. Very much like the vitalist physiologists of the Enlightenment, such as Haller or Fouquet in his article 'Sensibilité' for the *Encyclopédie*, Bichat held that 'animal sensibility is carried to the utmost degree in the skin'.[72] At the same time, he saw skin as a borderline, thus sharing a major aspect of the body ideal of neoclassicism; and he attached the idea of a beautiful skin to a dermis that is 'smooth on its external surface'.[73] This kinship with neoclassical aesthetics becomes even clearer in his discussion of the forms of the dermoidal system, where he explained that the skin, while hiding most parts of the body, articulates the most protruding parts. However, skin is not a clear cut and perfectly concealing membrane. The vital exchange processes between the environment and the internal body mediated by the skin necessitate a variety of vessels traversing the organ and transporting among others sweat and oily substances. While the latter can serve to a degree as protective ointments, in excess they swiftly turn into dirt and may attract cutaneous diseases. Chiming with the increasing concern with hygiene in the post-revolutionary period, Bichat – deploring the denaturalisation of contemporary French society and its reluctance to expose the body to water – considered bathing 'a natural costom' among men and animals and recommended regular baths in particular during the warmer season.[74] The modern body has to peel itself out of the *crasse* (grime) of the Ancien Régime, and its contour has to be constantly worked upon.[75] As has been elaborated by Philipp Sarasin, the modern discourse of hygiene is closely linked to the understanding of the body as a communicative medium that speaks the truth. One needs a clean canvas to properly read the signs of the body.[76] For Bichat the body is certainly a medium communicating via its external membrane. The movements of the muscles are transmitted to the skin thus becoming visible at the exterior. Unlike animals, whose whole bodies are involved in this externalisation, humans rely predominantly on the face, where all the 'passions paint themselves' [*les passions se peignent pour ainsi dire sur la face*].[77] The passions have in the face, he further explained, a triple means of expression. Besides the muscles of the face and of the eye that allow a more or less controlled transmission of emotions, the capillary system, carrying blood to the external zones of the skin, is the medium for involuntary blushing.

For Bichat, the dermis was an important model for thinking about the characteristics and demarcations of his systems, as the organ was simultaneously a distinct tissue structure and a boundary. To establish a distinction between functional systems and tissue structures, limits were crucial. What is more, Bichat himself associated limits with lines. In the case of the dermis he remarked that the divide between the inner mucous and the outwardly dermoidal system is not as pronounced in the organisation as in the colour and that the two systems 'blend together in an insensible manner', while simultaneously observing that the limits are 'constantly traced by a reddish line' as if someone had drawn demarcations into the body.[78] His notion of the skin accounted for the vital processes active within the organ, and the necessary communication between body and world, as well as its function as boundary. This multifaceted nature will serve, in what follows, as a framework for looking at portraits by David which were painted at the same time as Bichat's enquiries into the body. Artists and medics were equally concerned with the face and its skin. Shortly after the publication of Bichat's *Anatomie générale*, skin made its entry into artistic anatomy: Jean-Galbert Salvage's *Anatomie du Gladiateur* (which I will discuss in detail in chapter 6) paraphrased Bichat's account of the organ extensively. But more importantly, as already manifested in the *Encyclopédie méthodique*, there was at the time a heightened attention to the face and its skin as vital means of expression. During the Revolution and its immediate aftermath this visibility could hardly be separated from the deadly operations of the guillotine. David's portraits can equally be seen as defining life against the spectre of death – and they paint skin in a multilayered manner as a surface and transparent screen through which signs of vitality shimmer.

David's post-revolutionary portraits

David pursued quite distinct painterly strategies in his portraits. Some of them, especially portraits produced during the French Revolution, such as the one of Louise Trudaine, née Micault de Courbeton (ca 1791–92; Figure 4.2), or that of Louise de Pastoret and her son (1791), were executed with a fabric of evenly distributed brushstrokes that remain visible, but make no particular attempt to differentiate the textures represented. Richard Taws has convincingly associated this 'feathery, irresolute brushwork' with the provisionality of the political moment, and this way of working was indeed reserved to the revolutionary years.[79] Other portraits are more finished, especially in the rendering of the figures, their face, hands and clothes. Like Elisabeth Vigée-Lebrun in many of her portraits, among them the self-portraits with her daughter or the portrait of her friend and fellow painter Hubert Robert (1788; Figure 4.3), David generally used a surface textured by brushstrokes for the mostly monochrome backgrounds. In portraits like that of Mme Trudaine, however, the whole canvas features the marks of the painter's hand that work nevertheless in the interest of imitation. We recognise the woman seated on a simple chair, her body positioned in profile, while the head is turned towards us, catching the eye with an almost staring gaze. The painting as a whole is dominated by two fields of textured pigment: the rubiginous background and the lower part of the black dress which fully covers up the lower part of the sitter's body, giving no indication of its shape and position in space. No attempt is made to differentiate the fabric of the dress from that of the background – it is visibly a pictorially produced texture, which is, in the art theoretical terms of the time, neither a *signe imitatif* nor a *signe communicatif*. Watelet distinguished these two types of traces of the artist's pencil or brush in his article 'Touche' for the *Encyclopédie méthodique*,[80] defining the former as working in the service of imitating objects, and the latter as a sign of the artist's emotional state while working at a drawing or painting. David, however, who covered the entire canvas with brushstrokes applied in an even and repetitive manner, avoids their reading as a sign communicating his subjective state of mind or emotion and as those final *touches spirituelles* that were understood at the time as signs of liveliness (especially when applied to the imitation of a person's face) and traces of the artist's enthusiasm. In contrast to Fragonard's *portraits de fantaisie* there is barely any impasto, and little variation in the size and frequency of the brushstrokes. The texture produced is predominantly a sign of a systematic working process and the lacklustre materiality of paint. This overall effect diminishes the hierarchy of fore- and background, and depending on where the beholder's eye lingers, the ground seems to push forwards, confusing the spatial relations of before and behind. Simultaneously, the chronology of the painterly process is foreclosed, as no privilege is given to final touches that would light up the painting. T. J. Clark has likened these even ways of treating different objects in a painting, as if all made of the same raw material, to eighteenth-century debates around materialism and the relations of body and soul. In its most radical manifestation, Diderot's *Rêve de d'Alembert*, discussed in the previous chapter, the distinction between animate and inanimate matter is fully blurred, and even stone can potentially turn into flesh. If a painter, Clark suggests, took such thoughts seriously, he would, when painting a portrait, 'be inclined to handle stuffs and flesh in ways which borrowed the characteristics of one for the other or set up analogies between the two.'[81] Of course painters took such issues seriously as they transformed paint into the things they represented. What is special about the portraits

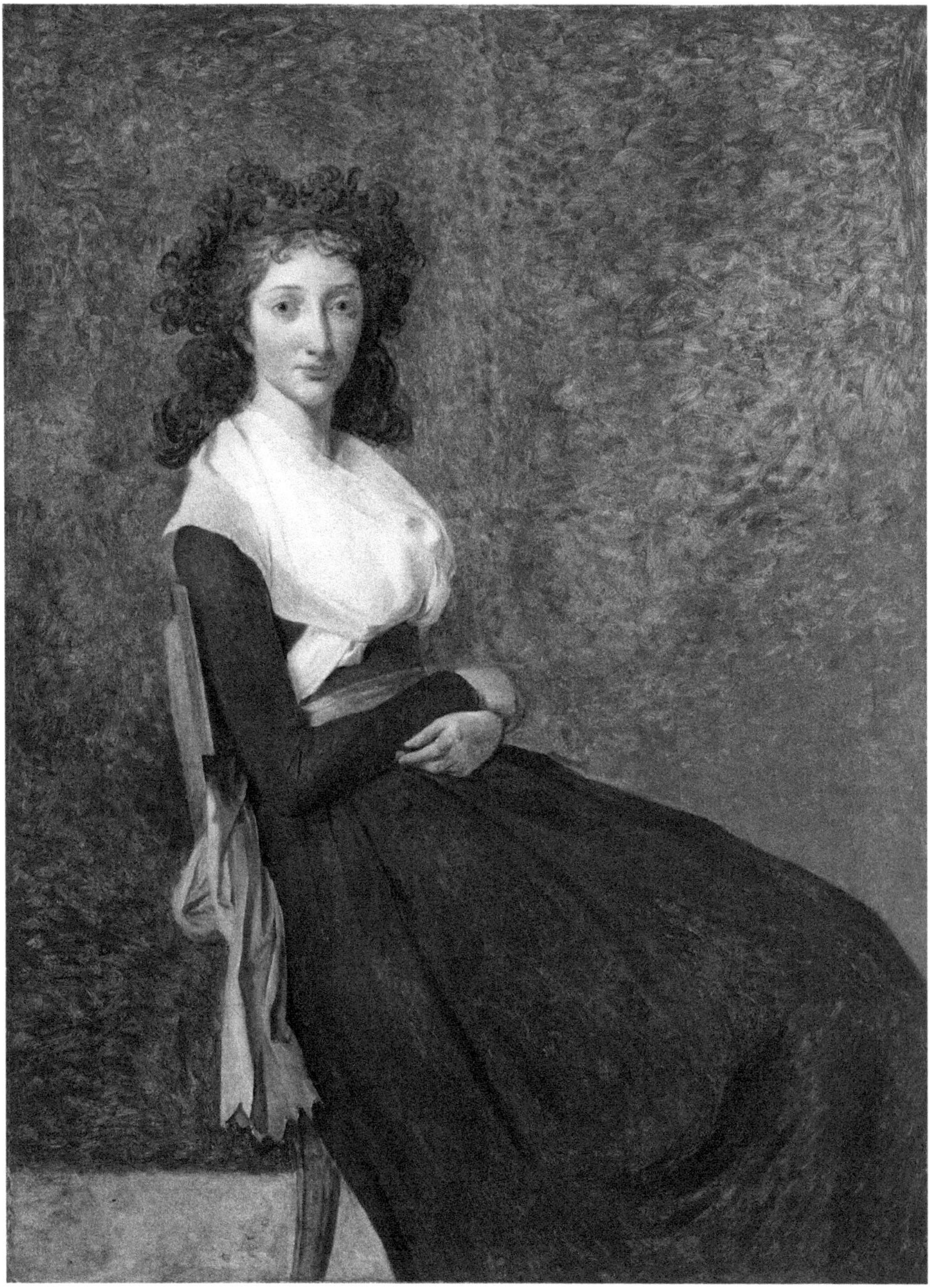

Jacques-Louis David, *Madame Trudaine*, ca 1791–92, oil on canvas, 130 x 98 cm. **4.2**

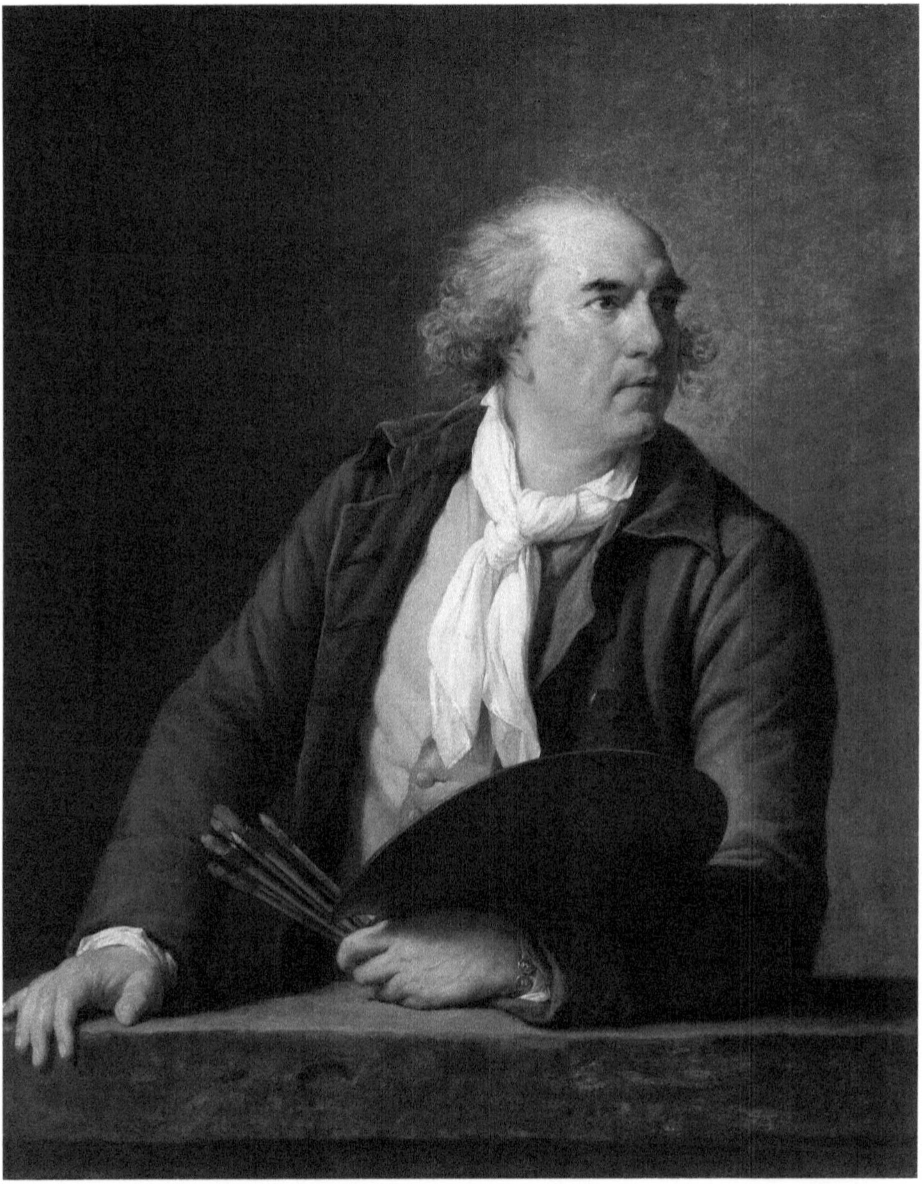

4.3 Elisabeth Vigée-Lebrun, *Hubert Robert*, 1788, oil on canvas, 105 x 84 cm.

in question is that they are, to a large extent, about the shared materiality of all things, rather than the visual illusion of distinct stuffs like skin, wooden furniture or muslin dresses.

Yet, the face still receives a special treatment in the portraits of Louise de Pastoret and Madame Trudaine. This area is painted in an equally dry manner, but the brushstrokes, applied with more density, are less apparent, setting the facial skin apart as of a slightly different materiality. Watelet had also singled out the head as a particular site of the artist's manual activity, as the site where the expression of the represented face and that of the artist's inspiration converge. However, this effect seems equally reduced in David's portrait of Madame Trudaine, as her expression is calm and rather non-descript. Worked evenly, with barely visible individual strokes, the painted skin is even and the reddish cheeks and lips seem generic indications of youth, health and aliveness, rather than signs of an animation resulting from the situation or a particular state of mind. Given the insistence on transparency and a language of truth (with which David's pre-revolutionary history paintings were associated) so prominent during the Enlightenment and even more during the Revolution,[82] it is remarkable that David refrained in the portrait from using the brushstrokes as expressive gestures and from that other form of physical expression, in which the represented body expresses their character or emotions. But skin was a tricky thing during the Revolution. While the quest for transparency might have favoured the kind of delicate skin Watelet described with regard to painting and Bichat for anatomy, a skin through which physiological and emotional processes shimmer, soft skin could be a dangerous sign of a privileged life protected from sun and physical labour.[83]

Among the portraits painted in the aftermath of the overthrow of the Jacobin government, resulting in the execution of Robespierre and other government members and the imprisonment of David, it is only his famous self-portrait in prison that works, in parts, with this painterly mode (Plate 8).[84] This self-portrait, on which Clark's article centres, also makes a point about the transformation of paint into 'stuffs and flesh' through the way the palette is represented. Showing it as a used wooden board, blotched with left-over paint, was highly unusual. Most (self) portraits of artists, such as the portrait of Noël Coypel by Florent de la Mare-Richart (Plate 1), or, to name a later example, Vigée-Lebrun's *Self-portrait with Straw Hat* (London, National Gallery), present the palette as a well-organised tool and symbol of their profession. Of course, we expect David to disrespect the rules of art institutions and artist's manuals, and his painting suggests that there is no room for such painterly etiquette in a self-portrait made in prison. But there is also a logic to it: the painting is finished and the paint is used up. It is about the completed painting, rather than potential new ones he would be offering to make. The palette is thus staged as the site from which the transformation of raw material into a representation originated. And the left-over colours are not accidentally chosen. They are flesh tones, mixed to paint the artist's own skin:[85] two shades of rose for painting the skin and giving the body relief, and a bit of vermilion to animate the cheeks but also the fringes of the coat. These spots of red and rose are literally the material residues of David's self-making, the matter of his restoration as a person and a painter.

With the portraits of Jacobus Blauw and that of David's sister and brother in law Émilie and Pierre Sériziat, all dating from 1795, the artist returned to more conventional modes of portrait painting (Figure 4.4 and 4.5; plate 9), and gave skin a different significance. These portraits are less concerned about the materiality of flesh and paint, than about skin as a translucent membrane that is rendered in a manner very much akin to Bichat's medical definitions of the organ. It is in these portraits that David re-established the kind of 'bodily legibility' and transparency that Amy Freund has associated with Revolutionary politics and portraiture.[86] Blauw is shown at his desk writing, in a pose familiar from many earlier eighteenth-century portraits, among them Van Loo's portrait of Diderot (Figure 3.10). But it lacks the sense of suddenness that this and other images of the period try to capture, as Blauw addresses viewers with an intense but still look. The figure is also more confined and compact, with the arms limited by the objects that are at hand. The handkerchief keeps Blauw's left arm in place, the hand holds on to the tobacco box, while the right wrist and writing hand lie neatly on the white paper and in line with its borders. If these objects indicate his position as an envoy, then he is rather more restrained by his situation than in command of it. This might also be caused by the ambiguous status of these things. The tobacco box and a handkerchief are both touching Blauw's skin, and the rose coloured cloth subtly echoes the more reddish parts of flesh tones. They are everyday objects connected to the body and involved in the physical exchanges of substances. While this might suggest an intimate relationship, it seems that these objects are not personal belongings at all, but studio props. They appear again, a good twenty years later, in a portrait of Emmanuel-Joseph Sieyès, painted in Brussels where painter and sitter were fellows in exile.[87] The objects, handed over from one portrait to the other and through time and space, thus link two former revolutionaries involved in the formation of the Dutch Republic.

Blauw was a Dutch patriot and committed republican, who officially became Ministre plénipotentiaire (a kind of ambassador) of the new Batavian Republic after the Treaty of The Hague signed on 16 May 1795. This treaty, negotiated by Jacobus Blauw and his compatriot Gaspard Meyer (whom David portrayed in the same year) on the Dutch side, and Emmanuel-Joseph Sieyès and Jean-Jacques Reubell on the French, was not favourable for the Netherlands: France, whose troops had supported the Dutch republicans, annexed large territories, while the rest of the Republic had the status of a protectorate.

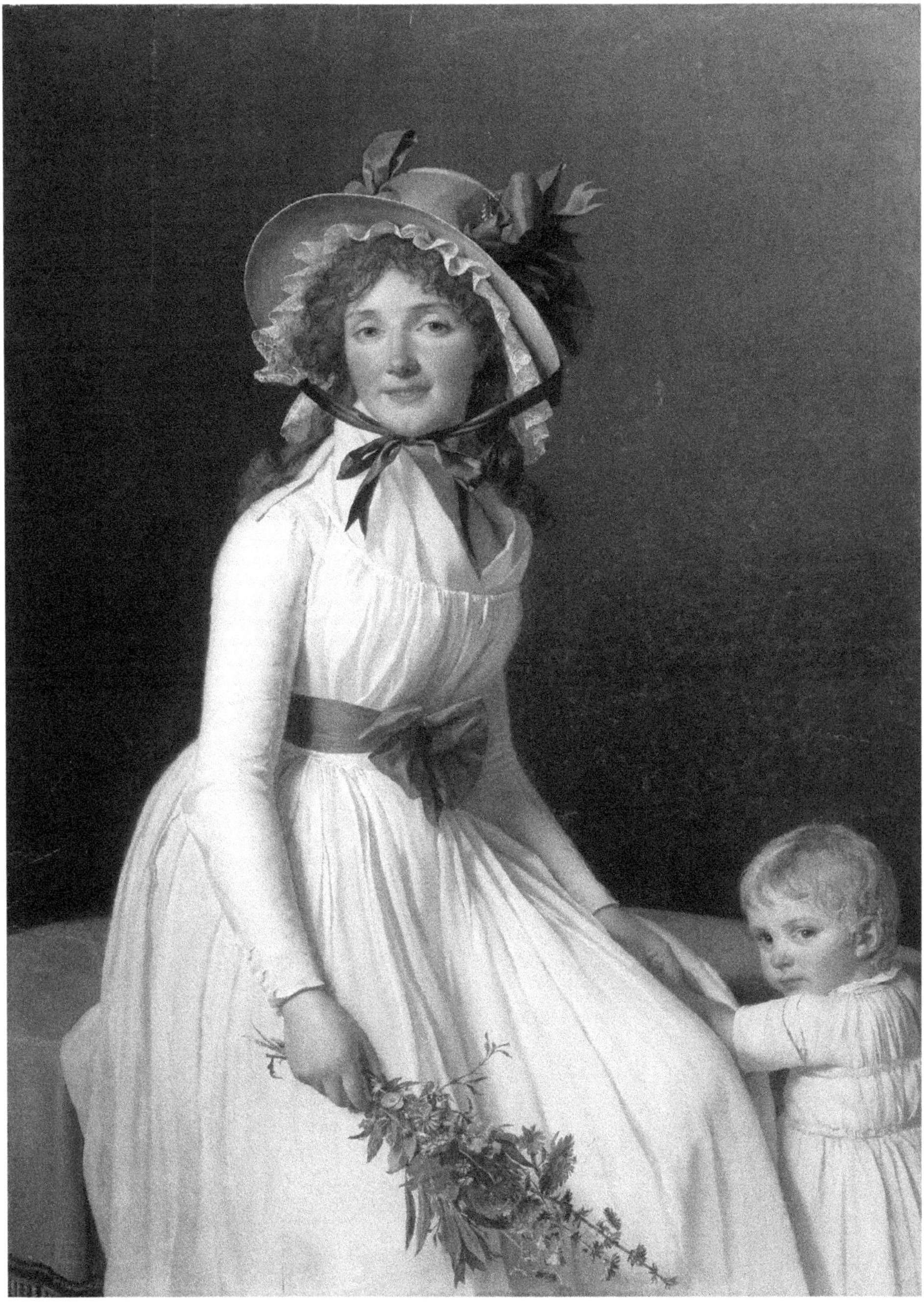

Jacques-Louis David, *Émilie Sériziat and her Son*, 1795, oil on canvas, 131 x 96 cm. **4.4**

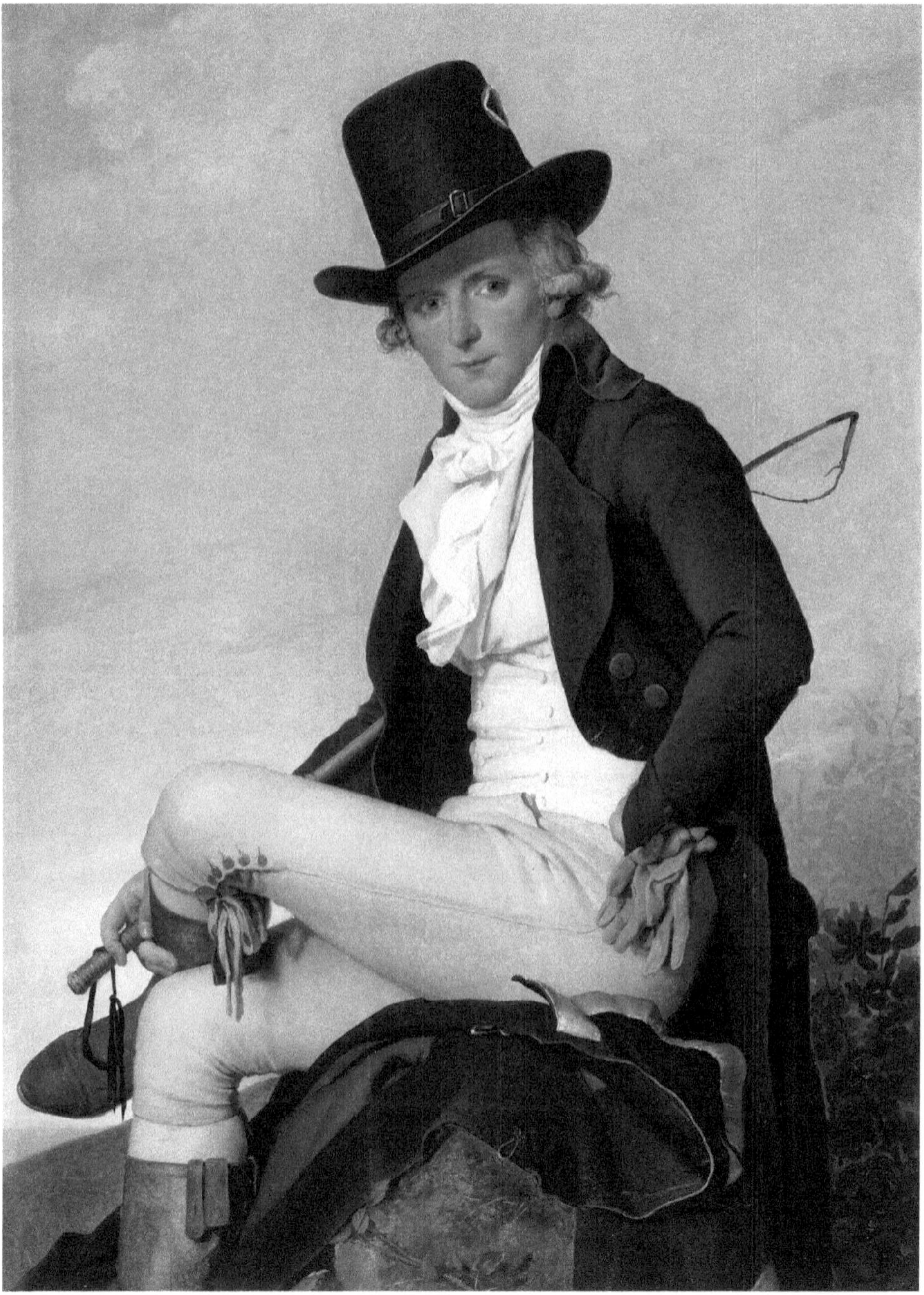

4.5 Jacques-Louis David, *Pierre Sériziat*, 1795, oil on canvas, 129 x 95 cm.

Both paintings were, in all likelihood, commissioned after Blauw and Meyer had been nominated Ministres plénipotentiaires – a position spelled out in the inscription on the sheet of paper on which Blauw is writing – and painted in autumn 1795, not long after David's release from his second stay in prison between the end of May and August of the same year. Judging from a letter written by Blauw to the artist on 29 November 1795 to acknowledge receipt of the portrait, the painting was finished by that date.[88] More importantly, this letter is a sign of the ties between the two men, as it goes beyond formulaic expressions of gratitude and respect for the artist whom Blauw calls 'Europe's first painter'.[89] The two men shared the commitment to the republican cause in France and the Netherlands respectively, and, at the very moment the portrait was made, probably also a frustration over the loss of more radical revolutionary ideals. The same Thermidor government that superseded Jacobin rule, with it ending David's immediate involvement in politics, made the Batavian Republic pay a very high price for France's support in their struggle for independence.[90] In his letter, Blauw explicitly referred to the role David played in the organisation of revolutionary festivals, while keeping silent about the artist's involvement in the Terror. As much as an allusion to their shared commitments and an evocation of the *fraternité* celebrated in these festivals, the note can also be read as an attempt to conceal the commercial character of the commissioning and exchange of a portrait, as Blauw wished to regard it as a token of male friendship rather than a purchase, declaring the sum paid humble in relation to the merits of the painting.[91] More than that, giving the old trope of the 'creation of life on canvas' a new twist, Blauw suggested that the painter not only animated but re-animated him on canvas, as if he had saved his life or given him a new post-revolutionary life.

The letter plays on the friendship between Blauw and his portraitist, and the painting itself suggests a certain intimacy. Unlike the larger, and more representative portrait of Blauw's fellow ambassador Gaspard Meyer who is shown sitting in a chair richly decorated with neoclassical ornament displaying self-confidence and a certain air of distance, the likeness of Blauw is more subdued, as the sitter addresses the viewer with an almost anxious, worried look, sharing in this respect aspects of David's *Self-Portrait in Prison*. At the same time, it is worked with a much more finished brush than the self-portrait subtly differentiating the texture of the fabrics and objects in view, from the velvety tablecloth and the dense fabric of the jacket, via the quilt and metallic sheen of the brass buttons and tobacco box to the powdered white hair. The painted surface is however not as uniform as it would later be in the portraits by David's student Ingres, as paint layers are employed in different densities from thinly painted areas indicating shadows to the highlights made of lead white applied in impasto.[92] The skin is painted as a fairly even surface, its ivory base is modelled with reddish nuances over the face and on the hands. The cohesive brushstrokes conceal the skin and make it at the same time susceptible to its environment. It is the skin as much as his facial expression that marks Blauw (who was reported by others to have been moody and prone to outbreaks of anger, much to the detriment of his diplomatic profession) as a man of sensibility with the pale complexion for which the art theoretical tracts of the time praised Dutch women. On the face and hands the colour is delicately nuanced, the skin tones ranging from ivory with touches of blue-grey here and there, to complex gradations of red and rose. This distribution of tones makes the skin seem transparent, a screen reflecting both organic life and psychological affect. On the side of the painter, these delicately rendered colours demonstrate the kind of observational sensibility that Watelet had described in his entry 'Chairs' when lauding those 'delicate and attentive eyes' able to discern the subtleties of flesh tones. He also highlighted the special talent needed to observe 'the imperceptible curves of the flesh and its transparency that makes the veins noticeable, spread on the half-tones ... slighly bluish nuances, which lead through soft gradations to the most radiant tones of the skin'.[93] In David's portrait, Blauw's body is indeed rendered legible and transparent through the manner in which skin is painted. The skin is turned into a contact zone where the susceptibility of the painter and that of the sitter meet. And it seems at its most radiant where David employed reddish-orange brushstrokes, at the underside of the hand, especially at the fingertips. These look like the glow of life itself, as if the very site of the re-animation Blauw talked about in his letter.

At the same time, the skin hints at the anatomical structure and materiality of the sitter's body. The reddish nuances along with the grey-blue shades give the face its relief and materiality, suggesting fleshiness at chin and cheeks, and a rather thin layer of skin stretched over the skull at the brow. On the hands, the ruddy tones indicate the knuckles and the bluish shadows not only contribute to the impression of volume, but also evoke the subcutaneous veins. The bodily surface thus refers to what is not directly visible, both the physical and psychic interior, while also reacting to its environment. The skin is also represented as a receptive organ, as the sitter is adjusted to his surroundings. Even the name (the Dutch word for blue) matches the colour of the coat, which again is reflected in the eyes of a slightly lighter blue while the white and rose chequered handkerchief echoes the flesh tones. The skin thus establishes a relation between the body and its exterior, the blue also reflecting the surrounding environment as it absorbs the colour of the vest. Using a conventional tactic in portrait painting – small highlights on the nose – the artist evokes the light apparently coming from outside the picture frame. As Norman Bryson has observed more generally, David's sitters tend to be situated within a socially and politically defined environment.[94] It is a relationship established not only via dress or accessories, but also via the physicality of the skin.

In another pair of portraits painted in 1795 – that of Émilie Sériziat née Pécoul, the sister of David's wife, and her husband Pierre – David employed equally subtle means to fit the sitters into their painted and lived environment. The portraits were done during the time David spent on the politically safe grounds of the country residence of his in-laws in Saint-Ouen near Tournon, to recover from his stay in prison. It is likely that the portrait of his sister-in-law was done during his one-month release from prison in May 1795 while her husband was painted after his second imprisonment, in all likelihood immediately before Jacobus Blauw sat for him and just in time to be displayed with its pendant in the Salon of autumn 1795.[95] Taking the advice of his wife, David re-entered the circle of professional painters with portraits of family members, thus publicly expressing gratitude for their support and manifesting the renewal of family ties. David and his wife had divorced during the Revolution due to political differences, but re-married for good after she stood by him during his imprisonment. Émilie Sériziat is shown indoors, wearing a simple but exquisitely painted white dress, in an informal pose with flowers in hand, as if just coming from outside and resting for a moment on a table while acknowledging her counterpart. David used a visual trope popular in eighteenth-century portraiture here: a simulation of a spontaneous encounter, evoking the moment of an initial look at a person often seen, for example, in portraits by Maurice Quentin de la Tour or Vigée-Lebrun. The latter also talked about the strategies the portraitist should use to preserve the freshness and interest of the model in order to avoid the expression of boredom caused by lengthy sitting. She recommended complimenting women on their beauty and their *teint frais*, as if simply mentioning it could maintain a fresh complexion.[96] David's portrait however meets this only half way. Mme Sériziat seems not quite open-minded as she ambivalently acknowledges her counterpart outside the picture frame with a restraint and timid smile. This counterpart is, of course, anybody looking at the painting, but it is initially the artist himself, who paints this look directed on to him as a potential intruder, someone accepted in with doubt. This links the portrait of his sister-in-law to the questioning mode of the self-portrait in prison.

Pierre Sériziat is granted a much more secure pose: outside, in riding outfit, firmly sitting on a rock, indicating in a very English manner the possession of the lands in which he is situated.[97] Despite this pronounced staging of gender difference via the contrast of inside/outside and the allocation of child rearing, another tradition distinguishing male and female characters with the means of paint is barely exploited: there is hardly any difference in their complexions. Both portraits emphasise the diaphanous quality and all three figures display equally reddish cheeks. Here (as in other portraits) David carefully indicated that this colour results from physiological processes and not from the external application of rouge, as the red seems to push through from inside showing on various regions of face and hands. It is, however, an indication not so much of the sensibilities and moral feelings associated with blushing,[98] as of the healthiness of well-to-do life, and in this particular case the benefits of the open air, the portrait again linking the body to its environment via skin.

David thus rendered skin in a manner that evokes the understanding of the organ as a *limite sensitive* regulating the relationship between body and environment. Both David and Bichat were concerned with the demarcation of the body and, especially during the troubled moment of Thermidor, with the status of the self. At the same time, through the subtle use of colour and layering of paint, the vital qualities and sensibility of the human's outermost organ are mimicked. Rather than a tissue re-enacted with the brushwork's texture – as suggested in mid-eighteenth-century art theory and probed in some of Fragonard's portraits – skin is turned into a light screen that is semi-transparent towards a physical and psychological interior.

Notes

1 Michel Foucault, 'Technologies of the self', in Paul Rabinow (ed.), *Michel Foucault. Ethics, Subjectivity and Truth: Essential Works of Foucault 1954–1984*, vol. 1 (London: Tavistock, 1988), pp. 223–51.

2 Jan Goldstein, *The Post-Revolutionary Self: Politics and Psyche in France, 1750–1850* (Cambridge/Mass.; London: Harvard University Press, 2005), p. 4; George Vigarello, *Le sentiment de soi: histoire de la perception du corps* (Paris: Éditions du Seuil, 2014), p. 80: 'Il [le mot soi] ouvre pourtant une manière toute à fait nouvelle de parler de l'individu'.

3 *Encyclopédie méthodique. Beaux-arts*, ed. Claude-Henri Watelet and Pierre-Charles Lévesque, 2 vols (Paris: Panckoucke, 1788–91); the work is mostly referred to as the *Dictionnaire des beaux-arts*; I am using the first edition which was part of the multivolume *Encyclopédie méthodique*, an enterprise by the publisher Panckoucke, which unlike d'Alembert and Diderot's *Encyclopédie* with its universal approach, divided knowledge into disciplines; see Tom Holert, *Künstlerwissen: Studien zur Semantik künstlerischer Kompetenz im Frankreich des 18. und frühen 19. Jahrhunderts* (München: Fink, 1998), pp. 162–75.

4 Étienne Jollet, 'Les rapports entre les sciences et les beaux-arts dans les écrits de C.-H. Watelet', *Revue du dix-huitième siècle*, 31 (1999), 217–31; Martial Guédron, *De chair et de marbre: imiter et exprimer le nu en France (1745–1815)* (Paris: Éditions Champion, 2003), pp. 87–9, 257.

5 Watelet is a good example for what Lilti has described as the mixture of wealthy *gens du monde* and *hommes de lettres* in the Parisian salons of the second half of the eighteenth century, focussing in particular on that of Madame Geoffrin. See Antoine Lilti, 'Sociabilité et mondanité: les hommes de lettres dans les salons parisiens au XVIIIe siècle', *French Historical Studies*, 28 (2005), 415–45.

6 George Levitine, *The Sculpture of Falconet*, with a translation from the French of Falconet's *Réflexions sur la sculpture* by Eda Mezer Levitine (Greenwich/Conn.: New York Graphic Society, 1972), p. 18

7 On the impact of European and in particular German art theory on Lévesque's entries Christian Michel, 'Deutsche Ästhetik und französische Kunsttheorie am Ende des Ancien Régime: die "Encyclopédie méthodique. Beaux-Arts"', in Uwe Fleckner et al. (eds), *Jenseits der Grenzen: französische und deutsche Kunst vom Ancien Régime bis zur Gegenwart* (Köln: DuMont, 2000), pp. 329–44.
8 Holert, *Künstlerwissen*, pp. 167, 175; see generally on the significance of Winckelmann's *History of Ancient Art* and on his notion of 'style' Alex Potts, *Flesh and the Ideal: Winckelmann and the Origins of Art History* (New Haven; London: Yale University Press, 1994). On Winckelmann's reception in the *Dictionnaire*, Philippe Bordes and Régis Michel, *Aux Armes et aux Arts! Les arts et la Revolution 1789–1799* (Paris: A. Biro, 1988), p. 169; and more generally in France Élisabeth Décultot, *Johann Joachim Winckelmann: enquète sur la genèse de l'histoire de l'art* (Paris: Presses Universitaires de Frances, 2000), pp. 76–8, and Édouard Pommier, 'Winckelmann et la vision de l'Antiquité classique dans la France des Lumières et de la Révolution', *Revue de l'art*, 83 (1989), 9–20.
9 *Encyclopédie méthodique. Beaux-arts*, vol. 1, p. 270, entry 'Estompe'.
10 Ibid., vol. 2, p. 804, entry 'Vessie'.
11 Ibid., vol. 1, entry 'Chairs', p. 100. See also the beginning of the entry 'Carnation', p. 97.
12 More generally on this conflict Holert, *Künstlerwissen*, pp. 165–6.
13 *Encyclopédie méthodique. Beaux-arts*, vol. 1, entry 'Carnation', p. 97.
14 Aubin-Louis Millin, *Dictionnaire des beaux-arts* (Paris: chez Descray, 1806).
15 This had already been the case in William Hogarth, *The Analysis of Beauty* (London: J. Reeves, 1753).
16 See on 'whiteness' in the eighteenth century, with a particular focus on British art, Angela Rosenthal, 'Visceral culture: blushing and the legibility of whiteness in eighteenth-century British portraiture', *Art History*, 27 (2004), 563–92.
17 *Encyclopédie méthodique. Beaux-arts*, vol. 1, entry 'Chairs', p. 100.
18 On the eighteenth-century artistic concern with the ways different surfaces reflect light see Michael Baxandall, *Shadows and Enlightenment* (New Haven; London: Yale University Press, 1995).
19 *Encyclopédie méthodique. Beaux-arts*, vol. 1, entry 'Chairs', pp. 100–1.
20 Ibid., entry 'Carnation', 'Chairs', pp. 97, 101.
21 Ibid., entry 'Couleur', p. 162.
22 Ibid., p. 163.
23 Ibid., p. 161.
24 Ibid., p. 164.
25 Ibid., vol. 2, entry 'Touche', p. 407.
26 Ibid., vol. 1, entry 'Peau', p. 630.
27 See extensively on this matter Hans Körner, '"Die Epidermis der Statue": Oberflächen der Skulptur vom späten 17. bis zum frühen 19. Jahrhundert', in Daniela Bohde and Mechthild Fend (eds), *Weder Haut noch Fleisch: das Inkarnat in der Kunstgeschichte* (Berlin: Gebr. Mann, 2007), pp. 105–32.
28 *Encyclopédie méthodique. Beaux-arts*, vol. 1, entry 'Peau', p. 629.
29 Ibid., entry 'Détail', p. 192.
30 See the footnote by the editor to the *Encyclopédie méthodique. Beaux-arts*, vol. 2, p. 372. Only an abbreviated version of Falconet's article was published in Diderot

and d'Alembert's *Encyclopédie ou dictionnaire raisonné des sciences, des arts et des metiers*: vol. 14, 1760 (17 vols, 1751–65, and 11 vols plates, 1762–72 (accessed via University of Chicago: ARTFL Encyclopédie Projet (winter 2008 edn), ed. Robert Morrissey, http://encyclopedie.uchicago.edu/)).

31 For the translation of Falconet's 'Reflections on Sculpture', see Levitine, *Falconet*, p. 64–75, here p. 70. *Encyclopédie méthodique. Beaux-arts*, vol. 2, entry 'Sculpture', p. 377.

32 See Körner, '"Die Epidermis der Statue"'; Klaus Herding, *Pierre Puget: das bildnerische Werk* (Berlin: Gebr. Mann, 1970), p. 20.

33 Levitine, *Falconet*, p. 70; *Encyclopédie méthodique. Beaux-arts*, vol. 2; entry 'Sculpture', p. 377. On the Milo see Klaus Herding, 'Schwindender Heroismus – gesteigerte Sinnlichkeit: Pugets *Milon von Kroton* als Ausdruck einer Krise der Männlichkeit im absolutistischen Zeitalter', in Mechthild Fend and Marianne Koos (eds), *Männlichkeit im Blick: Visuelle Inszenierungen in der Kunst seit der Frühen Neuzeit* (Köln; Weimar; Wien: Böhlau, 2004), pp. 137–59; and *Pierre Puget*, pp. 95–103.

34 Johann Joachim Winckelmann, *Reflections on the Paintings and Sculptures of the Greeks*, trans. Henry Fuseli (London: the translator, 1765), pp. 15–16; and 'Gedankenüber die Nachahmung der GriechischenWerke in der Mahlerey und Bildhauerkunst' [1755], in *Kleine Schriften, Vorreden, Entwürfe* (Berlin: de Gruyter, 1968), p. 36.

35 Potts, *Flesh and the Ideal*; Mechthild Fend, *Grenzen der Männlichkeit: der Androgyn in der französischen Kunst und Kunsttheorie zwischen Aufklärung und Restauration* (Berlin: Reimer, 2003), in particular pp. 27–43. For the same argument in the *Encyclopédie méthodique. Beaux-arts* see vol. 2, entry 'Sculpture', p. 328.

36 *Encyclopédie méthodique.Beaux-arts*, vol. 2, entry 'Sculpture', p. 328.

37 Irmela Marei Krüger-Fürhoff, *Der versehrte Körper: Revisionen des klassizistischen Schönheitsideals* (Göttingen: Wallstein, 2001), pp. 32–4.

38 Winckelmann, *Reflections*, pp. 9–10; and 'Nachahmung', p. 33; see further on this passage Whitney Davis, 'Winckelmann divided: mourning the death of art history', *Journal of Homosexuality*, 27 (1994), 141–59.

39 Krüger-Fürhoff, *Der versehrte Körper*, p. 9.

40 Norbert Elias, *The Civilizing Process: The History of Manners* [1939] (Oxford: Blackwell, 1978); Michael Bakhtin, *Rabelais and His World*, trans. Helene Iswolsky (Cambridge/Mass.: MIT Press, 1968); and reading Bakhtin in her cultural history of skin Claudia Benthien, *Skin: On the Cultural Border Between Self and the World* [1999], trans. Thomas Dunlap (New York; Chichester: Columbia University Press, 2002), pp. 38–9.

41 Dorinda Outram,*The Body and the French Revolution: Sex, Class and Political Culture* (New Haven: Yale University Press, 1989), in particular pp. 11–13; Fend, *Grenzen der Männlichkeit*, p. 9.

42 On hygiene see Philipp Sarasin, *Reizbare Maschinen: eine Geschichte des Körpers 1765–1914* (Frankfurt a. M.: Suhrkamp, 2001); and more particularly for France George Vigarello, *Concepts of Cleanliness: Changing Attitudes in France since the Middle Ages* [1987], trans. Jean Birell (Cambridge: Cambridge University Press, 1988).

43 Martial Guédron, *L'art de la grimace: cinq siècles d'excès de visage* (Paris: Hazan, 2011).

44 Fend, *Grenzen der Männlichkeit*, pp. 34–43.

45 Letter to the Comité d'instruction publique, 5 May 1795. Quoted from Philippe Comar in Philippe Comar (ed.), *Figures du corps: une leçon d'anatomie à l'École des beaux-arts* (Paris: Beaux-arts de Paris, 2008), p. 28. See on the anatomy theatre at the Louvre also Margaret A. Oppenheimer, '"The charming spectacle of a cadaver": anatomical and life study by women artists in Paris, 1775–1815', *Nineteenth-Century Art Worldwide*, 6 (2007), www.19thc-artworldwide.org/spring07/46-spring07/spring07article/142-qthe-charming-spectacle-of-a-cadaverq-anqthe-charming-spectacle-of-a-cadaverq-anatomical-and-life-study-by-women-artists-in-paris-17751815atomical-and-life-study-by-women-artists-in-paris-17751815.

46 Jean-Joseph Sue (the younger): *Élémens d'anatomie, à l'usage des peintres, des sculpteurs et des amateurs* (Paris: Méquignon, l'ainé 1788), p. 8.

47 Pierre-Jean-Georges Cabanis, *Rapports du physique et du moral de l'homme*, 2 vols (Paris: Crapart, Caille et Ravier, 1802), vol. 1, p. 12; Sarasin, *Reizbare Maschinen*, p. 35.

48 On the persistence of the theory of humours and temperaments in eighteenth- and early nineteenth-century France Tony Halliday, *The Temperamental Nude: Class, Medicine and Representation in Eighteenth-century France* (Oxford: Voltaire Foundation, 2010); and Sarasin, *Reizbare Maschinen*, pp. 34–42.

49 See Elizabeth Haigh, *Xavier Bichat and the Medical Theory of the Eighteenth Century* (London: Wellcome Institute for the History of Medicine, 1984).

50 Ibid., p. 4.

51 Daniel Arasse, *The Guillotine and the Terror* [1987] (London: Lane 1989), here in particular pp. 8–9.

52 Haigh, *Bichat*, p. 11; she is referring to Bichat in 1799.

53 Ibid., p. 13.

54 Xavier Bichat, *Physiological Researches upon Life and Death*, trans. Tobias Watkins (Philadelphia: Smith and Maxwell, 1809), p. 1; see also Haigh, *Bichat*, p. 10.

55 Caroline Hannaway and Ann La Berge (eds), *Constructing Paris Medicine* (Amsterdam; Atlanta: Rodopi, 1998), pp. 32–3, stress how much Foucault identified with Bichat.

56 According to Andrew Cunningham, *The Anatomist Anatomis'd: An Experimental Discipline in Enlightenment Europe* (Farnham; Burlington/Vt.: Ashgate, 2010), pp. 162–3, the expression was used for the first time in Jean-Joseph Sue (the younger), *Recherches physiologiques, et expériences sur la vitalité* (Paris: chez l'auteur, An VI [1797]).

57 Arasse, *Guillotine*, p. 37; Ludmilla Jordanova, *Nature Displayed: Gender, Science and Medicine, 1760–1820* (London; New York: Longman, 1999), p. 120.

58 Grégoire Chamayou, 'La querelle des têtes tranchées: les médecins, la guillotine et l'anatomie de la conscience au lendemain de la Terreur', *Revue d'histoire des sciences*, 61 (2008), 333–65 (pp. 339–41).

59 Sue, *Recherches physiologiques*, p. 57.

60 Jordanova, *Nature Displayed*, p. 119.

61 Arasse, *The Guillotine*, p. 134.

62 Michel Foucault, *The Birth of the Clinic: An Archaeology of Medical Perception* [1963], trans. A. M. Sheridan Smith (London: Tavistock, 1973), p. 127.

63 Ibid. I am not using the notion of the 'surface gaze' or of the 'medial gaze' that has, following Sheridan Smith's 1973 translation, dominated the reception of Foucault's *Naissance de la clinique* in anglophone countries, and has to my mind interpreted the clinician's eye too one-dimensionally as a cold and dominating gaze, while the French word 'regard' can mean look, attention and concern. See on this issue also Hannaway and La Berge's introduction to their *Paris Medicine*, p. 34.

64 Xavier Bichat, *A Treatise on the Membranes in General, and on Different Membranes in Particular*, trans. John G. Coffin (Boston: Cummings and Hilliard; Cambridge/Mass.: Hilliard & Metcalf, 1813), p. 35; *Traité des membranes en général et de diverses membranes en particulier* (Paris: Richard, Caillé et Ravier, 1799), p. 22. See also Laura Otis, *Membranes: Metaphors of Invasion in Nineteenth-Century Literature, Science, and Politics* (Baltimore; London: Johns Hopkins University Press, 1999), a study that mainly considers the later nineteenth century, but briefly discusses Bichat, pp. 11–13.

65 Xavier Bichat, *General Anatomy, applied to Physiology and the Practice of Medicine*, trans. Constant Coffyn. Revised and corrected by George Calvert. 2 vols (London: Printed for the Translator, 1824), vol. 1, p. 2; *Anatomie générale, appliquée à la physiologie et à la médecine*, 4 vols (Paris: Brosson, Gabon et Cie, 1801), part 1, vol. 1, p. 12.

66 Haigh, *Bichat*, p. 118.

67 John Forrester, 'The homoeomerous parts and their replacement by Bichat's Tissues', *Medical History*, 38 (1994), 444–58 (p. 454).

68 The hostility towards medical images is most explicitly expressed in Xavier Bichat, *Traité d'anatomie descriptive*. New edn, revised and corrected, vol. 1 (Paris: Gabon, 1829), pp. xxiii–xxiv.

69 See more extensively on this problem Goldstein, *The Post-Revolutionary Self*.

70 For the potential social and political dimension of Bichat's notion of organisation see still John Pickstone's provocative article, 'Bureaucracy, liberalism and the body in post-revolutionary France: Bichat's physiology and the Paris School of Medicine', *History of Science*, 19 (1981), 115–42.

71 Bichat, *General Anatomy*, vol. 2, p. 744; *Anatomie générale*, part 2, vol. 4, p. 640.

72 Bichat, *General Anatomy*, vol. 2, p. 827; *Anatomie générale*, part 2, vol. 4, p. 711.

73 Bichat, *General Anatomy*, vol. 2, p. 775; *Anatomie générale*, part 2, vol. 4, p. 667.

74 Bichat, *General Anatomy*, vol. 2, p. 790, and generally on 'The Action of Water', pp. 790–6; *Anatomie générale*, part 2, vol. 4, pp. 680–5.

75 See Sarasin *Reizbare Maschinen* and, for a more Lacanian reading of the practices of washing, his article 'Vom Realen Reden? Fragmente einer Körpergeschichte der Moderne', *RISS. Zeitschrift für Psychoanalyse*, 14:2 (1999), 29–62, in particular pp. 133–4.

76 Philipp Sarasin, 'The body as medium: nineteenth-century European hygiene discourse', *Grey Room*, 29 (2007), 48–65.

77 Bichat, *Anatomie générale*, part 2, vol. 4, p. 645; *General Anatomy*, vol. 2, pp. 748–9.

78 Bichat, *General Anatomy*, vol. 2, p. 745; *Anatomie générale*, part 2, vol. 4, p. 641.

79 Richard Taws, *The Politics of the Provisional: Art and Ephemera in Revolutionary France* (University Park/Penn.: Pennsylvania State University Press, 2013), p. 4. The oft-debated question whether these portraits are finished the way they are or left in

the stage of an ébauche, a painted sketch, is not relevant for my argument. For an opinionated view of their 'wholeness' see Timothy J. Clark, '"Gross David with the swoln cheek": An essay on self-portraiture', in Michael S. Roth (ed.), *Rediscovering History: Culture, Politics, and the Psyche* (Stanford Cal.: Stanford University Press, 1994), pp. 243–307, 483–93 (p. 269). Both portraits were never claimed by their commissioners due to the circumstances of the French Revolution, and David kept them in his studio until his death. See Antoine Schnapper and Arlette Sérullaz, *Jacques-Louis David: 1748–1825*, exh. cat., Musée du Louvre (Paris: Réunion des musées nationaux, 1989), cat. no. 116 and 117, p. 278 and p. 280.

80 *Encyclopédie méthodique. Beaux-arts*, vol. 2, p. 409; see also Mary D. Sheriff, *Fragonard: Art and Eroticism* (Chicago; London: University of Chicago Press, 1990), p. 147, and chapter 3 of this book.

81 Clark, 'Gross David', p. 253.

82 Thomas E. Crow, *Painters and Public Life in Eighteenth-Century Paris* (New Haven; London: Yale University Press, 1985), pp. 2, 27.

83 On masking and transparency during the French Revolution see James H. Johnson, 'Versailles, meet Les Halles: masks, carnival, and the French Revolution', *Representations*, 73 (winter 2001), 89–116.

84 Clark, 'Gross David' and Ewa Lajer-Burcharth, *Necklines: The Art of Jacques-Louis David after the Terror* (New Haven; London: Yale University Press, 1999).

85 Ewa Lajer-Burcharth has made a similar observation in *Necklines*, p. 39.

86 Amy Freund, *Portraiture and Politics in Revolutionary France* (University Park/Penn.: Pennsylvania State University Press, 2014), pp. 16–23.

87 Ewa Lajer-Burcharth, 'The self in exile: David's *Portrait of Emmanuel-Joseph Sieyès*', in Mark Ledbury (ed.), *David after David: Essays on the Later Work* (Williamstown/Mass.: Sterling and Francine Clark Institute and New Haven; London: Yale University Press, 2007), pp. 232–51.

88 John Leighton, *Jacques-Louis David: Portrait of Jacobus Blauw* (London: National Gallery Publications, 1987); and Michael Wilson, 'A new acquisition for the National Gallery: David's Portrait of Jacobus Blauw', *Burlington Magazine*, 126 (1984), 694–8; and Schnapper and Sérullaz, *David*, cat. no. 143, p. 318.

89 See for the full letter Leighton, *Portrait of Blauw*, p. 694, and Daniel Wildenstein, *Documents complémentaire au catalogue de l'œuvre de Louis David* (Paris: Fondation Wildenstein, 1973), p. 135.

90 Leighton, *Portrait of Blauw*; for the history of the Batavian Republic see Jonathan Israel, *The Dutch Republic: Its Rise, Greatness and Fall, 1477–1806* (Oxford: Clarendon Press, 1995).

91 This thought was inspired by Sarah Monks's talk 'Slippery blisses: same-sex desire in Thomas Lawrence's male portraiture', given on 3 November 2011 at the UCL History of Art research seminar.

92 As the infra-red photographs made by the National Gallery suggest, David used a fair amount of lead white in various areas of the painting: besides the skin, also the powder on the jacket, the white scarf around the neck (where impasto is employed) and the highlights on the metal objects. Leighton, *Portrait of Blauw*, p. 22, and oral communication by Morvenna Blewett, 3 October 2011.

93 *Encyclopédie méthodique. Beaux-arts*, vol. 1, entry 'Chairs', pp. 100–1.

94 Norman Bryson, *Tradition and Desire: From David to Delacroix* (Cambridge: Cambridge University Press, 1984), especially p. 163.
95 Lajer-Burcharth, *Necklines*, pp. 66–7; see also Schnapper and Sérullaz, *David*, pp. 312–13.
96 ElisabethVigée-Lebrun, *Souvenirs de Madame Louise-Elisabeth Vigée-Lebrun*, 3 vols (Paris: Librairie de H. Fournier, 1835–37), vol. 3, p. 357.
97 On the pendant landscape see Freund, *Portraiture and Politics*, pp. 181–2.
98 As elaborated by Rosenthal, 'Visceral culture'.

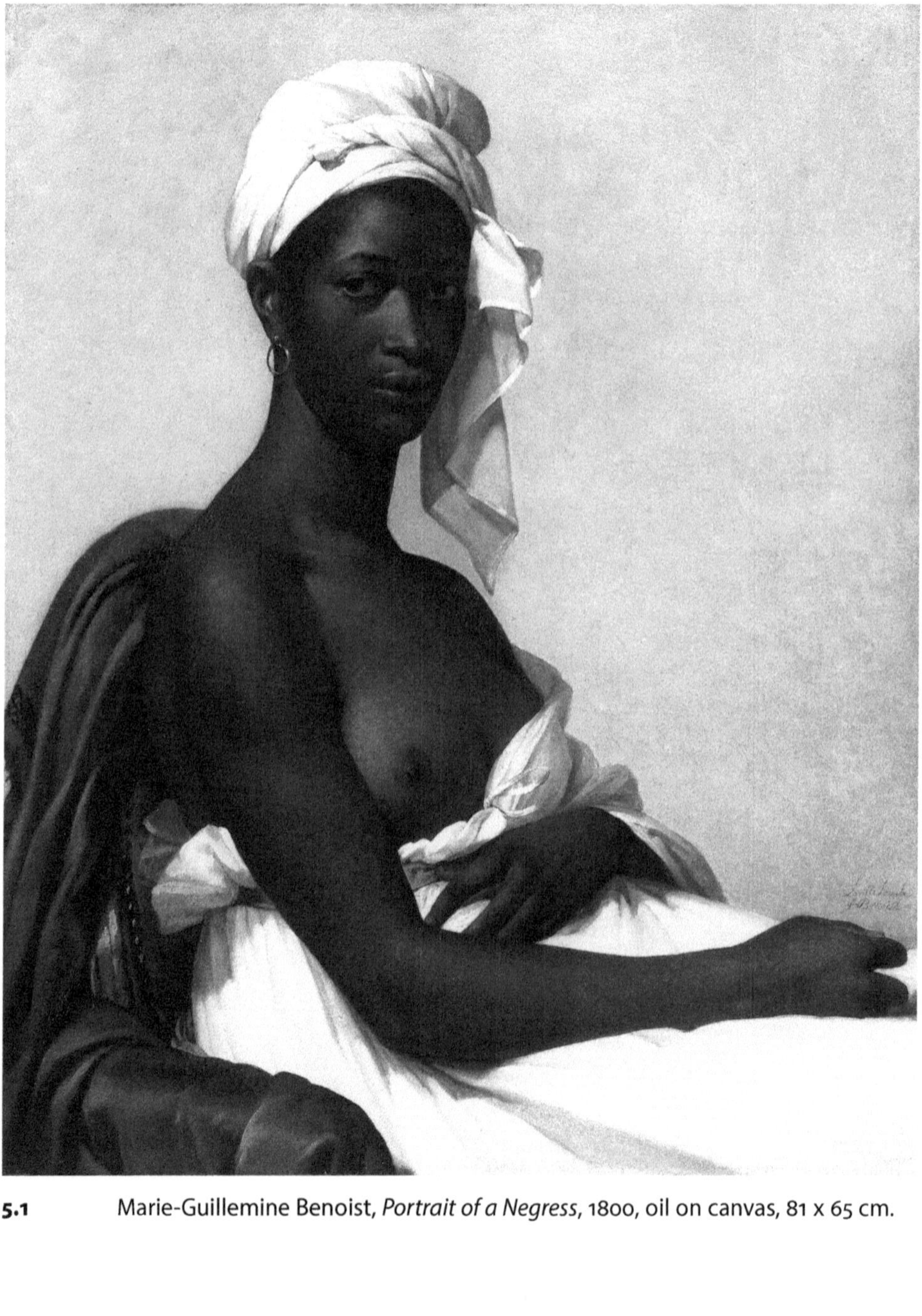

5.1 Marie-Guillemine Benoist, *Portrait of a Negress*, 1800, oil on canvas, 81 x 65 cm.

Skin colour 5

The culture of neoclassicism centred around the ideal of a body in close borderlines. Based to a large extent on an appreciation of ancient sculpture and a fantasy of actual Greek bodies, it envisaged a body well shaped according to the contemporary ideals of femininity and masculinity, soft and rounded on the one side, athletic with moderate relief of muscles on the other, but in any case contained. In the eyes of the period, the ideal ancient sculpture was made of white marble even though there was an awareness that the material had, at least initially, often been bronze, and sculptures made of polychrome stone were known. The whiteness of the marble was frequently confounded with the imaginary whiteness of their models. Resulting assumptions about the supremacy of whiteness became interlinked with the emerging discipline of racial anthropology, which was in many respects an aesthetic endeavour as it was largely based on the visual perception of the markers of difference among humans.

As shown in my previous discussions, the art literature of the period declared the white skin of northern European woman to be a universal beauty ideal more explicitly than ever before. Within this aesthetic framework some portraits stood out. Displayed at the Salons of 1798 and 1800, in the midst of mythological paintings, landscapes and other portraits, the works by two students of David must have been perceived as singular: Anne-Louis Girodet's *Jean-Baptiste Belley* and Marie-Guillemine Benoist's *Portrait of a Negress* (Plates 10 and 11, figure 5.1). The company of the other paintings must inevitably have raised the visibility of the works' skin colour. The portraits themselves contribute to highlighting skin colour by employing strong contrasts of black and white: Benoist shows her model in a white gown and headdress and Girodet contrasts the colour of Belley's face and hands not only with a white scarf and cuffs but also with a bust of the then recently deceased abolitionist philosopher Abbé Raynal made in white marble. Skin colour becomes visible through contrast and discrimination, and is as much an issue of artistic media and materials (in this case marble versus paint). Skin colour is thus introduced not simply as a faithfully imitated physical feature but as a representational problem and as a matter of perception.

Artists had of course painted, drawn and sculpted people of dark skin before, but – as I argue in what follows – what they saw and visualised when engaging with this aspect of human appearance was not always the same. Skin colour is not simply a somatic phenomenon the existence of which can be taken for granted. This chapter will engage with the seventeenth- and eighteenth-century scholarly debates and anatomical enquiries into the location and materiality of the colour of humans, and examine the links between the medical and artistic explorations of colour. It will argue that the increasing visibility of skin and its colour resulting from these enquiries gained significance in conjunction with the developing discourse of racial anthropology and within the aesthetics of neoclassicism with its implicit ideals of whiteness. Returning to Girodet's and Benoist's painting in the final section, it raises the question of what it meant to paint skin colour – in painterly, aesthetic and political terms – in the wake of the French Revolution.

Complexions

Skin colour or *couleur de peau* as a compound word only gradually emerged during the eighteenth century. Nowadays mostly associated with rather abstract distinctions of 'white' and 'black' for people with a multitude of appearances and ethnic affiliations, it has become much more a political term than an account of a physical feature. But even as such the colour of a person was not always visible or understood in the same way. Historian Valentin Groebner has argued that 'skin colour' has indeed a history, elaborating that skin colour only gradually became an attribute of the body that was associated with collectives and people from specific geographic locations.[1] In medieval and early modern Europe, the colour of a human was mostly referred to as 'complexion', a term still used in the English and French languages (in particular in the realm of cosmetics) to designate a combination of sanitary condition, texture and tint of the skin. The *complexio* played an important role in medieval perceptions of a person and their temperament, but not so much as skin than as *body* colour which was itself considered as produced by a mixture of bodily fluids.[2] Its understanding was closely connected with the writings associated with the ancient physicians Hippocrates and Galen which had, as is well known, a strong impact on European medicine from the late Middle Ages onwards and remained influential throughout the eighteenth and nineteenth centuries.[3] Humorism considered well-proportioned bodily liquids as the basis of a healthy condition in conjunction with a balanced temperament; and a person's outer appearance – including the degree of moisture, texture and tone of the skin – was indicative of this general state of health and mood. The complexion could change depending on external influences like climate or nutrition, and changing conditions such as age or health. Even though people were roughly categorised in four temperamental groups (the sanguine with a reddish skin tone, the phlegmatic whose complexion turns white from the slime, the choleric who is tinted from the yellow bile and the dark melancholic whose dominant humour is the black bile), complexion is a relational term and not an essentialist category, and each individual was thought to have their own specific, and at the same time changeable, complexion. A harmonious mixture of colours – rather than white – was considered as the ideal tint of flesh and skin.

How this ideal colour was described depended on the individual authors and often on their country of origin; Italian and French treatises, for example, tended to be quite negative about the white complexion and excess of phlegm attributed to the people of the North, which were associated with the cold, moist conditions of their bodies and the climate they were exposed to. In any case, it would have seemed absurd at the time to perceive of all Europeans as *one* race distinguished by *one* skin colour and to think of them collectively as 'white'.[4] These questions were also discussed in speculations about the complexion of Christ or the Virgin Mary and it was often deduced that they must have had a balanced complexion reflecting an ideal character.[5] Artists striving to give a good likeness of the Virgin would have tried to produce such an ideal tone with a mixture of colours. The particular hue of that tone might have been different depending on regionally and historically specific beauty ideals; however, not many European paintings show Mary as dark.

In any case, the painterly production of flesh tones and the composition of complexions were understood in the same terms, and this association was deeply ingrained in the tradition of European painting. Painting flesh tones was never considered an issue of finding the one and only right pigment to match the tint of a person's flesh, but always one of finding the right mixture, distribution and layering of pigments. What artists produced when painting human faces or other undressed body parts was body colour and not skin colour. From the Middle Ages onwards painters' manuals describe the right mixture of pigments as *the* secret for a lifelike representation of skin. Classicists have suggested that the technique for a differentiating imitation of flesh tones, that is, the use of mixtures rather than a single pigment, had already been developed in ancient Greek painting, and in close relation to Hippocratic theories of humours and their impact on skin colour.[6] This technique and understanding of the mixing of colours for the rendering of skin was taken up in medieval tracts such as Theophilus's *De diversis artibus*, where these mixtures of colours are literally referred to as 'temperaments'. According to Theophilus the 'skin colour resembling flesh' should be composed of white, red and yellow to which a dark green might be added for paler skin. These colours corresponded with the basic colours Hippocrates and Galen associated with the four humours (with the exception of black, which was substituted by a dark green also used as a primer).[7] For centuries, the proper blending of colours remained the key to lifelike rendering of flesh and the emphasis put on the chemistry of the painted flesh tones has to be understood in relation to the complexities of the notion of 'complexion'. In rendering a body's material substance, painters had not only to get the coloured appearance right, but also to match the consistency of flesh with their conglomerates of pigments and binding materials.

The matter of the body's colour

The perception of people's colour changed gradually from the sixteenth century, and this shift was related to the colonial expansion of European nations, the increase of the transatlantic slave trade and the exploitation of African slaves in America and the Caribbean. 'Black' became a synonym of slave and a discriminative marker in the colonial politics of slave labour. Along with it, body colour slowly migrated into the outer zones, and became – as skin colour – a potentially essential category and a marker of racial identity. Initially, this locating of the colouring matter in the skin was not part of the attempt to classify humans in sets of species or of racially defined groups, but of medical investigations into the organ itself. The same anatomists and naturalists interested in the build-up and texture of skin where also curious about the location of the colouring matter. Questions regarding the colour of the 'Ethiopians' (a term used both for the inhabitants of Ethiopia and generically for sub-Saharan Africans) – where it comes from, what it consists of and where in the human body it resides – were frequently asked throughout the seventeenth and eighteenth centuries.[8] The Parisian anatomist Jean Riolan had argued early on (in 1618) that the colouring matter sits in the outer layer, the cuticle, and does not even go as deep as the dermis.[9] He observed that 'Ethiopians' were born 'with their blackness' and concluded that this colour is innate.[10] Riolan combined Hippocratic humorism with a hereditary explanation of blackness. While stating that the 'colour of the body, the way it appears in the face and on the surface of the skin' is an indication of the humour that dominates in a human, he argued that the epidermis of 'negroes' did not receive its colour from the 'true skin' (and hence the humours) but resided solely in the 'surpeau', the superficial layer of the human envelope.[11] For authors like Riolan, human colour could be both innate and skin deep.

Later seventeenth-century studies of the microstructure of the organ of touch approached the question of human colour with new procedures for the analytical de-composing of the dermis. In his *De externo tactus organo* Malpighi described a procedure often repeated by later seventeenth- and eighteenth-century anatomists and naturalists: he separated the skin of dissected subjects, soaked it in chemicals which helped to disintegrate the sample and then carefully peeled it layer by layer observing the components and their structure with the help of a loupe and microscope.[12] He corrected prevailing assumptions, stating that both the outermost layer and the dermis were white in all humans, and concluded that the colouring matter must reside in an intermediate stratum, the reticular layer. Malpighi's hypothesis was confirmed by most of the relevant anatomists of the eighteenth century who had taken up his account of the location of the colour of humans. Skin and the question of human colour was, during this period, the main anatomical interest when black bodies were dissected.[13] In France, Alexis Littré, already mentioned for his early use of the term *tissu* in a medical context, continued the research on the composition and colour of skin. He reported the dissection of a 'moor' and the isolation of pieces of his skin which he macerated in a number of 'strong dissolvents' none of which were capable of severing the 'black sap' from the reticular layer to which it adhered.[14] Without explicitly using the compound 'skin colour', anatomists like Littré firmly tied the human colouring matter to a layer in the skin. Colour was now no more distributed throughout the flesh, but concentrated in the outer part of the dermis.

Despite the increasing interest in the location of skin colour, there were – as far as I can see – no visual images concerned with this phenomenon before the eighteenth century. Lairesse's illustrations of the skin and its components for Bidloo's 1685 *Anatomia humani corporis* (Figure 2.1), demonstrate no interest in this issue. In his *Anatomy of Blackness* Andrew Curran has recently brought an illustration from Riolan's 1649 *Encheiridium anatomicum et pathologicum* into relation with the anatomist's early localisation of the colour in the skin. It is doubtful though whether this image is concerned with skin colour at all, or with something Curran calls 'African anatomy'.[15] The full page of illustrations into question shows on the left a male nude serving as the universalised 'anatomical man' and at his side, the same man opened for dissection. Showing the first step of an anatomical aperture, the unfolded skin lays bare the well-structured and graphically textured muscles of the abdomen (Figure 5.2).[16] This image does indeed demonstrate a then still unusual interest in the skin and makes a point about its layering. At the cut edges the skin delaminates in four sheets denominated in the legend of the English translation as A. the 'Scarf-skin' (epidermis), B. 'the Skin', C. 'the Fat' and D. 'the fleshy Membrane'.[17] The varying depth of the three inner coats is indicated with outlines of different thickness. In contrast, the blank epidermis lacks an outline becoming only discernible against the textured dermis. In order to render these coats – and in the case of 'B' its upper and under sides – discernible, the printer used white and differently textured surfaces. The relative darkness of these textures does not represent skin colour, but serves as a graphic means of discrimination. It will take a further step before the anatomical method of separating out parts of the human body and illustrating this graphically merge with the move to

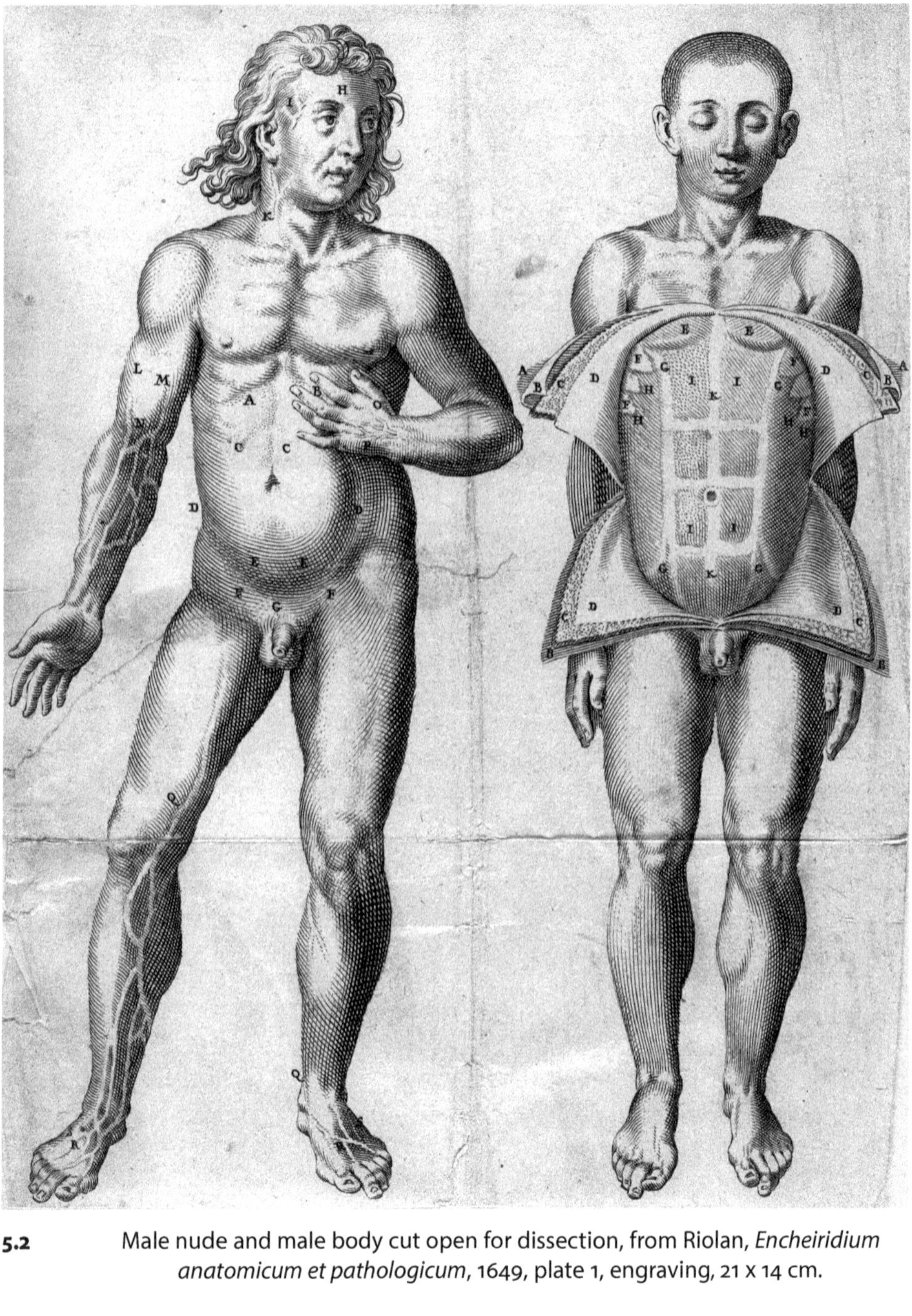

5.2 Male nude and male body cut open for dissection, from Riolan, *Encheiridium anatomicum et pathologicum*, 1649, plate 1, engraving, 21 x 14 cm.

discriminate people as black and white. In this process the black colouring matter became a tool of discrimination and the signifier of difference.

Just over half a century later, an image of skin from Frederik Ruysch's *Thesaurus* is already an entirely different matter (Figure 5.3). 'Fig. III', top right, is an engraving of a piece of skin taken from the sole of the foot of an 'Ethiopian', which was preserved in a jar with alcohol in the anatomist's famous cabinet. Even though similar graphic strategies are employed to distinguish inner and outer aspects, as well as the cut edge, of a piece of a skin, this is very different. The image, that abstracts from the container and liquid in which the specimen must have been kept, shows the piece suspended with a thread, and curved around itself. By the means of variation in hatching, the outer surface ranges in tone from light to dark grey, while the more densely worked inner side looks black in colour and furry in texture. Here, the black

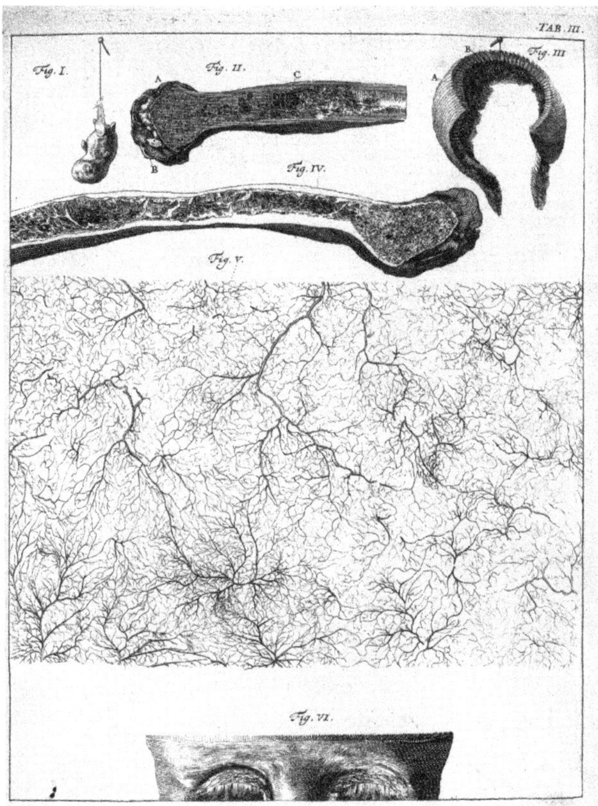

Various specimens, including the fragment of skin taken from an 'Ethiopian', from Frederik Ruysch, *Thesaurus anatomicus primus* [– *decimus*], part 10, 1716, table 3, engraving, 21.3 x 16 cm (platemark). 5.3

ink clearly represents the colouring matter in an Ethiopian's mucous layer. The dark colouring matter in an actual body thus took on a similar function to the printer's black ink in its ability to render the structure of the skin more easily visible. For a prominent visitor to Ruysch's cabinet in Leiden, the philosopher Voltaire, the specimen was a material proof for the essential blackness of the 'negro'. The little piece of skin was of great service to him in an argument against Buffon and in favour of the division of humans into 'entirely different races', a difference he believed to be plainly visible.[18]

While the two engravings and their commentators, Riolan and Ruysch, addressed the layering and, in the latter case, also the coloration of the skin as a matter of black and white, there is one exceptional medical illustration which brings colour into the image (Plate 12). It is a colour mezzotint dealing not only with the microscopic structure of skin but also with the issue of skin colour. It accompanies a 1737 treatise by Bernard Siegfried Albinus the title of which translates as 'Dissertation on the seat and cause of the colour of Ethiopians and other humans'. In this text on black skin, the famous Leiden-based anatomist whose name ironically designates 'white', confirmed earlier observations according to which both dermis and the most external parts of the skin are white in all humans, and that the colour must reside in the reticular body.[19] Following the methods already employed by Malpighi, Littré and others, he managed to dissolve the mucous layer and the colouring material, and specified that the colour is more densely distributed in the interstices of the reticular tissue and less so at the margins of the papillae. He carefully described the varying intensity of the colouring matter, which he held responsible for the fact that 'Ethiopians' are not uniformly dark.[20]

The layering and the distribution of colour is also at the heart of the illustration for Albinus's treatise printed by Jan Ladmiral after his own gouache. For the print the artist employed the then still relatively new technique of the colour mezzotint, using inks that mix when several plates are superimposed. As discussed earlier, this procedure introduced by Le Blon and promoted in his 1725 *Coloritto; or the Harmony of Colouring* was particularly affiliated with the visual imitation of flesh of one kind or another. Jan Ladmiral had worked with Le Blon in London before returning with the technical knowledge to the Netherlands where he specialised in the production of anatomical illustrations mainly for Ruysch and Albinus.[21] Given that this particular technique of colour printing had itself been only recently developed and still involved the experimentation with various inks, it certainly did not allow taking colour and its materiality for granted. In addition, Albinus's tract is the first text dedicated to the causes of human coloration that is accompanied by an illustration engaging with the colour of the skin. Nothing was thus self-evident when the image was made: the exploration of the colour in the skin and the ink with which it was reproduced literally went hand in hand.

For the print in question, Ladmiral actually employed a combination of mezzotint and aquatint techniques, also using the burin for retouching the plate.[22] Engraved are the letters forming the artist's name and those indicating the anatomical parts, the shadows cast by the specimens, and the pins holding them in place. The intervention of the artist, recalled through his name and present through his decision to use shadows to produce a *trompe l'œil* effect on the one hand, and the cutting and explanatory intervention of the anatomist on the other are thus marked via the incisions of the printer's burin. In contrast, the mezzotint technique itself produces a soft gradation of tones rather than clear-cut lines. It defines forms through distinct colours, and, especially in one fragment represented in this print, the anatomical cut is emphasised through the highlighting of the transverse section in white set against the swarthy colour of the surface. Cutting, peeling and segregation as well as layering and mixing are what the print is all about. It lays out the skin as dissected fragments. As the accompanying explanation of the image explains, they were taken from the breast, heel and thumb of an 'Ethiopian woman'. The three specimens are neatly arranged in the centre of the plate: two square-cut fragments of similar size are lined up next to each other and the tip of the thumb is placed in the middle underneath. On the small (ca 12 x 16 cm) plate the thumb is more or less life-size and as an easily recognisable body part it serves as a point of reference and orientation – it relates back to the viewer's own physique and sense of dimensions – and simultaneously as a guide into the image. The preparations are displayed on a ground of saturated green also employed by Ladmiral in other anatomical illustrations. As a transformation of yellow and blue, green showcases the most stunning effect of the mixing of colours, and in its velvety, intense quality also the refined work with the rocker used to roughen the plate.[23] On a representational level, it contrasts with the anatomical preparations, as it doesn't occur in a healthy human body, and is not used in anatomical imagery for the body and its parts. As with some of Lairesse's drawings for Bidloo, Ladmiral suggested that he was representing actual specimens by including pins fixing the organic fragments on the support. This choice of props makes a claim for the authority of the image as much as for that of the anatomist: it suggests that both the draughtsman and the physician have based their work on their own observations, dissections and analytical preparation of the body part in question. At the same time, this emphasis on the specimen, on the actual organic piece of matter that might change shape and colour as it deteriorates and thus needs fixing, thwarts the diagrammatic aspect of the image.

The analytical character of the dissection is matched by the almost abstract quality and organised set-up of the print, and especially of figure one (on the top left side). The figure is divided into four fields in an almost chequered distribution, each representing the skin in a different state of undoing. The lower left segment still shows the skin in its integral thickness, the tegument's un-dissected prospect with its outermost coat displaying a mixed brownish tone. At the left corner of this quarter the epidermis is slightly bent upwards thus hinting at the process of the organ's unfolding; on the right edge it slightly overlaps with the layer underneath, indicating that these strata normally stick together. The composition and decomposition of the organ, its functionality and the analytical process of the dissection via which it is known are simultaneously kept present in the figure. The other quarters, representing the strata beneath, are visualised via a clear-cut separation of black and white. The lowest stratum is designated in the explanations as 'cutis nuda' (naked dermis) and appears in the print as white with the reflections a white object would show, very much in the manner Le Blon had stressed in his treatise on the colour mezzotint. The second layer is displayed and described as the part of the reticulum that adheres to the dermis containing some colouring substance, and the third as the entire reticulum thick with dark colour and sprinkled with white dots signifying roots of hair.

The second fragment, taken from the heel of the woman, is meant to demonstrate the uneven colouring of this part of the body which, as most anatomists of the time observed, tended to be lighter than the rest of a black person's body. In rendering the transition between a darker and a lighter brown so smoothly, the print simultaneously displays the subtlety of the anatomical observation and the capacities of the printing technique.

Skin colour is treated in the print both in the form of an almost abstract contrast of black and white – in the squared distribution of black and white skin sections – and as complexion, because any part of the imitation of these body fragments is a result of the mixing of tints. As the test prints of the three individual plates in single colours, kept today at the Amsterdam Rijksmuseum, demonstrate, each segment of skin in the illustration consists of a mixture of various degrees of all three colours used.[24] No black ink was involved in the printing of the black layer of skin as it consists of the superimposition of the most intense blue, yellow and red in equal proportion. The divided printing process runs parallel to the analytical approach of the anatomist dissecting the skin; at the same time the build-up of the organ is re-enacted through superimposition, a layering through which the mixing of colours is achieved. This very process, and the particular knowledge of colour it entails, also brings with it a particular understanding of skin colour. Even though represented as an abstracted contrast of black and white which tied it to the symbolic and political dimensions this division had during the period of the trans-atlantic slave trade and the exploitation of slave labour in the colonies, it is simultaneously produced as complexion, the result of a complex mixture of coloured liquids the proportion of which can vary. In this sense skin colour is not only represented but mimicked here in all its complexity as the superimposition of semi-transparent, tinted inks. The print demonstrates through its very process how the intense dark colouring matter – which Albinus still referred to as 'sap' or 'humor' – is toned down by the non-coloured outer part of the epidermis, resulting in a brownish hue, produced through mixtures of less intense colours. It also recreates the semi-transparency of skin, an aspect to which the art literature of the later eighteenth century would pay so much attention, mostly as an attribute of white skin. In this print, however, any attempt at a neat distinction between black and white is undermined by the fact that the dark colouring matter is made with all three primary colours as is the 'cutis nuda' which needs small amounts of colour to appear like a white surface reflecting light. This colour mezzotint of skin colour thus suggests that any skin of a living human person is colourful in one way or the other. It grants an exceptional insight into the simultaneous madeness and materiality of the concept of skin colour.

Among the various French eighteenth-century treatises on skin and its colour, none is illustrated with an image comparable to those by Lairesse or Ladmiral. It is not until Gaultier's 1809 *Recherches sur l'organisation de la peau de l'homme et sur les causes de sa coloration* that there is a representation of the layers of skin and the location of the colour in a French context (Figure 5.4). Printed in black and white and far less detailed than Lairesse's engraving it is more diagrammatic than the earlier Dutch prints. Spelling out the elements of the mucous layer, their function and the precise seat of the colouring matter, Gaultier treated the black substance more explicitly as a heuristic tool than had previous tracts on skin colour. Earlier anatomical studies, for example those of Littré and to some degree also Albinus's tract (after all dedicated to the 'colour of Ethiopians *and other humans*') used black skin to research the layering of human skin as such, but because the distinct visibility of one layer was enhanced by the dark substance, Gaultier made an explicit point about this when he stated that his observations were 'helped by the anatomy of the skin of negroes'.[25] The dark colouring matter worked for him like the dyes already brought into play by early modern anatomists for injecting bodily vessels during dissection in order to highlight certain functional parts. Or, for a more recent example, it worked like the contrast-medium utilised in radiology and other modern medical imaging technologies to enhance the visibility of certain inner body parts. In the medical attempts to discriminate and pin down the colouring matter, black became the most discernible and visible colour, and the one that sticks most tightly to the body.

There is however a French eighteenth-century treatise that was particularly concerned with the substance that colours the skin: the 1765 *Traité de la couleur de la peau humaine* by Claude-Nicolas Le Cat, a surgeon and anatomist working in Rouen. This thorough and comprehensive medical study of the location and chemical composition of the colouring matter has no anatomical illustrations. Its frontispiece features an allegorical representation of the 'three species of mankind' with a European woman at the centre surrounded by a black page and an American Indian.[26] The frontispiece affirms Le Cat's view that the variation of human appearance allows the division of humankind into different species. The focus of the book is however not the diversity or classification of humans but the anatomy of the organ including the location and nature of its colouring matter. Le Cat most explicitly situated the issue of colour in the skin as he argued: 'When talking about the colour of human beings, it is the skin that is at stake.'[27] He started with a discussion of the structure of the human body's 'general envelope' in which he agreed with the by then largely accepted view of skin as consisting of various interconnected layers one of which, the mucous layer, is the site of the colour. Following the research methods of his predecessors in the analysis of skin, he claimed to have conducted numerous dissections of black and white subjects, as well as animals of the same species but of different colour, such as black and white

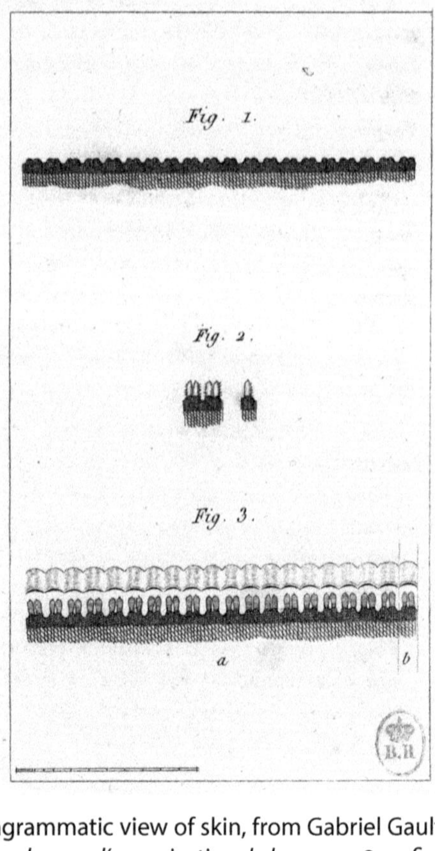

5.4 Diagrammatic view of skin, from Gabriel Gaultier, *Recherches sur l'organisation de la peau*, 1809, figure 1.

sheep. By means of deductive reasoning Le Cat ruled out that the black bile is the cause of the colour in blacks, an argument deriving from humoral theory and still widespread in the eighteenth century. For him, black bile is as little responsible for the colour of 'negros' as the white bile for the colour of whites. The bile only makes the latter look sick and 'spoils the whiteness terribly'.[28] Since the structure of the skin is the same in all humans, and the layers look the same except for the mucous layer, the latter must be the seat of the colouring substance. As this region of the skin is – as late seventeenth-century anatomists had already observed – also the location of the papillae responsible for the feeling of touch, and since there are no other vessels in the mucous layer, Le Cat concluded that the colour must be a juice produced by nerves.[29] Published in the same year as the *Encyclopédie* article 'Sensibilité', which regarded skin as a 'nervous canvas', Le Cat's text confirmed Enlightenment medicine's view of skin as a privileged site of nervous and sense activity. It discusses skin colour less as a matter of temperaments and humours than as a fluid circulating through nervous activity and serving the body as a communicative medium.

> We are looking for the colour of the skin [*couleur de la peau*], of which we know all the parts: what then is the one among them that makes the colour? Where does it reside? We are white, the Africans are black; it is thus only a matter of researching which part of this skin, or of the liqueurs it contains, is permanently white in us and black in the Moor.
>
> The arterial blood turns us vermilion, and it also communicates a little bit of that colour to the Ethiopian, all Ethiopian as he is. Our injections subtly coloured by vermilion still produce this in the Negro after his death. But on either side, one can well see that the vermilion, be it natural or artificial, is but an addition to the natural white or black.[30]

Again organising his research around the abstract opposition of black and white, Le Cat clearly posited the 'natural' (that is, inborn) character of the colour and firmly placed it in the skin. Unusually, he treated white as a colour too, and equally explored the material causes of the whiteness of white people, but the degree of coloration is not the same: black people seem entirely defined by their colour, as despite the colouring matter's location in just one layer of the skin, black as colour fuses with the identity of the black, as the denomination 'Ethiopian' becomes for Le Cat and other authors of the period a term equally employed for the people and their colour, so that the Ethiopian can be described as 'all Ethiopian as he is'.

What is unique about the *Traité de la couleur de la peau* within the eighteenth-century discourse on this issue is the concern with the material properties of skin colour. Anne Lafont has argued that, in the work of Le Cat and during the eighteenth century more generally, the medical and anthropological studies on the colour of Africans joined artistic enquiries into colour.[31] Le Cat identified a colouring matter he called 'ethiopis', today understood as the pigment melanin, and found it not only in human skin, but also in the iris and the dark ink of the sepia (an observation only taken up in the nineteenth century and still accepted by today's life sciences).[32] Sepia is of course a substance also used by artists or as ink in writing, but this is not the only overlap between Le Cat's observations and practices, and artistic usages of colour. In the passage quoted above, the tint of the blood allowed Le Cat to distinguish between artificial and natural colour both logically and in the material practice of his preparations. He described the colour of blood as vermilion, thus alluding to the pigment which had been – for centuries – one of the major ingredients of flesh tones in painting and was also frequently in use for anatomical preparations.[33] Understood as a colour, and hence as something perceived uniquely with the eyes, blood or its artificial substitute became a signifier, rendering the layering of skin visible in medical experimentation in a similar way as it signifies, in varying degrees, physical and emotional processes in the living body of any colour.[34] These processes were explicitly understood as communications. They thus turn the body into a medium that works like the imitation made of it in painting, when the circulation of blood is mimicked via a layering of paints. Beyond Le Cat's treatise, questions of body and skin colour were often understood in artistic or artisanal terms, for example when the colouring matter is referred to as a dye. Even the word 'pigment', gradually introduced from the late eighteenth century onwards to denominate the colouring matter in the skin, derives from the Latin *pigmentum*, referring to a colouring matter, paint or dye, a word itself stemming from *pingere* (to paint).[35]

Race and skin colour

Le Cat brought issues of skin colour and race together, in so far as he began his essay with two chapters on human diversity and its origins. And yet, after summarising various modes of classification or theories addressing the causes for the differences in colour, he ended with the conclusion that the question of origins has to be left to theology or mythology, and can't be answered from an anatomical point of view. This indicates that the attempt to order humans in a set of species or races was not generally accepted by the mid-eighteenth century, and that conflicting views still prevailed a century after the term 'race' was first applied to humans in France.

It is the physician, philosopher and traveller François Bernier who is credited for using the term 'race' with regard to humans for the first time. In a short text printed in 1684 in the *Journal des sçavans* and dedicated to the 'New division of the Earth', he described groups of humans classified according to their geographical distribution and physical appearance as 'races'.[36] The word as such entered the French language in the fifteenth century, but was initially used in relation to animals, in particular horses, in the context of breeding. Eventually applied to humans with reference to genealogy or the nobility of a family, it was not a value-free term, but lacked the connotations it gained in Bernier's text.[37] Using 'species' ('espèces') and 'race' interchangeably, Bernier applied the term to larger groups of humans not related by kinship but by shared physical features which he considered hereditary.[38] In French (and German), it retained a variety of meanings linked to its etymological history, and can refer to family lineage and breeds of one animal species as well as to groups of humans whose physical attributes are perceived as significantly different.

Bernier divided the earth's population as follows: the 'first race' is the largest group comprising not only people living in Europe, North Africa, the Middle East, Persia and India, but also all the native inhabitants of the Americas. The second species consists of sub-Saharan Africans, distinguished by the forms of their faces as well as by the dark colour of their bodies. The third species included East Asian populations and was, in Bernier's eyes, 'actually white' but too distinct in the physical features to form part of the 'first race'. Finally, the author singled out the 'Lapps' who he describes, building on a long tradition of vilifying this relatively small group of inhabitants of northern Scandinavia, as not conforming to the beauty ideals indirectly defined by his account of the 'first race'.

While distinguishing four species of men, Bernier's classification is predominantly organised by the contrasting of an assumed 'we' against which all other people are judged, and the most pronounced non-we are, from his perspective, sub-Saharan Africans.[39] Although colour is not at all the main criterion for his classification and aesthetic judgement – he can be relativist with regard to colour when a body's shape is perceived as beautiful – it is crucial for the ways sub-Saharan Africans are singled out. Even though describing other physical features, Bernier called only their colour explicitly essential. Unlike the various gradations of olive and brown found among the populations of Asia and the Mediterranean region, this 'noirceur qui leur est essentiel' was, for Bernier, not caused by exposure to the sun; but inherited, passed on by parents to their offspring and stable even if a black person moved to a colder climate.[40] Writing decades before the wave of anatomical studies on the location of colour in the skin, colour remained body colour for Bernier. When mentioning skin as one of the distinguishing physical features of Africans, he described the 'oily, smooth and shiny'[41] quality of the external organ, but not its chromatic appearance. His body colour is however not complexion in the Hippocratic sense either, as it is innate and permanent. This led Bernier to a generalising juxtaposition of 'blacks' and 'whites', which complied with the significance of this division for the contemporary colonial domination and exploitation of slaves. In France, the holding of slaves in the plantations of the French Caribbean colonies and the Atlantic slave trade were regulated in the *Code Noir*, an edict promulgated by Louis XIV in 1685, just a year after Bernier's 'Nouvelle division de la terre'. The *Code Noir* firmly established the equation of 'nègre' and slave and the political hierarchy of black and white.[42] Or, as Dian Kriz and Geoff Quilley have put it, the 'economy of colour was drawn in black and white'. And, building on Homi Bhabha's *Location of Culture*, they point out that 'questions of colonial authority are invariably bound up with the visualization of difference that is not a transcription of the Real but a representation having material effects'.[43] Both the medical attempts to discriminate layers of skin and localise skin colour's material substrate and imagery from the visual arts contributed to this visualisation of difference.

A particularly striking example is one of the portraits of a woman with her black page, so popular during the seventeenth century: the portrait of Louise de Kéroualle, the French mistress of Charles II turned duchess of Portsmouth, painted by Pierre Mignard in Paris during a visit of the duchess in 1682 (Plate 13). The portrait strongly contrasts the differing skin colours of the duchess and the servant girl, who is offering her corals and a shell full of pearls. The darkness of the pages highlights the immaculate and – so it seems today – artificially white skin with the rouged cheeks of Kéroualle and certainly brings seventeenth-century ideals of female beauty to the fore.[44] But it does so by enhancing the beauty and desirability of both the servant girl and her mistress, who are entwined through multiple inversed contrasts: white pearls on black skin and black hair set against white skin.[45] Mignard's strategy of working with contrasts is quite different from the suggestions for portraits made, not much earlier, in Antoine Le Blond's 1669 *Instructions touchant la Peinture* (see chapter 3). This manual suggests, in an unusually explicit manner, that 'to express the traits of a beautiful princess, queen or empress' the artist should include an entourage of 'rather brownish women and old Moors [*des femmes un peu bazannées & de vieilles moresques*], pages with unruly gestures or deformed dwarfs, in order to give more grace and majesty to the principal subject'.[46] Even though no less hierarchical, difference has multiple faces here, and is manifested by rank, behaviour and various physical features including complexions, while Mignard's portrait of Louise de Kéroualle makes distinctions in black and white and directs the focus on to skin colour.

Although physically ingrained, such difference was not yet unanimously defined as racial. Bernier's method of ordering humans according to a set of physical characteristics did not immediately find followers, and the classification of humans generally remained a contested issue in pre-revolutionary France, or Enlightenment Europe more broadly speaking.[47] The Swedish naturalist Linnaeus, for example, provoked as much mockery as praise for his classifications. In the first of the many editions of his *Systema naturae*, published in 1735, he ranged the humans together with the apes and the sloth among the anthropomorphic quadrupeds and subdivided them neatly into four 'varieties' ordered geographically and chromatically. In later editions he added, besides other attributes, the predominant temperaments: he characterised the Americans as ruddy and choleric, the Europeans as white and sanguine, the Asians as yellow and melancholic, and the Africans as black and phlegmatic.[48] He thus grounded human coloration again in the theory of humours, but one that was not necessarily in accordance with earlier associations, for example, of the black bile with the melancholic temperament and dark body colour. More importantly, it lacked the fluidity of previous Hippocratic approaches as it allocated one dominant temperament to the population of an entire continent. Diderot and the French naturalist and long-standing (1739–88) intendant of the Jardin du Roi in Paris, George-Louis Leclerc de Buffon, were among the prominent opponents of Linnaeus's approach rejecting the whole classificatory frenzy and the essentialism it entailed. The *Encyclopédie*, although itself a gigantic enterprise of enlightened ordering of knowledge, generally followed this scepticism.[49] For Buffon, there was no way in which the multitude of nature could be fitted into a fully consistent man-made system.[50] Buffon and authors affiliated with him, argued that the groups interpenetrate and that the demarcations between them are not clearly defined. Engaging with human diversity in the third volume of his *Histoire naturelle* (1749), he acknowledged that humans vary according to the climates they traditionally lived in and considered 'colour the most remarkable of these varieties', but stressed that internal variations could be more pronounced than those between members of different varieties.[51] Following up from this mode of thinking, Pierre Cabanis, also a friend of Girodet, argued in his 1796–97 lectures on the *Rapports du physique et du moral de l'homme* that the 'progress of commerce tends to confound all the races, all the forms, all the colours'.[52]

In pre-revolutionary France, the classification of humans into races whose distinctive marker is skin colour was thus by no means generally accepted. Reading eighteenth-century approaches to the question of human variation (as it was mostly called at the time) as immediate forerunners of the nineteenth-century science of race is, as Claude Blanckaert has argued, in itself a problematic way of genealogical thinking and means overlooking the complexities as well as the political insights of the Enlightenment debate.[53] During the eighteenth century, theories of human variety were not a homogeneous field at all, and race was not a generally accepted category, far less a clearly defined one. The hereditary nature of the markers of human variety was equally contested. Major controversies existed between polygenists like Voltaire, who believed that humans existed in different races from the start, and monogenists, such as Buffon or Petrus Camper, who argued that humans derived from one prototype and had developed (or 'degenerated' as Buffon saw it) over extended periods of time due to the influence of climate and conditions of life. Skin colour was one of the attributes that was subject to change in this process. It was only during the nineteenth century that race became the dominant concept for the division of humans and predominantly seen as a hereditary, essentialist category.[54] As a highly visible marker of race, skin colour became a biopolitical concept in which differences in colour marked social differences thus naturalising inequality and hierarchies.

What further complicates the picture of the Enlightenment debate is that several of the scholars who produced what seem today the most absurd and objectionable assessments of physical difference, such as Johann Friedrich Blumenbach in Germany, were outspoken abolitionists. Others, like Camper in the Netherlands, used anatomical arguments to dismiss discrimination based on skin colour.[55] In a lecture 'On the origin and colour of blacks' held at the anatomy theatre in Groningen in 1764 (and published in French translation in 1802), Camper built on the work of his teacher Albinus, as well as that of Littré, Le Cat and others, to confirm that the colour of all healthy humans resides in the reticular layer of the skin and explicitly rejected contemporary medical theories according to which blacks are black through and through. Instead, he used an anatomical dissection to demonstrate that beyond the coloured layer just below the epidermis, humans all look fairly alike, thereby convincing his audience that 'we are white Moors, or rather; we are people similar to Blacks in every way except that we have the middle layer less tanned'. He concluded: 'you will no longer raise any objections to joining me in holding out the hand of brotherhood to Negroes and Blacks, and in recognizing them as true descendants of the first man whom we recognize as our Father!'[56]

Camper continued to work on human variety and later developed a way of distinguishing humans based on a less changeable element of the human body: the form and bone structure of the head. Interestingly, Camper developed his comparative approach to the exterior form of men and animals, including his notorious theory of the facial angle, in a series of lectures held in 1770 at the Amsterdam Drawing Academy. Published in 1791 in Dutch, they were quickly translated into French, German and English. The questions regarding the 'natural difference of features in persons of different countries and periods of life' were thus initially raised as an aesthetic and representational problem.[57] The aim was to develop an anatomically more accurate method of recording human variety in artistic practice, as he accused artists of having painted Africans without properly studying their physique, making them look like 'painted black men' and not like 'Moors'.[58] Camper, who had himself received artistic training and remained an amateur painter, draughtsman and sculptor, also provided the illustrations for the publication of the lectures in question.[59] The anatomist framed his first lecture by bringing his own early interest in painting into play; it came, he suggested, with a visual attentiveness to the physical features of men and animals. He recounts how he was 'particularly struck with the figure and colour of Moors; and with the differences in features and complexion between the East Indian-blacks and the natives of Africa'.[60] The text subtly distinguishes between attentive contemplation and the heightened and sudden visual attention triggered by the sight of 'Moors'. Introduced as a highly visible phenomenon, blackness becomes the prime marker of difference that initiates the more nuanced observation of colour variation and the main topic of the book, which is – unlike in his earlier lecture – not skin colour but disparity in human shape and bodily structure. Camper moves indeed swiftly away from skin colour and towards the realm of art. Mentioning 'the best models of the Ancient Greeks', praising the works of Winckelmann and stating his preference for classical over Flemish and contemporary French artists he sets up a neoclassical framework in which form is privileged over colour and drawing is valued as the chief observational tool of artists and basis of all art forms.[61] This art theoretical position goes hand in hand with the anatomist's assessment of skin colour as a rather accidental physical attribute and his focus on the hard structure of the skull as synecdoche of human difference. Besides this neoclassical underpinning, Camper's methodic grasp on human variety owes much to artistic studies of human proportions. Measuring and calculation dominate this approach in which Camper used the varying backward slant of the forehead ('facial angle') as a short cut for recording human difference. Various diagrams of skulls and sculptures, animal and human heads, accompany the exercise. They make their own visual arguments and are more ambiguous than their empirical premise might suggest. A frontal view of craniums and fleshed out faces of what is explained as an ape, an Angolan, a Kalmuck, an European and the *Apollo Belvedere* could be seen as two non-humans – the animal and an ancient sculpture – framing three varieties of humans with the largest head taking centre stage (Figures 5.5–5.6). The Kalmuck's head thus interrupts an increase in size and with it the reading of the diagram as a genealogical progression and makes it more likely that the head of the ancient sculpture is seen to be as distant from the trio of humans as the ape, as Camper also stressed in the text that 'antique beauty … is not in nature; but to use the term of Winckelman, it is an ideal beauty'.[62]

Camper's lining up of heads in profile invites a different comparative approach and hardly prompts a neutral assessment. Even though the 'assemblage of craniums' was meant to demonstrate 'the boundary that the Creator has placed' between animals and humans despite the 'striking resemblance between the race of monkies and of blacks', the illustration brings precisely this visual similarity to the fore and has proven more effective than the accompanying warning. However much Camper intended to draw a line between apes

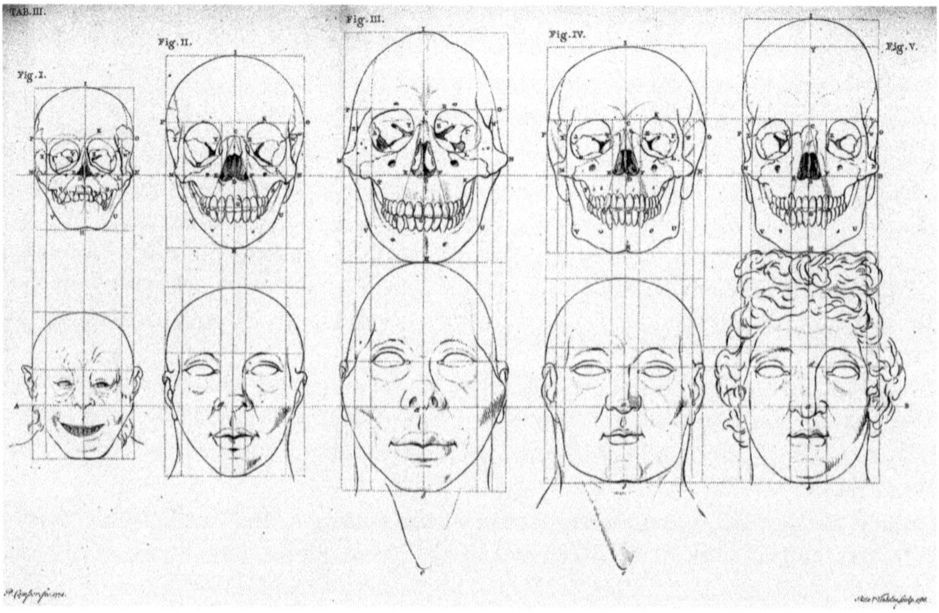

5.5 Rein. Winkeles after P. Camper, Skulls and heads of a monkey, humans and the *Apollo Belvedere*, frontal view, from Petrus Camper, *Dissertation physique sur les différences …*, 1791, table 3, engraving, 27 x 43 cm (platemark).

and humans and claimed (with Buffon) the unity of humans in distinction from animals, his line-up of heads was easy to read in the tradition of the 'great chain of being', as a progression towards perfection which assumes a hierarchy of different kinds of humans.[63] Only a few years after the publication of the lectures, the French naturalist and anthropologist Julien-Joseph Virey pushed Camper's theory and illustrations in this direction (Figure 5.7). Taking up the comparative line up of profiles with different facial angles, the illustration for his treatise makes a significant alteration in reducing the number of profiles to three and by blending the European with the ideal appearance of a Greek sculpture. The head of an orang-utan, a 'negro' and the mask-like profile (reminiscent of ancient images of Zeus) representing 'l'espèce blanche' are arranged in a vertical row more clearly indicating an ascending ladder and suggesting that the black is as far from the white as he is close to the ape. Virey, publishing his *Histoire naturelle du genre humain* in 1801, a time when Napoleonic France was seeking legitimisation for the re-introduction of slavery after its abolition during the French Revolution, reinforced earlier arguments according to which nature had made Africans natural slaves and correlated (unlike Camper) anatomy with character and intelligence.

Camper's lectures departed from the anecdotal prose of travel writers

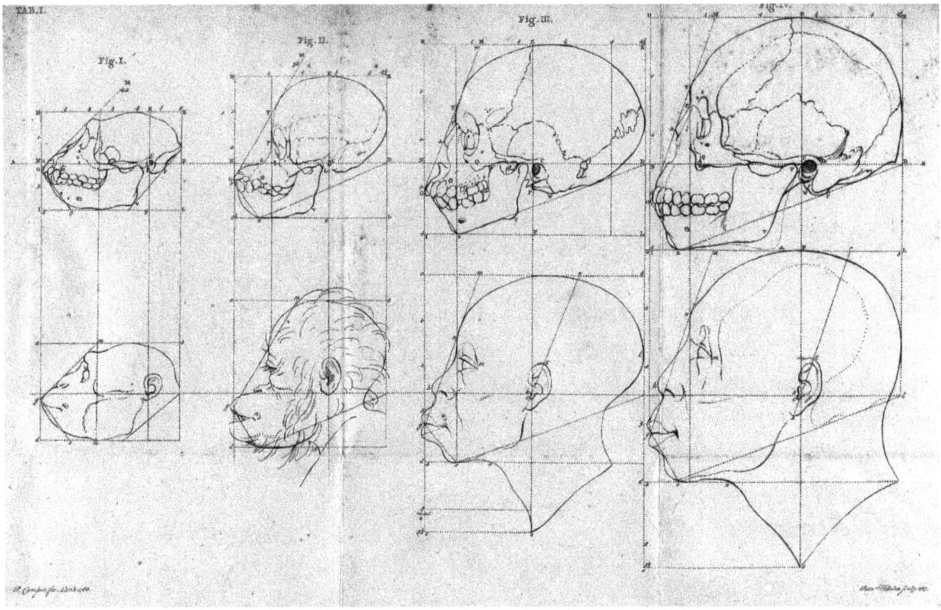

Rein. Winkeles after P. Camper, Skulls and heads of apes and humans in profile from Petrus Camper, *Dissertation physique sur les différences …*, 1791, table 1, engraving, 27 x 43 cm (platemark). 5.6

responsible for many early narratives of human diversity, which mixes physical descriptions with accounts of habits and customs. Explicitly written from the perspective of a European cosmopolitan observing the 'concourse of people assembled together in a large commercial city',[64] his works move towards an account of variety grounded in a combination of aesthetics and mathematics and the solid structure of physical appearance. Explicitly addressing artists, he draws their attention to physical difference rather than attributes, clothes and habits among humans, and flags it as a representational task, while providing terms for the engagement with the multi-ethnic populations of cities like Amsterdam and Paris. The universal human – as incarnated by the male academic life model and the nudes drawn from it, and reinforced by the neoclassical 'beau ideal' – was both reasserted and compromised in this venture.

Neoclassical ideals and a world of brownish people

Camper was not the only anatomist who spoke to this newly foregrounded representational task. In 1797, during the period he was lecturing on artistic anatomy in a theatre installed at the Louvre, Jean-Joseph Sue (the younger), published an *Essai sur la physiognomonie des corps vivans, considérée depuis l'homme jusqu'à la plante* which equally addresses artists as one of its key audiences and engages with the issue of human variety. The non-illustrated and text-heavy essay argues forcefully that anatomical and physiognomic study is a necessity for artists, and gives a detailed description of the ideal human body, and an overview of the prevalent theories regarding physiognomy and the expressions of passions. As the focus on physiognomy suggests, the treatise marks a shift in attention within artistic anatomy (which will be discussed in more detail in the next chapter): the internal conformation of the body is now treated predominantly in relation to its impact on the living body's exterior. Under the physiognomic paradigm attention is directed towards the outer appearance and the entire body is turned into a 'face' which the reader shall learn to read.[65] Sue postulated on the one hand a universal anatomical man whom he projected, fully in line with neoclassical aesthetics, as the ideal

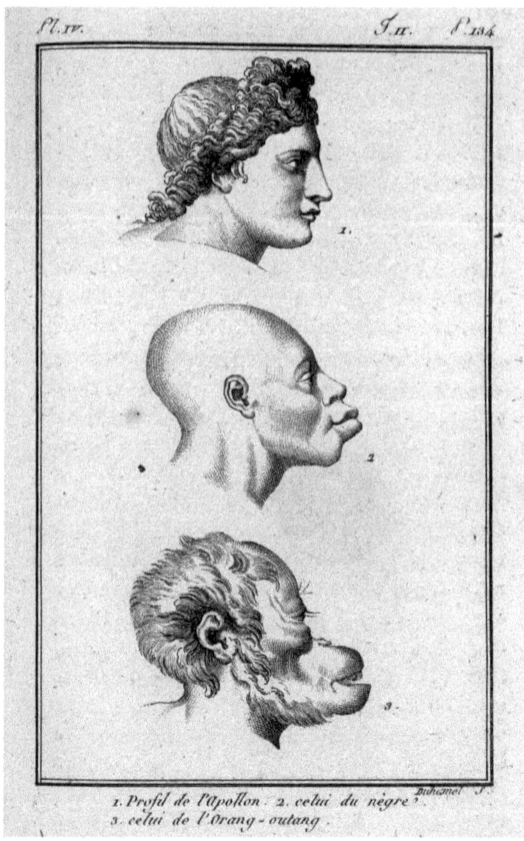

5.7 Heads of 'Apollo, negro and orang-utan', from Julien-Joseph Virey, *Histoire naturelle du genre humain*, 1801, vol. 2, plate 4, engraving, ca 20 x 12 cm.

body, living in the temperate climate of Greece, well exercised and nourished, with muscles covered by a pleasing envelope of skin and flesh. On the other hand he engaged with the multiple appearances of individual physiognomies as they also form a crucial facet of the bourgeois notions of the subject and, in the same vein, of the portraiture of the period. Finally, he confronts the infinity of human variation and nuances of skin colour in the world, but also in the multitude of the French body politic. To stress the importance of this aspect of painterly representation, he imagined young artists whose task is 'to draw or paint a seaport where men of different countries can be found, ... or a battle that normally involves two nations'.[66] Following most eighteenth-century natural histories he accounted for human diversity in the same manner as for variety in plants and animals, but, similarly to Cabanis, not so much with regard to the allegedly natural distribution of humans in various parts of the world, but to mixture and conflict brought about by commerce and civilisation.

Published in the very year when Talleyrand, Ministre des relations extérieures, presented the project of turning Egypt into a colony in a lecture at the Institut national,[67] the *Essai sur la physiognomonie* anticipated an artistic challenge that painters would face in the aftermath of Napoleon's Egyptian campaign. This endeavour ended, as is well known, in a military disaster which did not hinder the political rise of the emperor to be, and a number of history paintings by students of David such as Antoine-Jean Gros's *Battle of Aboukir* (1806) or Girodet's *Revolt of Cairo* (1810), commemorated the (from a French perspective) more successful episodes in a heroic light. In these battle scenes, the artists paid much attention to the multi-ethnic composition of the Egyptian troops, rendering differences in skin tone and dress with care. Similarly to Vivant Denon's drawings produced on site during the campaign itself, the battle paintings tried to capture the diversity of Egyptian physiognomies and a variety of emotional expressions. As Melanie Ulz has argued in her study of the imagery of the Egyptian campaign, such images were predominantly not about constructing ethnic types, but about unfolding the diversity of the North African population. The large-scale battle scenes by Gros and Girodet paint the enemies as diverse and disorderly in contrast to the more uniform French soldiers thus underlining the unity and dominance of the French army. The paintings helped constitute the modern identity of the French body politic by contrasting it with a manifold other.[68] Besides and independent of his *Revolt of Cairo*, Girodet explored the diversity of skin tones in a group of portraits and oil sketches of North Africans and Indians and in particular Mamelukes (soldiers who had been fighting for the Ottoman Empire in Egypt) who came to live in Paris in the wake of Napoleon's Egyptian campaign and the creation of an imperial Mameluke corps. Besides the interest in colourful costume, Girodet carefully rendered the distinct physiognomies and variations in skin tone of his models.[69]

In Sue's physiognomy for artists, similar attention is paid to the 'Variétés de l'espèce humaine', as the author spent just two pages on theories of racial classification, referencing Camper's theory of the facial angle, mentioning Kant's distinction of four or Exleben's division into six races and repeating, at least for the Asians, Europeans and Africans, Linnaeus's association of skin colour and temperament.[70] Far more detailed are his considerations on the differences in skin colour where a classificatory mode and one of nuanced observation collapse from the outset: 'The complexions of different peoples of the earth vary from white to black. There is an infinity of nuances between these two extreme colours, and they are blended with pale, yellow or red tones. These variations can be reduced to four principal colours, which are white, yellowish, swarthy and black.'[71] Like most of the anatomists previously discussed, Sue treated the question of the materiality and seat of the colour in a section on peoples with *teint noir* and substantiated his arguments with reference to his own dissections and preparations. He thus confirmed the dominant opinion that the colouring matter resides in the mucous layer underneath the epidermis.

In the other three sections, dedicated to one complexion each, things seem more complicated and confused. Although geography and climate played a role for Sue, the peoples of one colour cannot be confined to one continent (as Linnaeus had suggested), and the majority of 'whites' are not actually white. While most Scandinavians deserve this qualification, this hue gets gradually darker the further south one goes, but on the other hand there are 'whites in some islands of Asia' and in other parts of the world. The most precarious group though were the 'peuples qui ont le teint basané', a swarthy or brownish complexion. This range of tones is not only the most frequently found in all parts of the world, it is also not clearly defined as it forms 'the majority of all intermediary nuances between the fresh and vermilion colour of the peoples that live in moderate climates, and the black complexion of those exposed to the most burning heat of the sun, but it also belongs to climates where excessive cold reigns'.[72] While the black colour of people originating from sub-Saharan Africa – and Sue particularly referred to places like Senegal that were centres of the transatlantic slave trade – could be simply described as 'deep and radiant black like ebony or polished jet',[73] *basané* requires a multitude of descriptive attempts that finally collapse. Evoking various degrees of brown ranging between the olive-greenish and the deep black, at times mixed with red or approaching the hue of 'rusty iron mixed with oil',[74] Sue admits that 'one can only approximate a matter the observation of which is so delicate, and where language lacks expressions that could paint such nuances with precision; even the arts that speak to the eye can only imperfectly imitate them'.[75]

Addressing artists as his main audience, Sue turned the question of skin colour into a matter of delicate observation and into the proper business of artists, thus also heightening the visibility of skin colour as both a physical phenomenon and artistic concern. While sticking to some degree to the universal (implicitly male and white) body which had served for centuries as the basis of anatomy and as the model for artistic engagement with the human body, Sue, drawing as much attention to the external appearance of the body as to its internal formation, raised the awareness of human variety, thus challenging the ideals of universal manhood as they were performed in the practices of life drawing. Sue published his essay in the same year as Girodet painted his portrait of Belley and only shortly before Benoist embarked on her *Portrait d'une négresse*. The three must have been aware of each other's works, since, during the years 1796 to 1798 Girodet and Benoist both occupied studios at the Louvre,[76] while Sue was giving his public anatomy lectures for artists at the same place. Rather than taking a ready-made system of racial classification and fitting their models into it, as some scholars have suggested, Girodet's and Benoist's paintings were part of their attempts to understand skin colour. And it was a challenging task, as their training within the neoclassical framework of David's studio is unlikely to have provided them with the skills to render flesh tones beyond the range usual for North European artists. Both might have taken up the challenge to advertise their skills as colourists, but even so, the making of skin colour in paint was – at the time the portraits were produced and exhibited – equally a political issue. Girodet and Benoist, in making their portraits with brush and paint, had to come to terms with the complexity the problem of skin colour had both politically and aesthetically in revolutionary and post-revolutionary France and within the culture of neoclassicism.

Girodet's *Jean-Baptiste Belley*

When Girodet's *Jean-Baptiste Belley* was first shown, there was even an uncertainty about what to call the portrayed subject (Figure 5.8; plate 10). Initially displayed in a private exhibition at the Elysée in October 1797 it came under the lengthy title: *Portrait d'un Nègre. Le costume dénote un Représantant du Peuple Français. Le buste du celèbre Raynal, philosophe et historien, est un tribut de reconnaissance que les hommes de couleur doivent au premier apôtre de la liberté des Américains français*. It was only during its second display at the Salon 1798 that it became *Portrait du citoyen Belley, ex-représentant des Colonies* thus lending the living model a name while omitting that of the recently deceased Raynal.[77] The first subject Girodet chose to paint after his return from Rome (where he had stayed after having been awarded the Rome prize), was an unusual one: the first and only black delegate in the revolutionary parliament. Belley was one of three deputies of Saint-Domingue, the present day Haiti, and during the eighteenth century France's most prosperous

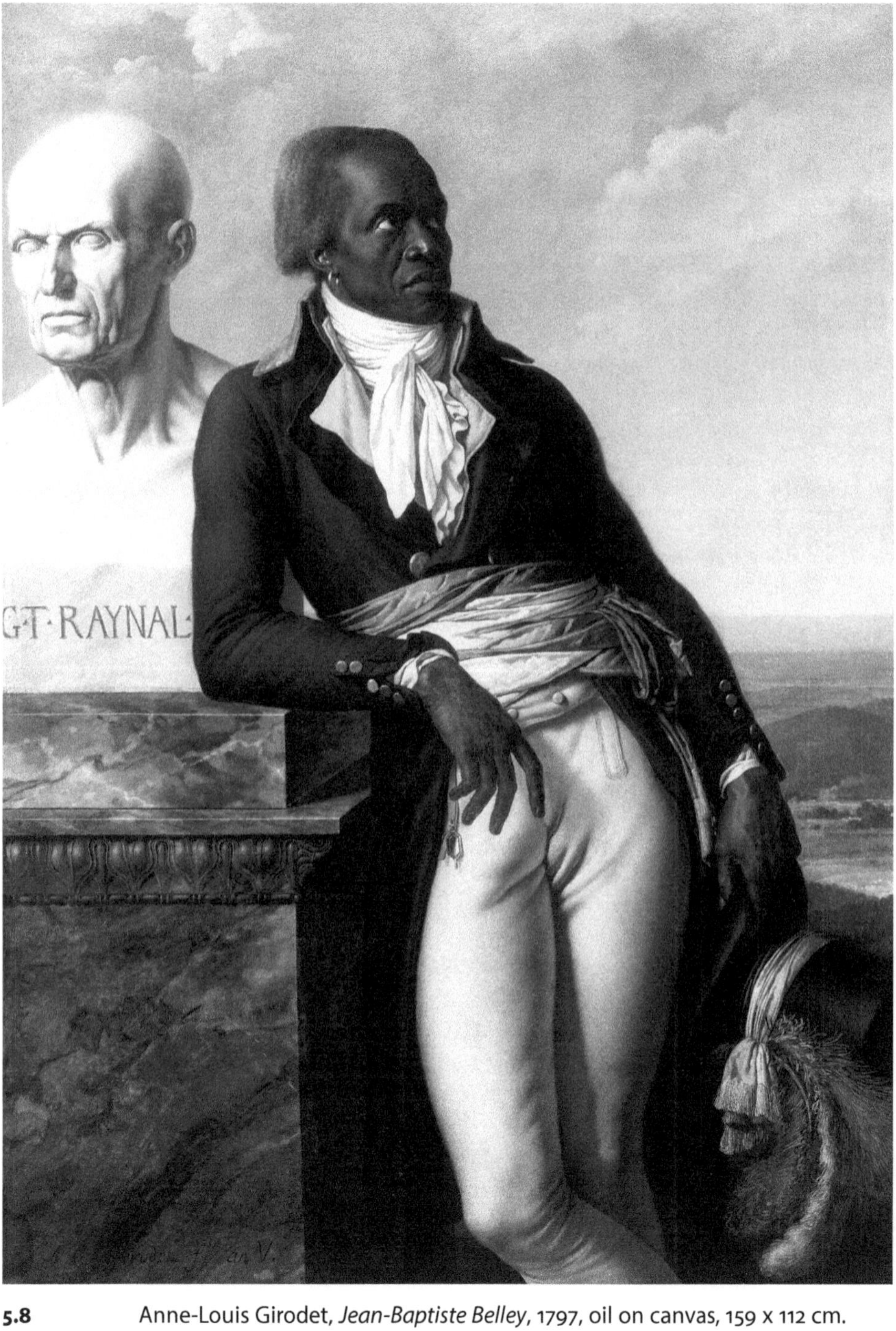

5.8 Anne-Louis Girodet, *Jean-Baptiste Belley*, 1797, oil on canvas, 159 x 112 cm.

colonial settlement with a population of circa 500,000 slaves working to provide nearly half of the world's sugar and coffee.[78] Slave uprisings that began in August 1791 forced the local French authorities in Saint-Domingue to abolish slavery in the colony, a development that initiated what is now recognised as the Haitian Revolution, the only successful slave revolt in world history, leading, in 1804, to the country's independence. The events in Saint-Domingue thus pre-empted abolition in France, and elected delegates from the colony were sent to France to seek endorsement for the general emancipation of slaves.[79] Besides Belley, a white man, the colonist Louis Dufay, and a mulatto named Jean-Baptiste Mill, arrived in Paris in February 1794, the three of them representing the colony's multi-ethnic population (by no means proportionately given that the vast majority of the colony's inhabitants were black), and its classification into three skin colours that had been also symbolic of their social status: black equalled slave, liberated slaves and their descendants were typically referred to as people of colour or mulattos and white signified a colonist and usually slave owner. This tripartite symbolism did not match the more complex realities of colour. Although representing the black population of Saint-Domingue, Belley was socially a man of colour: born in Senegal, he had been brought to Saint-Domingue as a slave and gained his liberty by joining the French army. By the time he embarked for France he had served many years, and would continue his military career in parallel to his political functions, first in the national convention and after the fall of the Jacobin government in the Conseil des Cinqs-Cents where he remained until May 1797. When Girodet painted him, Belley might have already handed over his mandate, while he was at the peak of his military career, and would have been in the position to commission a portrait.[80] He is represented in the costume of the revolutionary convention, thus commemorating the moment when the deputies from the colonies put the seriousness of the revolutionary claims for universal freedom and equality to the test, and made their mark in the meetings that decided the abolition of slavery.[81] Shortly after their arrival, the national convention, accepting a final speech by their spokesmen Dufay, decided that 'slavery of the blacks is abolished in all the colonies'[82] and that all men, irrespective of their 'colour', are French citizens. Slavery was abolished (a decision that was by no means uncontested at the time given the economic interests tied to slave labour in the colonies), by bringing skin colour – its very basis – to the fore. The three delegates from Saint-Domingue made their plea for inclusive equality by staging difference with their bodies' colour. As Darcy Grimaldo-Grigsby has argued, they presented themselves and were perceived as *tricolore*, thereby embodying a new symbolic meaning of the revolutionary *tricolore*.[83] Belley's singular presence in the parliament and the fact that he metonymically both embodied slavery and represented the colonies' black population, heightened the visibility of blackness.

Girodet's painting engages with these issues as it addresses skin colour and its representation with regard to its visibility and embodiment. Placing Belley next to a white marble bust of Guillaume Thomas (called Abbé) Raynal, an imitation in paint of a bust shown at the Salon of 1796, the year of the philosopher's death,[84] Girodet juxtaposed two pronouncedly different physiques. Contrasting black and white in a manner similar to the many portraits of white women with their black page especially popular in seventeenth- and eighteenth-century Britain and France, Girodet emphasised difference. At the same time the portrait brings the black subject to the fore. Leaning on the pedestal on which the bust of Raynal sits, Belley's body is put forward, slightly covering the bust. Their heads are not quite in the same scale, that in marble being larger, but they are situated at equal height, and scholars have focused on either the first, interpreting it as the marking of a difference and hierarchy between the two, or the second, preferring to see a formal arrangement which stresses their equality.[85] First of all, however, this lining up of the heads is an invitation to look in a certain way, tempting viewers into the comparative mode and judgemental connoisseurship of eighteenth-century physiognomies. But, rather than seeing the heads displayed in strict profile like the silhouettes and outline drawings illustrating Johann Kaspar Lavater's *Physiognomical fragments* or Camper's line-up of 'counterfeits' demonstrating different facial angles, we are looking at each head from a different angle, a different degree of obliqueness hindering a straight comparison. How we look at Raynal and Belley is a question of a point of view. It is possible to see in this encounter of a marble bust and the portrait of a black man a mockery of the uneven comparisons between monkeys, men and statues in which a drawing of the *Apollo Belvedere*'s head stood in for the ideal human.

The two personalities in Girodet's painting occupy different levels of reality within the image; while Belley is simply painted, Raynal is evoked via the representation of a representation. The contrast between the two is thus mediated – Raynal's whiteness is that of marble and Belley's colour that of paint – and evokes the juxtaposition of marble and flesh in many late seventeenth- and eighteenth-century art theoretical texts, especially those written by advocates of colour like de Piles. As discussed in more detail in chapter 2, de Piles declared colour the distinguishing quality of painting, and gauged its skilful use specifically around the ability to render flesh in a lifelike manner. In a good painting, stone should resemble a natural stone, while the carnations should 'appear true flesh'.[86] Girodet's painting adheres to this advice as it showcases the artist's ability to imitate materials according to their physical properties as well as his mastery of monochrome whites and monochrome shades of black, in a colourful painting overall. While Raynal is a dead philosopher commemorated in a marble bust, Belley is quite emphatically in the flesh – an aspect further emphasised by the stressing of his sexuality, his index finger pointing to the genitals showing through the tight leather trousers.[87]

The whiteness of Raynal is not that of his skin but that of the marble of which his bust is made, and the painting makes this difference very apparent as the material is mimicked very faithfully. The marble head is not simply white, but captures the marble's yellowish tone which is different from the white of the scarf around Belley's neck. Nor could the face of Belley simply be black, as the pigments used range from white for the shiny areas of nose and ear, via a yellowish tone around the temples and parts of the hairline, to brownish hues on which black is applied to form more receding parts of the face.[88] The painting emphasises both the shape of the head and the materiality of Belley's skin.

Within neoclassical aesthetics the whiteness of marble was often confounded with that of skin. It was Winckelmann who first associated the alleged whiteness of ancient marble sculptures with the ideal beauty of Greek male bodies, hence interpreting the whiteness of the stone as a marker of the physical, moral and social superiority of the ancient Greeks and by extension of the Europeans now viewed as a unified group of white people. Winckelmann credited the blossoming of the arts in ancient Greece not only to a favourable climate but also to the freedom that reigned there, an idea rather vaguely defined by Winckelmann, yet one in which revolutionary France was heavily invested.[89] Girodet himself had engaged with that imaginary ideal male beauty in his *Sleep of Endymion*, an academic nude painted while in Rome but sent to Paris for display at the only Salon under Jacobin government in autumn 1793. The sleeping nude, his beautifully drawn contours and a smooth surface undisturbed by muscles evoking the subdued eroticism of a skin touched by moonlight, embodies the ideal of 'noble simplicity and quiet grandeur' but in lacking any agency questions the politicised interpretation of Winckelmann's ideals of Greek masculinity.[90] When the portrait of Belley and the reclining nude were put next to each other at the 1797 exhibition, the paintings thus recalled, in very different ways, the moment of the radical Revolution, and cast some doubt on universal ideals of freedom, equality and Revolutionary agency, in presenting, as Viktoria Schmidt-Linsenhoff has argued, two versions of male alterity.[91] Shown side by side with both the *Endymion* and the painted bust of Raynal, Belley's physicality and colour stand out, prompting the question of how integrative the French body politic and the aesthetics of neoclassicism actually were.

In order to think about the latter, it is worth reading the *History of Ancient Art* in a more oblique way, focusing not so much on Winckelmann's predilection for the simple and smooth forms in ancient images of youthful gods, or for that matter on his depreciative remarks on the physiognomy of 'Moors'. There is a passage in which a discussion of colour and polychromy led Winckelmann to an approach to beauty more interesting from today's perspective.[92]

In Girodet's painting, neither Raynal nor Belley feature the perfect forms of ideal beauty; both are represented with the marked features of individuals, of what Winckelmann called the 'particular' as opposed to the ideal. Except for the white marble, the Raynal of this bust shares nothing with the ancient sculptures of Gods, as his physiognomy is carved pronouncedly into the stone. In Girodet's painted version even more than in the bust on which it was based the features are cut deeply into the face, making Raynal's head and neck look almost like an écorché with muscles and bones showing.

'Color contributes to beauty, but it is not beauty itself', begins Winckelmann, fully in keeping with the privileging of form over colour in idealist aesthetics, conceding that colour 'enhances beauty and its forms'. However, he continued with a praise of white, thus initially following theories of colour and light prevalent in the eighteenth century: 'Since white is the color that reflects the most rays of light, and this is most easily perceived, a beautiful body will be all the more beautiful the whiter it is, and nude it will thereby appear larger than it actually is, just as newly formed gypsum figures seem larger than the statues from which they were cast.'[93] This optical grandeur of whiteness is counterbalanced in Girodet's portrait by the black Jean-Baptiste Belley.

Winckelmann's text moves from actual persons and a praise of whiteness of skin as a physical distinction, to the whiteness of sculptures and their reproduction in plaster. Paradoxically, plaster, the underdog in the hierarchy of materials which also played such an important role in Le Blon's consideration of the reflective qualities of different materials, makes figures seem larger. While considering colour as an accessory element of beauty, and the reflective qualities of colours and materials, the attention shifts from essential qualities of things and forms to issues of their perception. In this context Winckelmann pondered the potential relativity of beauty ideals:

> A Moor can be called beautiful when his facial features are beautiful, and a traveler assures us that daily contact with Moors diminishes the untoward quality of their color and reveals what is beautiful in them. Similarly, the color of the metal or of the black or green basalt is not detrimental to the beauty of ancient heads. The beautiful woman's head in the Villa Albani would not be more beautiful in white marble; the head of Scipio [Africanus] the Elder in dark basalt in the Palazzo Rospigliosi is more beautiful than three other heads of him in marble ... A knowledge of the beautiful thus reveals itself to us even when it is in an unusual guise and in a color that in nature is displeasing: beauty is thus different from agreeableness.[94]

Of course, Winckelmann was, in the end, making an idealist argument claiming that beautiful sculptures are pleasing for their forms while colour is accidental. More than that, colour can be unpleasant and a proper appreciation requires one to see beyond colour and material. But this distinction is hard to maintain, and Winckelmann would not mention ebony, ivory, dark metal or stones in relation to skin colour if the use of non-white stone was completely arbitrary and looking beyond colour was an obvious mode of perception. The use of black marbles in European sculpture strengthened the equation between the colour of stones and that of bodies. In particular since the seventeenth century, polychrome sculpture became popular for the imagery of Africans, or, in a more allegorical sense, Africa.[95] The continent and its inhabitants were thus associated both with the precious colourfulness of the polychrome stones and the artistic skills which enhanced them, and with the solid darkness of the black marbles. In a seventeenth-century Italian pair of busts of a male and female 'Moor' for example, which entered the collections of the Louvre during the Revolution, pure black marble is used for the heads, white marble for the clothes and dark veined portoro marble for the socle (Figure 5.9). The marble is thus used somatically as the blackness of the material and that of the carved

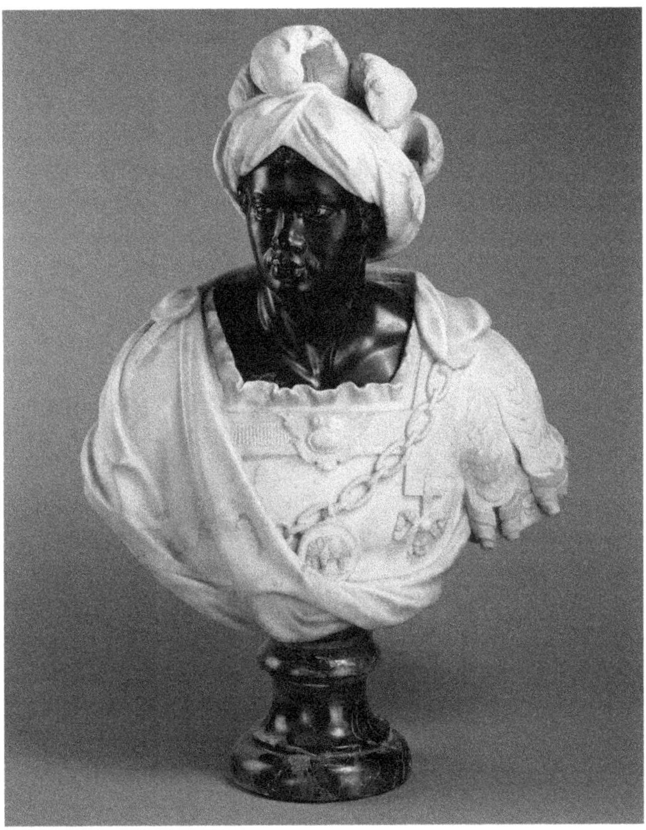

Bust of a '*Maure*', Italian seventeenth century, black and white marble, portor, 93.7 cm. 5.9

bodies blur. Even though there are ancient sculptures that deploy coloured marbles in a similar way, Winckelmann interestingly chose the example of a bust of Scipio Africanus, the sculpted head of a man whose byname does not refer to his place of origin but to the battles he won in North Africa during the second Punic War. In this case, the dark stone is used in a non-essential way, that is, to represent a person whose skin colour is different from that of the stone. What Winckelmann drew attention to is that colour is a matter of visibility, and of the way it is seen – asking us to see the beautiful 'even in unusual guise'. The text thus poses the question of how to adapt to something uncommon within a given pattern of perception. In my view, Girodet raised the same issue in presenting the audience of the 1797 and 1798 exhibitions with the challenge of looking at the image of Belley, the first and only black deputy in revolutionary France and outstanding member of the small black population in late eighteenth-century Paris.[96] The painting makes blackness as much a question of political representation as a matter of visual representation, of colour and its materiality, as it is hard not to actively see the colours in this painting. The juxtaposition with the marble Raynal makes Belley all the more colourful, highlighting the intense black and sheen of his skin, and the dashing uniform of the deputies with its sash in tricolour colours the fadedness of which adds an element of temporality. In all their differences Raynal and Belley are united as both rest on the pedestal of the bust.[97] Supporting them both, it seems a mediator between black and white – as it is painted as brown marble with striking veins and as such reminiscent of the brown marbles often used for socles in European polychrome busts of Africans.

By displaying colour in relation to various artistic media – white and coloured marble as well as paint as such, all of which had complex cultural meanings with regard to skin and flesh and its artistic imitation – the portrait of Belley makes its viewers aware of the fact that they are dealing with a representation. It emphasises Belley's liveliness almost paradoxically via the way it evokes the old art theoretical trope of the competition of painting and sculpture or colour and drawing. Made of paint and colour the figure of Belley evokes a body of flesh and blood. This painting is not just colourful but about colour, both in the sense of skin colour and colour in art theoretical terms. It is precisely via this connection that it has the potential to question prevalent neoclassical aesthetics and associated body ideals with their privileging of form and outline which co-ordinated all too well with the emphasis on physiognomy. The painting of Belley challenges neoclassical or anthropological norms of ideal beauty, as it asked the Parisian audience looking at it whether it was prepared to adapt to the sight of a black citizen. Unlike the kneeling and enchained black slave in abolitionist images, such as the 1788 seal of the Société des Amis des Noirs, who submissively begs for liberation and integration in asking 'Am I not your brother',[98] the figure of Belley in Girodet's painting has the potential to ask: 'Are you prepared to adapt to my presence?'

This possibility of changing one's view while looking at the image of Belley, was probed in a low-brow vaudeville critique, where a female figure – as was often the case in this type of art critique of the time – stands in for the spontaneous and naïve point of view and has to serve for a didactic demonstration. The woman initially exclaims: 'Oh! My God! How black he is!', to which her male companion replies: 'Wait a moment, … let's get closer: one must not judge people from their looks.' As they advance, she is prompted to concede:

> Yes, black, but not so much a devil.
> Seeing him closer I find him admirable …
> How mistaken I was.
> Yes, learned Giraudet [sic]
> This tableau pleases me![99]

This takes up a French proverb of a person who is 'pas si diable qu'il est noir' to say that they are, as the English adage goes, 'not as black as they are painted'.[100] This works with the long-standing negative associations of black with the obscure, wicked or even the devil,[101] indicating at the same time that prejudice upon first sight can be misleading. But it also shifts the meaning of 'noir', which in the proverb is an adjective for any person who looks sinister, to the designation of a person of black skin colour. If the painting pleases in the end, it is because representation and represented have managed to challenge the canon of classical beauty.

Benoist's *Portrait d'une négresse*

The fuelled reactions to Marie-Guillemine Benoist's *Portrait d'une négresse* (Figure 5.1; plate 11) shown at the Salon of 1800 take a different turn from the comments in the vaudeville critique of Girodet's portrait: the dialogue in *Le nouveau Arlequin et son ami Gilles au museum* does not result in a changed perspective:

> GILLES: Good heavens! I don't want to stay here, I have seen the devil.
> ARLEQUIN: Where that?
> GILLES: Look. …
> ARLEQUIN: What on earth can we trust,
> after such shock
> It is a white and pretty hand
> who made us this blackness.[102]

Repelled by such a terrifying sight they move on to the next painting, a mythological scene with Venus and Adonis (by Nicolas-André Monsiau), and exclaim with relief: 'There, at least a white skin. Ah! What a beautiful woman! How she caresses this beautiful tanned man who is right next to her'.[103] Together the comments on the two paintings evoke a scenario of acceptable and unacceptable touches. What made the sight of Benoist's painting so irreversibly horrible for the *Critique en vaudeville* was apparently the fact that it was painted by the hand of a woman whose skin colour did not match the blackness of her subject. A fear of contamination is induced by the thought alone of a white woman's hand touching black paint with her brush in order to make what cannot even be described as a person but is an entity entirely defined by darkness. The next painting leads back to a sanctioned arena of touches: a white male painter who made the white skin of a beautiful white woman caressing a man within a painting that establishes gender difference via a gradation of flesh tones. The way gender is mobilised in this response suggests that the diminished willingness to accept a portrait of a black person was not only due to shifts in the political atmosphere in turn-of-the-century France where pro-slavery arguments were regaining support since Napoleon had come into power, preparing the reintroduction of slavery in 1802.[104] The painting also provoked such anxieties and critical defence mechanisms because it was painted by a woman, and because of the particular ways the image of the anonymous black woman with her exposed breast addresses the viewer.

Recent scholarship has frequently discussed Girodet's Belley and Benoist's *Portrait d'une négresse* along with each other, and the comparison has often been to the detriment of the woman painter and her portrait. One of the reasons for the unfavourable assessment is that Benoist denied her model a name, thus, it is argued, denying her the status of a subject.[105] This argument though, is not without inner contradiction, because this granting of subjecthood or identity is expected from the portrait otherwise regarded (and to some extent dismissed) as the most bourgeois of genres of post-revolutionary culture.[106] How would that subjecthood be gained, other than through subjection under the paradigms of bourgeois portraiture?[107] In addition, Benoist's alleged political convictions and more so those of her family are generally taken as an indication that the black woman could hardly have been painted with an egalitarian attitude. Benoist came from a prosperous family, with a father, René Laville-Leroux, who made his career in various royal institutions. Less conventional with his daughters' education, he enabled two of them to train as artists with Guillemine initially studying with Vigée-Lebrun and in the mid-1780s along with her sister in the studio of David.[108] Her husband, Pierre-Vincent Benoist, whom she married in 1793, was a lawyer and dedicated royalist; during the post-revolutionary period he translated English novels and travel accounts while his wife supported the family with her artistic work. After Napoleon's 1799 *coup d'état* he made a career as a government official. It has been reasonably assumed that Guillemine Benoist became acquainted with the travel literature her husband translated in the year immediately before she embarked on her *Portrait d'une négresse*, for example with Mungo Park's *Travels in the Interior Districts of Africa* which appeared in Benoist's French translation in the same year his wife's painting was shown in the Louvre. This account would have made her familiar with the Scottish explorer's description of the region around the Niger river, with a largely sympathetic view of the people and their commerce, but clearly with the prospect of exploitation in mind.[109] But whatever Leroux-Benoist might have learned from this book, it is hard to say how it relates to the person and task she faced when painting the portrait of a black woman in Paris. It is assumed that the artist met her model in the household of her brother-in-law, Benoist-Cavay, where she might have been a house servant and former slave whom he had brought back from his travels to Guadeloupe. The association of the sitter with this region is supported by the painting itself, since the woman's headdress was well known from the imagery of Caribbean women slaves.[110] Benoist-Cavay was immediately involved in the administration of the French colonies, and spent long periods of time travelling.[111] The artist's family directly benefited from France's colonial enterprise, yet it is impossible to deduce the artist's attitude towards slavery and her sitter from that. Nor can it help to explain the provocation the painting presented when publicly shown.

The salon critic's hostile reaction to what they saw in the painting had little if anything to do with the family background and possible political affiliation of the artist, but rather stemmed from the simple fact that she had put a black subject on canvas. The fact that the model had no name, added, I argue, to the painting's provocation. Portraying a personality of contemporary history, as Girodet had done with Belley, was one thing, painting an anonymous black woman another. This act in itself states that a black person was worthy of a painting as such. Since the image does not take on an anthropological view representing a generic 'négresse' alongside representatives of other human varieties, this was tantamount, within the framework of neoclassical aesthetics, to stating that the sitter was beautiful. Highlighting the beauty of black people could at the time been understood as a political statement in itself, as it frequently served as an abolitionist argument.[112] Such aesthetic reasoning also worked from the other end of the political spectrum though. Jean-Baptiste Boutard, writing for the *Journal des Débats*, and the most vitriolic critic of the painting, was, it seems, so blinded by the sheer thought of a black woman represented in portrait-like manner, that he could not see its qualities of colour. He commented on the painting and in particular issues of colour almost entirely in categorial rather than specific terms, suggesting that the subject as such was not favourable for the artist's career because African faces did not offer themselves to art. They are not favourable to the 'art of the colourist', the critic continued, because 'such a figure can neither be detached from a brown ground nor be placed in harmony with a light ground; it is

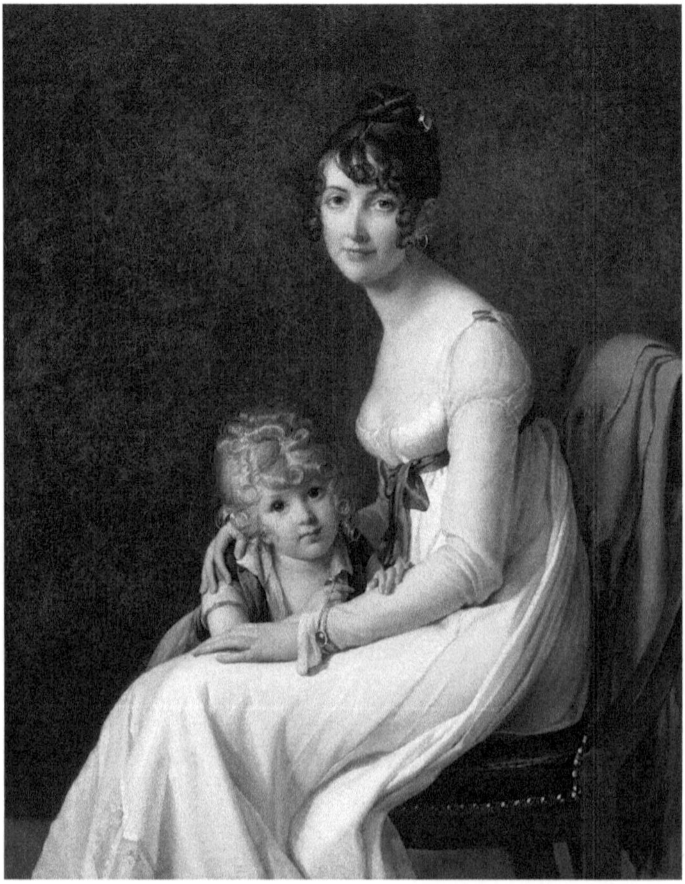

5.10 Marie-Guillemine Benoist, *Jeanne Eglé Desbassayns de Richemont, née Mourgue*, ca 1802–3, oil on canvas, 117 x 89 cm.

impossible to make the air circulate around it, because it does not lend itself to the gradation of colour and light necessary to produce this effect.'[113] In contrast to these generic reflections, Boutard became more specific and appreciative with regard to the colour blind aspects of the painting, that is, to everything that relates to drawing and composition rather than colour, lauding the way the artist posed the model and arranged the headdress as well as the rendering of the arm. It is in the execution of these elements that he saw the heritage of the artist's teacher, David. Another critic, Charles-Paul Landon, was able to make a different assessment, by hiding the subject under the formulaic language of art criticism: 'the artist knew how to take something advantageous out of the opposition of lines and flesh tones [*carnation*]. This portrait has a lot of relief.'[114]

Boutard, on the other hand, acknowledged the challenge painting a black person posed for the artist, but failed to recognise the ways it was taken on. While painting her black sitter, Benoist both embedded and extended, or even inverted, the Davidian tradition. She deployed a monochrome sand-coloured background against which the model is set rather than the grey or muddy colours she and her former teacher would use in portraits. Examples are David's 1799 *Portrait of Madame Verniac* or the *Portrait of Jeanne Eglé Desbassayns de Richemont*, now considered a work by Benoist and in all likelihood the same painting shown at the Salon of 1802 as *Portrait d'une dame*,[115] interestingly also without disclosing the name of the sitter (Figure 5.10). In the latter portrait the skin of the sitter seems exaggeratedly white, animated only by the slightly reddish cheeks, competing with the whiteness of the dress and strongly contrasted with the black hair and dark background. In the *Portrait d'une négresse* the neck and shoulder lines are drawn sharply, almost creating a silhouette against the buff background. The head is wrapped in a white cloth modulated with grey in the manner of a grisaille, framing and bringing out the face. But the juxtaposition of black and white is less pronounced than in Girodet's portrait of Belley, where the white neck scarf forms a stark contrast with Belley's black skin, as the black woman's own head casts a shadow on the white cloth, draped to dangle on one side, thus moderating the contrast. The white dress brings forth the warm tonality of the flesh tones especially around the breast where the fabric is painted in pure white. The body – posed in semi-profile with the face and exposed breast turned towards the viewer – is modulated via the gradation of tones with a yellowish brown used for the lit parts. A fairly muscular arm is put in relief by the means of this shading with the gradation of tones generally adding to the palpable physicality of a woman who can well be imagined as someone whose body is shaped by physical labour.

The exposed breast, framed by the sitter's arm and dress and pointed directly towards the viewer, is a prominent and ambiguous feature of the painting. Art historians have listed a number of associations for this motif that were within the visual horizon of the time, ranging from allegories of liberty to Raphael's *Fornarina*,[116] a painting of another woman lacking a proper name (Figure 5.11). *La Fornarina* (the baker) was thought at the time to be a portrait of Raphael's beloved and thus certainly considered an ideal beauty. The association with the *Portrait d'une négresse*, evoked by the exposed breast as well as the posing of the arms, not only compares Benoist to one of the most highly regarded artists in France but also embeds her black sitter into the European canons of ideal beauty and grace, thus questioning the implicit association of neoclassical ideals with whiteness. For those drawing this comparison, it would have been as much an aesthetic as a political provocation. This is precisely the point Boutard seemed to get, when, instead of seeing the actual painting, he denied black people the right to figure in art. The painting presented contemporary

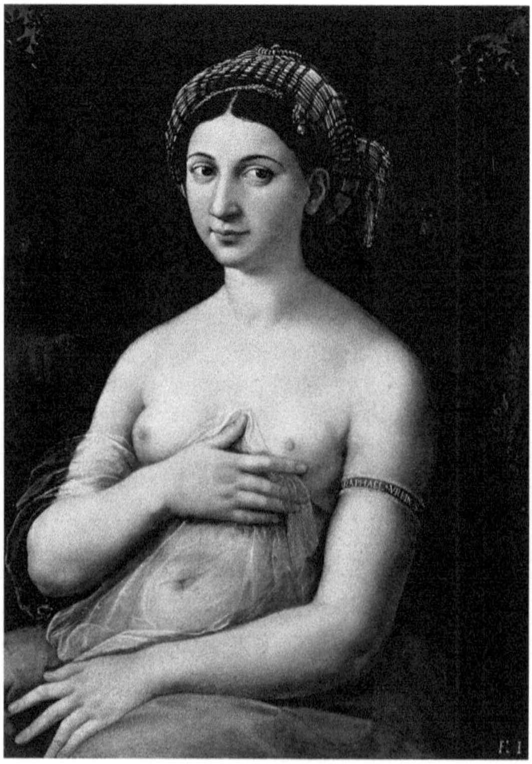

5.11 Raphael (Raffaelo Sanzio of Urbino), *La Fornarina*, ca 1516–20, oil on panel, 87.3 x 60 cm.

viewers with the question of whether they were prepared to face the presence of black men and women not only as servants but as subjects of paintings.

On a more abstract level the painting also raises the question of the integration of black women (and men) into the French national body.[117] This is evoked by the allegorical aspect of the painting that is supported by the sitter's drapery-like gown à l'*antique*, the reference to the *tricolore* (the white dress, the red belt and the blue shawl around the chair), but also the headwrap. Well known from images of the Caribbean colonies, this garment would have been associated by contemporary viewers with the West Indies and with slavery. In a pair of prints, probably issued in 1794 in response to the abolition of slavery and possibly also reacting to the slave revolts in Haiti, this headscarf takes on a significant role (Figures 5.12 and 5.13). The prints show a black man and a black woman in profile with the inscription 'Moi libre aussi', which can be understood as a statement of freedom or a plea for liberation. The female figure is even more complex, as liberation concerned not only her status as slave but also that as woman, since women – no matter what colour – were never given full

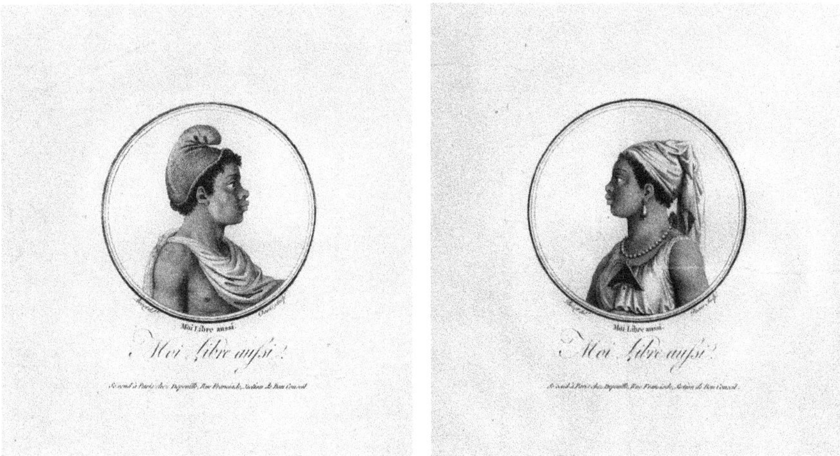

Louis Darcis after Louis Simon Boizot, 'Moi libre aussi', ca 1794, stipple engravings, 16.2 x 15.5 cm. 5.12–13

citizenship during the French Revolution. This is underlined by the prints in so far as, despite the parity in the formal arrangement within the roundel, the male figure is much more integrated into the cultural symbolism of the *French* Revolution: dressed with a chlamys (exposing his breast) and a Phrygian cap he takes part in the revolutionary adaption of antiquity. In contrast, except for the symbol of justice and equality suspended from her necklace, the black woman's dress and jewellery mark her as different on multiple levels and stress her origins from outside France. Still, the pairing of Phrygian cap and Caribbean headscarf is remarkable as it turns the latter into both a symbol of slavery and the liberation from it, like the former.[118] If the Caribbean headdress as liberty cap is a potential connotation of the *Portrait d'une négresse* then the allegorical aspect of the portrait has a liberating potential.

The exposed breast equally links the portrait to contemporary allegorical imagery. Revolutionary allegories of liberty or of the *Republique* often had one or both breasts exposed emphasising the desirability of the key revolutionary value or the nourishing quality of mother nation often conflated with *La nature*. One such allegory of nature, in an anonymous print probably issued around 1793–95, is breastfeeding a white infant on her right and a black on her left suggesting that the nation cares for people of all colours. Like the abolitionist imagery of a slave waiting to be liberated, this patronisingly stresses the generosity of the Republic in the guise of 'mother nature' represented by a white figure (Figure 5.14). A black allegory of France feeding both white and black children would have been harder to imagine, and – to my knowledge – did indeed not exist. This prompts the question what kind of offer the gesture of the frontally exposed breast of a black woman painted by Benoist actually is. It has

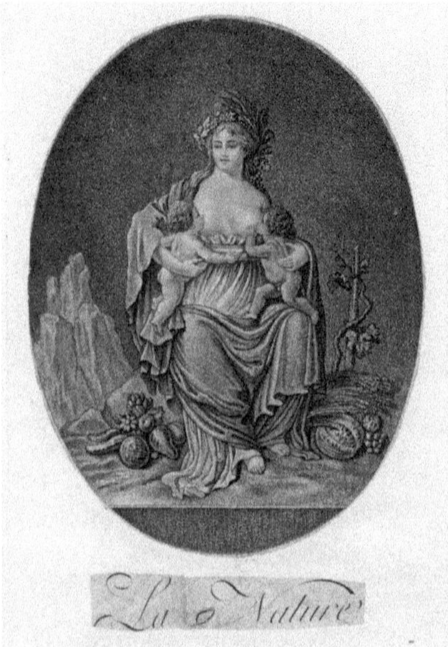

5.14 'La Nature', ca 1793–95, stipple engraving, 16.5 x 15.5 cm, printed 'chez Basset (à Paris)'.

occasionally been suggested that the laying bare of the breast might indicate the sitter's potential function as a wet nurse. It is well known, however, that wet-nursing was a highly contested issue in eighteenth-century France. In the French colonies, this Enlightenment debate and shift in attitude had its own significance and twist as it entailed, in addition, the issue of interracial wet-nursing. While the latter practice was initially regarded as beneficial for the health and robustness of the children of white colonists, it became over the course of the eighteenth century a practice condemned, not only as maternal neglect but also as a threat of racial contamination. The sixteenth-century surgeon and anatomist Ambroise Paré still thought that wet nurses should have a balanced temperament and that those with a brownish complexion – in terms of humoral theory a sign that they had more heat and vigour than women with a white complexion – were preferable, which made women from the countryside particularly well suited.[119] Similar arguments were made in the colonies where African women slaves were thought throughout the seventeenth century to be the best nurses for the colonists' offspring, as their milk was believed to foster the suckling's general health and to immunise children against tropical diseases. This attitude changed over the course of the eighteenth century, when the notion of the temperament acquired a different meaning, as a *tempérament maternel* transmitted in an almost hereditary way by the mother's milk in order to guarantee national and racial cohesion. The anxiety that came with this shift in understanding was that the child might 'Africanise' through the milk from a black wet nurse and incorporate not only the slave mentality but eventually also the colour.[120] Colonial wet-nursing thus evoked the spectre of hybridisation – which had of course (with different causes) long been a reality of the Caribbean colonies,[121] a reality that could not be domesticated so easily as the images of a harmonious tricolour union in the French motherland that circulated during the French Revolution suggest.

The vaudeville critique of the Salon, evoking the artist's white hand which made this 'noirceur', conjures a similar fear of contamination by a transmission of painterly rather than bodily fluids during which the artist took the risk of being tainted by the black paint that made her subject. The reference to the artist's hand is all the more interesting as there is something deeply unsettling about the right hand of the woman *in* the painting. Resting on the woman's lap, the fingers are flexed with the index and middle finger forming a cleft and making it look deformed. It is impossible to say whose hand is clumsy here. Has the painter got the anatomy wrong or did she skilfully paint a misshaped hand?[122] The hand, for centuries a symbol of human agency, skill and perfection, raises the question of authorship, which asserts itself in this painting just above the painted hand: the signature 'Laville-Laroux femme Benoist', naming both the artist's father and husband, is placed right above the hand of the portrayed and painted in her skin colour.[123] In order to make it discernible on the light-coloured priming, the 'white hand' had to dip her brush in dark paint again. To stand her ground, the artist had to adapt to a colour scheme determined as much by the sitter's appearance as by her own design.

In the *Portrait d'une négresse* the colour of the sitter's skin and the paint with which it was brought on to canvas are inextricably linked. And the contemporary critics seemed to perceive it exactly that way, and suggested that you couldn't possibly treat the subject without getting your hands dirty. Skin colour in both Girodet's and Benoist's portraits was simultaneously a painterly and a political matter. Rather than representing a pre-existing physical appearance, the portraitists were literally making skin colour and contributed to the fabrication of the modern perception of skin colour as an over-determined marker of difference. This understanding had gradually evolved since the seventeenth century, when the colonial exploitation of slavery, for which the contrasting division of black and white was crucial, coincided with a growing medicalisation of the question of the colour of humans. As this chapter has shown, anatomists and natural philosophers increasingly tied the body's colour to the dermis. But what this colouring matter physically consisted of – how it could be made visible and be visualised – remained an open question often still tied to the notion of complexion. How exactly skin colour and the attempts to classify humans into different races were to be mapped on to each other and how these attempts were to be squared with quests for abolition also remained issues of debate during the Enlightenment. And as much as racial classification was based on physical appearances, questions of bodily form and colour were often intersected with those of image making through drawing and colour. The arrival of emancipated slaves in the revolutionary parliament and the actual abolition of slavery between 1794 and 1802 gave those discussions a new urgency and put the revolutionary ideals of freedom and equality to the test. Confronting their audiences at this very moment and as outstanding presences in the Salon, both paintings inevitably brought skin colour (in its multiple senses) to the fore and, as the critics understood, for better or for worse, put the pressure of adaptation on those looking at them.

Notes

1 Valentin Groebner, '*Complexio*/complexion: categorizing individual natures, 1250–1600', in Lorraine Daston and Fernando Vidal (eds), *The Moral Authority of Nature* (Chicago; London: University of Chicago Press, 2004), pp. 361–83; and 'Haben Hautfarben eine Geschichte? Personenbeschreibungen und ihre Kategorien zwischen den 13. und 16. Jahrhundert', *Zeitschrift für historische Forschung*, 30 (2001), 1–17; and the chapter 'Complexio', in Steven Connor, *The Book of Skin* (London: Reaktion Books, 2004), pp. 9–48.

2 Joseph Ziegler, 'Skin and character in medieval and early Renaissance physiognomy', *Micrologus. Nature, Sciences and Medieval Societies*, 13 (2005), 511–35 (p. 532), Special issue: *The Human Skin*.

3 On colour and humoral theory in antiquity see Adeline Grand-Clément, *La fabrique des couleurs: histoire du paysage des Grecs anciens* (Paris: de Broccard, 2011), pp. 219–20; on complexions, humoral theory and eighteenth-century theories of race see Roxanne Wheeler, *The Complexion of Race: Categories of Difference in Eighteenth-Century British Culture* (Philadelphia: University of Pennsylvania Press, 2000), in particular, pp. 21–3. Elsa Dorlin discusses the significance of humoralism and the notion of 'temperament' in theories of gender difference in her *La matrice de la race: généalogie sexuelle et coloniale de la Nation française* (Paris: La Découverte, 2006) (in particular p. 24) and race (in particular pp. 229–30); in relation to art history see also Toni Halliday, *The Temperamental Nude: Class, Medicine and Representation in Eighteenth-century France* (Oxford: Voltaire Foundation, 2010).

4 Groebner, '*Complexio*/complexion', p. 379.

5 See for an interesting example, a sermon by the fifteenth-century Italian Dominican monk Gabriel de Barletta, quoted and discussed in Michael Baxandall, *Painting and Experience in Fifteenth-century Italy: A Primer in the Social History of Pictorial Style*, p. 57.

6 Wilhemina Lepik-Kopaczyńska, 'Das antike Inkarnat in der Überlieferung der mittelalterlichen Humanisten', in Johannes Irmscher (ed.), *Renaissance und Humanismus in Mittel- und Osteuropa* (Berlin: Akademie Verlag, 1962), pp. 76–83; and more recently Yvonne Schmuhl, 'Das Inkarnat in der griechischen Malerei', *RIHA Journal* 0061, 26 November 2012 www.riha-journal.org/articles/2012/2012–oct-dec/schmuhl-inkarnat.

7 Lepik-Kopaczyńska, 'Das antike Inkarnat'; Theophilus Presbyter, *De diversis artibus*, ed. and trans. C. R. Dodwell (Oxford: Clarendon Press, 1961), p. 5; see also chapter 2, pp. 21–2. On the specific pigments see Esther Pia Wipfler '"Color humanus": das Inkarnat in den Quellenschriften des Mittelalters', *Kunsttechnik und Kunstgeschichte* (2012), 48-65 (pp. 50–1).

8 With a particular clustering of studies from the 1730s onwards, see Renato Mazzolini, 'Anatomische Untersuchungen über die Haut der Schwarzen (1700–1800)', in Gunter Mann and Franz Dumont (eds), *Die Natur des Menschen: Probleme der physischen Anthropologie und Rassenkunde (1750–1850)* (Stuttgart: Gustav Fischer 1990), pp. 169–87 (p. 169). See for a short overview also Sidney Klaus, 'A history of the science of pigmentation', in James J. Nordlund (ed.), *The Pigmentary System: Physiology and Pathophysiology* (Oxford: Blackwell, 2006), pp. 5–10.

9 See on Riolan and skin colour also Klaus, 'A history of the science of pigmentation', p. 5; and Andrew S. Curran, *The Anatomy of Blackness: Science and Slavery in an Age of Enlightenment* (Baltimore: Johns Hopkins University Press, 2011), pp. 120–1.
10 Jean Riolan (the younger), *Anthropographia ex propriis et novis observationibus collecta, concinnata* (Paris: Ex officina Plantiniana, apud H. Peter, 1618), p. 139; see also the French version of this text in his *Œuvres anatomiques*, trans. Pierre Constant (Paris: Denys Moreau, 1629), p. 191.
11 Jean Riolan (the younger), *Manuel anatomique et pathologique: ou, abrégé de toute l'anatomie, & des usages que l'on en peut tirer pour la connoissance: & pour la gueri-son des maladies* (Paris: Gaspard Meturas, 1661), pp. 89 and 106.
12 See Mazzolini, 'Die Haut der Schwarzen'; Klaus, 'A history of the science of pigmentation'.
13 Mazzolini, 'Die Haut der Schwarzen', p. 175; Klaus, 'A history of the science of pigmentation', p. 6; for the British context see Cristina Malcolmson, *Studies of Skin Color in the Early Royal Society: Boyle, Cavendish, Swift* (Farnham: Ashgate, 2013).
14 Alexis Littré, ['De la structure de la peau'] in *Histoire de l'Académie Royale des Sciences*, Année MDCCII (Paris: chez Gabr. Martin, Jean-Bapt. Coignard, et les Frères Guerin, 1743).
15 Curran, *Anatomy of Blackness*, pp. 120–1.
16 A similar illustration was also used in Thomas Bartholin's *Anatomia reformata* (Leiden: Apud Franciscus Hackium, 1651), tabula II, p. 19. See in relation to the first steps of a dissection Andrew Cunningham, *The Anatomist Anatomis'd: An Experimental Disci-pline in Enlightenment Europe* (Farnham; Burlington/Vt.: Ashgate, 2010), pp. 60–2.
17 Jean Riolan (the younger), *Encheiridium anatomicum et pathologicum, in quo ex naturali constitutione partium, recessus a naturali statu demonstratur* (Leyden: A. Wyngaerden, 1649), explanation of table 1, figure 2; and its English translation *A Sure Guide, or, the Best and Nearest Way to Physick and Chyrurery … Being an Anatomical Description of the Whol Body of Man, and its Parts, with their Respec-tive Diseases*, trans. Nich. Culpeper (London: Peter Cole, 1657), p. 35.
18 François-Marie Arouet de Voltaire, 'Essai sur les mœurs et l'esprit des nations', in *Œuvres complètes de Voltaire*, new edn, ed. Louis Moland, 54 vols (Paris: Garnier frères, 1883–85), vol. 11, p. 5; see also Mazzolini, 'Die Haut der Schwarzen', p. 176; Curran, *Anatomy of Blackness*, pp. 146–7.
19 Bernhard Siegfried Albinus, *Dissertatio secunda de sede et caussa coloris Aethiopum et caeterorum hominum* (Leiden: Theodore Haak; Amsterdam: Jacobum Graall & Henricum de Leth, 1737), p. 4.
20 Mazzolini, 'Die Haut der Schwarzen', p. 176.
21 Florian Rodari (ed.), *Anatomie de la couleur: l'invention de l'estampe en couleurs* (Paris: Bibliothèque nationale de France, 1996), p. 81.
22 Ibid., p. 84.
23 Ibid.; see for a brief account of the print also Madeleine Pinault Sørensen, 'La peau de l'homme noir', *Lumières*, 14 (2009): Dossier: *L'invention et la représentation des races au 18ème siècle*, 101–14 (p. 102).
24 Rodari (ed.), *Anatomie de la couleur*, p. 144.
25 Gabriel-Antoine Gaultier, *Recherches sur l'organisation de la peau de l'homme et sur les causes de sa coloration* (Paris: chez Gabon, 1809), pp. 11–12.

26 Anne Lafont, 'Étrange étrangeté: la science au cœur de la répresentation de l'Africain', in Anne Lafont (ed.), *L'artiste savant à la conquête du monde moderne* (Strasbourg: Presses Universitaires de Strasbourg, 2010), pp. 141–56 (pp. 154–5); Londa Schiebinger, *Nature's Body: Gender in the Making of Modern Science* (New Brunswick/N.J.: Rutgers University Press, 2004), p. 196; Victor Stoichita, *L'image de l'Autre: Noirs, Juifs, Musulmans et 'Gitans' dans l'art occidental des Temps modernes 1453–1789* (Paris: Hazan and Musée du Louvre, 2014), pp. 80–1.

27 Claude Nicolas Le Cat, *Traité de la couleur de la peau humaine en général, de celle des negres en particulier et de la métamorphose d'une de ces couleurs en l'autre, soit de naissance, soit accidentellement* (Amsterdam [s. n.], 1765), p. 24.

28 Ibid., p. 74.

29 Ibid., p. 73.

30 Ibid., p. 40.

31 Lafont, 'Étrange étrangeté', p. 143.

32 Mazzolini, 'Die Haut der Schwarzen', p. 177.

33 See on this matter also the treatise by Le Cat's contemporary Jean-Joseph Sue (the elder), *Anthropotomie, ou l'art d'injecter, de disséquer, d'embaumer et de conserver les parties du corps humain* (Paris: chez l'auteur, & chez Cavellier au Lis d'or, 1765), p. 25.

34 Other eighteenth-century scholars did not look that hard and denied black people the ability to blush and with it the emotional and moral sensibility which was associated with this physical process. See Angela Rosenthal, 'Visceral culture: blushing and the legibility of whiteness in eighteenth-century British portraiture', *Art History*, 27 (2004), 563–92.

35 According to the *Oxford English Dictionary* (www.oed.com/Oxford University Press, 2015) the term was first used in the English language for the colouring matter in plants in the late eighteenth century and for humans in the 1820s. In France, it was, as far as I can see, not in use in this context before the 1830s. See for an early study Pierre Flourens, 'Recherches anatomiques sur le corps muqueux, ou appareil pigmental de la peau, dans l'Indien Charrua, le nègre et le mulatre', *Comte rendu hebdomodaire des séances de l'Académie des sciences*, 3 (1836), 700–6.

36 See on Bernier and the introduction of the modern concept of race in particular Stiep Stuurmann, 'François Bernier and the invention of racial classification', *History Workshop Journal*, 50 (2000), 1–21; and Pierre H.Boulle, 'François Bernier and the origins of the modern concept of race', in Sue Peabody and Tyler Stovall (eds), *The Color of Liberty: Histories of Race in France* (Durham/N.C.; London: Duke University Press, 2003), pp. 11–41.

37 Boulle, 'François Bernier and the origins', p. 11; see for this use of the term the entry in Jean Nicot's 1606 *Thresor de la langue francoyse, tant ancienne que moderne* (Paris: David Douceur). For a similar early use of 'race' as stock see Malcolmson, *Studies of Skin Color in the Early Royal Society*, p. 3.

38 Wheeler, *Complexion of Race*, p. 96.

39 François Bernier, 'Nouvelle division de la terre, par les differentes espèces ou races d'homme qui l'habitent', *Journal des* sçavans, April 1684, 133–40 (p. 133); and Stuurman, 'François Bernier', p. 6.

40 Bernier, 'Nouvelle division de la terre', p. 135.

41 Ibid.

42 The full title is: *Code Noir ou recueil d'edits, declartions et arrets, concernant la Discipline & le Commerce des Esclaves Nègres des Iles Françaises de l'Amérique.* See Sue Peabody, *'There Are No Slaves in France': The Political Culture of Slavery in the Ancien Regime* (New York; Oxford: Oxford University Press, 1996), here in particular p. 11; Christopher Miller, *The French Atlantic Triangle: Literature and Culture of the Slave Trade* (Durham/N.C.; London: Duke University Press, 2008).

43 Geoff Quilley and Kay Dian Kriz (eds), *An Economy of Colour: Visual Culture and the Atlantic World, 1660–1830* (Manchester; New York: Manchester University Press, 2003), pp. 9 and 2; Homi K.Bhabha, *The Location of Culture* [1994] (London; New York: Routledge, 2004).

44 Rosenthal, 'Visceral culture', p. 569; Katja Wolff, 'Schwarz-Weiß-Malerei: Beobachtungen zum Inkarnat in Bildnissen mit Mohrenpagen', in Annegret Friedrich (ed.), *Die Freiheit der Anderen: Festschrift für Viktoria Schmidt-Linsenhoff zum 21. August 2004* (Marburg: Jonas Verlag, 2004), pp. 137–44 (p. 141).

45 Viktoria Schmidt-Linsenhoff, *Ästhetik der Differenz: Postkoloniale Perspektiven-vom 16–21.Jahrhundert*, 2 vols (Marburg: Jonas Verlag, 2010), vol. 1, pp. 262–3.

46 Antoine Le Blond de la Tour, *Lettre du Sieur Le Blond de La Tour, à un de ses amis, contenant quelques instructions touchant la Peinture* (Bordeaux: P. Du Coq, 1669), p. 59.

47 As is forcefully argued by Wheeler. Focusing on British culture her *Complexion of Race* also touches upon the French debates; for Benier see p. 96.

48 Carl Linnaeus, *Systemae naturae sive regna tria naturae systematice propostia per classes, ordines, genera, & species*, 1st edn (Leiden: Theodorum Haak, 1735), and 10th edn (Stockholm: Salvi, 1758), pp. 20–2; Staffan Müller-Wille, 'Linnaeus, Carl', in *New Dictionary of Scientific Biography*, ed. Noretta Koerge, vol. 4 (Detroit; London: Thomas Gale, 2008), p. 316.

49 For Buffon, French natural history and the Jardin du Roi in the eighteenth century see Emma Spary, *Utopia's Garden: French Natural History from Old Regime to Revolution* (Chicago; London: University of Chicago Press, 2000); also Curran, *Anatomy of Blackness*, pp. 158–9.

50 Georges-Louis Leclerc, Comte de Buffon, *Histoire naturelle, générale et particulière, avec la description du Cabinet du Roy*, 15 vols (Paris: Imprimerie Royale, 1749–67), vol. 1, p. 36. See also Claude Blanckaert, 'La classification des races au XVIIIe siècle: l'anthropologie naturaliste entre méthode et anti-méthode', *Lumières*, 14 (2009), pp. 3–41', p. 26, Special issue: *L''invention et la représentation des races au XVIIIe siècle.*

51 Buffon, *Histoire naturelle*, vol. 3, p. 371. See Blanckaert, 'La classification des races', pp. 26–7.

52 Pierre Cabanis, *Rapports du physique et du moral de l'homme*, 2 vols (Paris: Crapart, Caille et Ravier, 1802), p. 478. See Blanckaert, 'La classification des races', p. 27.

53 Blanckaert, 'La classification des races', in particular, p. 41; and further Wheeler, *Complexion of Race.*

54 See Curran, *Anatomy of Blackness*, pp. 169–76; as well Isabelle Baudino's introduction to the special issue *L'invention et la représentation des races au XIIIe siècle* (*Lumières*, 14 (2009)), p. 7; and, in the same issue, Blanckaert, 'La classification des races', pp. 13–14; David Bindman, *Ape to Apollo: Aesthetics and the Idea of Race in the 18th Century* (Ithaca/N.Y.: Cornell University Press, 2002), pp. 11 and 17.

55 This is also pointed out by Schmidt-Linsenhoff, 'Klassizismus und Sklaverei',

p. 180; Bindman, *Ape to Apollo*, pp. 12 and 202–5; and specifically for Camper, Miriam Claude Meijer, *Race and Aesthetics in the Anthropology of Petrus Camper (1722–1789)* (Amsterdam: Rodopi, 1999), pp. 55–61.

56 I am quoting from Meijer's translation of the lecture in *Race and Aesthetics*, pp. 190 and 192. See for the French translation Petrus Camper, *Œuvres qui ont pour object l'histoire naturelle, la physiologie et l'anatomie comparée*, 3 vols (Paris: H.-J. Hansen, 1803), vol. 2, unpaginated.

57 Hence the title of the lecture in the English edition: *The works of the late Professor Camper on the Connexion between the Science of Anatomy and the Arts of Drawing, Painting, Statuary, in two books*, trans. T. Cogan (London: C. Dilly, 1794). The French edition is: *Dissertation physique de Mr. Pierre Camper, sur les differences réelles que présentent les traits du visage chez les hommes de différents pays et de différents ages; sur le beau qui caractèrise les statues antiques et les pierres gravées*, trans. from the Dutch by Denis Bernard Quatremere D'Isjonval (Utrecht: B. Wild et J. Altheer, 1792).

58 Camper, *The works of the late Professor Camper*, p. 2.

59 See on Camper's 'artistic background' and his lectures at the Amsterdam Drawing Academy Meijer, *Race and Aesthetics*, pp. 87–100.

60 Camper, *The works of the late Professor Camper*, p. 1.

61 Ibid., pp. 1–7. See also Bindman, *Ape to Apollo*, p. 208; and in more detail Nicholas Grindle, 'Our own imperfect knowledge: Petrus Camper and the search for the "Ideal Form"', *RES: Anthropology and Aesthetics*, no. 31 (spring 1997), 139–48.

62 Camper, *The works of the late Professor Camper*, p. 99.

63 Meijer, *Race and Aesthetics*, in particular, p. 46; Bindman, *Ape to Apollo*, pp. 205–9.

64 Camper, *The works of the late Professor Camper*, p. 13.

65 Jean-Joseph Sue (the younger), *Essai sur la physiognomonie des corps vivans, considérée depuis l'homme jusqu'à la plante* (Paris: l'auteur, 1797), pp. i–ii.

66 Ibid., p. vii.

67 Melanie Ulz, *Auf dem Schlachtfeld des Empire: Männlichkeitskonzepte in der Bildproduktion zu Napoleons Ägyptenfeldzug* (Marburg: Jonas, 2008), p. 18.

68 Ibid., in particular pp. 123–38; Darcy Grimaldo Grigsby, *Extremities: Painting Empire in Post-Revolutionary France* (New Haven; London: Yale University Press, 2002), pp. 105–63.

69 Sylvain Bellenger (ed.), *Girodet 1767–1824* (Paris: Gallimard; Musée du Louvre Éditions), pp. 384–97; Grimaldo Grigsby, *Extremities*, pp. 105–63.

70 Sue (the younger), *Physiognomonie*, pp. 57–8.

71 Ibid., p. 75.

72 Ibid., p. 80.

73 Ibid., p. 86.

74 Ibid., p. 82; for the varieties of *basané* see pp. 80–5.

75 Ibid., p. 81.

76 See Astrid Reuter, *Marie-Guilhelmine Benoist: Gestaltungsräume einer Künstlerin um 1800* (Berlin: Lukas Verlag, 2002), pp. 55 and 113–14.

77 Bellenger (ed.), *Girodet*, p. 322; Helen Weston, 'Representing the right to represent: the portrait of citizen Belley, ex-representative of the colonies by A.-L. Girodet', *RES: Anthropology and Aesthetics*, no. 26 (autumn 1994), 83–99 (p. 83).

78 Jeremy Popkin, *A Concise History of the Haitian Revolution* (Malden/Mass.: Wiley-Blackwell, 2012), p. 2.

79 Ibid.

80 Even though there is (as yet) no conclusive answer to the question whether Belley might have commissioned the portrait, Anne Lafont has suggested that it is quite plausible; see her article 'Les rencontres hypothétiques du peintre et de son modèle: clefs sociales dans l'interprétation du tableau', in Anne-Lise Desmas (ed.), *Les portraits du pouvoir: actes du colloque organisé par Olivier Bonfait et Brigitte Marin* (Paris: Somogy, 2003), pp. 115–25 (pp. 123–5).

81 For the biography of Belley see Bellenger (ed.), *Girodet*, pp. 327–8; Lafont, 'Rencontres hypothétiques', pp. 120–3.

82 Quoted from Popkin, *Concise History of the Haitian Revolution*, pp. 66–7; more comprehensively on the three delegates and the abolition of slavery Jeremy Popkin, *You Are All Free: The Haitian Revolution and the Abolition of Slavery* (Cambridge: Cambridge University Press, 2010), here in particular pp. 327–73.

83 Grimaldo Grigsby, *Extremities*, pp. 14–16.

84 Bellenger (ed.), *Girodet*, p. 328.

85 See in particular Grimaldo Grigsby, *Extremities*, pp. 37–8; and Helen Weston, 'Girodet's *Portrait of C. Belley: Ex-Representative of the Colonies*: in remembrance of "Things Sublime"', in Adrian Forty and Susanne Küchler (eds), *The Art of Forgetting* (Oxford: Berg, 1999), pp. 75–92 (p. 82).

86 Roger de Piles, *Dialogue upon Colouring*, trans. Mr. Ozell (London: printed for Daniel Brown and Bernard Lintott, 1711), p. 39, see in more detail chapter 2, pp. 23–9. On the contrast between marble and flesh in the painting see also Viktoria Schmidt-Linsenhoff, 'Klassizismus und Slaverei: zum Funktionswandel kultureller Differenz in A. L. Girodet's *Portrait du Citoyen Belley* und M. G. Benoit's *Portrait d'une Négresse*', in Hansjörg Bay and Kai Merten (eds), *Die Ordnung der Kulturen: zur Konstruktion ethnischer, nationaler und zivilisatorischer Differenzen 1750–1850* (Würzburg: Könighausen & Neumann, 2006), pp. 173–93 (p. 174); Grimaldo Grigsby, *Extremities*, pp. 37–42.

87 Grimaldo Grigsby, *Extremities*, pp. 55–6; Weston, 'Representing the right to represent'; also Lafont, 'Étrange étrangeté', p. 151; Bellenger (ed), *Girodet*, pp. 331–2.

88 For other detailed descriptions of the rendering of the skin, see Lafont, 'Rencontres hypothétiques', p. 116; and Grimaldo Grigsby, *Extremities*, p. 46.

89 Alex Potts, *Flesh and the Ideal: Winckelmann and the Origins of Art History* (New Haven/Conn.; London: Yale University Press, 1994), in particular p. 225.

90 See more extensively on the *Endymion*, Mechthild Fend, *Grenzen der Männlichkeit: der Androgyn in der französischen Kunst und Kunsttheorie zwischen Aufklärung und Restauration* (Berlin: Reimer, 2003), pp. 60–76; as well as Whitney Davis, 'The renunciation of reaction in Girodet's Sleep of Endymion', in Norman Bryson, Michael Ann Holly and Keith Moxey (eds), *Visual Culture: Images and Interpretations* (Hanover; London: University Press of New England [for] Wesleyan University Press, 1994), pp. 168–201.

91 Viktoria Schmidt-Linsenhoff, 'Male alterity in the French Revolution: two paintings by Anne-Louis Girodet at the Salon of 1798', in Ida Blohm, Karen Hagemann and Catherine Hall (eds), *Gendered Nations: Nationalism and Gender Order in the Long Nineteenth Century* (Oxford; New York: Berg, 2000), pp. 81–105, wrongly refers to the Salon of 1798, although the paintings were displayed together only in the Elysée exhibition; this does however not derogate her overall argument. See

Ann Lafont, 'Un portrait entre cliché racial et émancipation sociale', in Desmas (ed.), *Les portraits du pouvoir*, pp. 110–13 (p. 111).

92 See on both these aspects also Potts, *Flesh and the Ideal*, pp. 158–64.

93 Johann Joachim Winckelmann, *History of the Art of Antiquity*, trans. Harry Francis Mallgrave, introd. Alex Potts (Los Angeles/Cal.: Getty Research Institute, 2006), p. 195.

94 Ibid., p. 195. See also the comments on this passage in Johann Joachim Winckelmann, *Schriften und Nachlaß*, ed. Akademie der Wissenschaften und der Literatur, Mainz; Akademie der gemeinnützigen Schriften zu Erfurt; Winckelmann-Gesellschaft, vol. 4.3 (Mainz: Philipp von Zabern, 1996), pp. 207–8; and Reuter, *Benoist*, p. 206.

95 See for further examples and discussion David Bindman and Henry Louis Gates (eds), *The Image of the Black in Western Art*, 5 vols (Cambridge/Mass.: Belkap Press, 2010–14), vol. 3, part 1–3.

96 For official numbers see Peabody, *'There Are No Slaves In France'*, in particular pp. 72–87; more subjective accounts suggest however that numbers could be perceived as much higher and some scholars stress the public visibility of black servants in cities like Paris, see Reuter, *Benoist*, p. 198.

97 While the bust itself was inspired by Espercieux's bust of Raynal, the pedestal of brown marble seems to be Girodet's addition. See on the brown marble Grimaldo Grigsby, *Extremities*, p. 23, who associates it with the mulatto.

98 Ibid., pp. 28–9; Schmidt-Linsenhoff, *Ästhetik der Differenz*, vol. 1, pp. 167–8; Susan H. Libby, 'The color of Frenchness: racial identity and visuality in French anti-slavery imagery, 1788–94', in Adrienne L. Childs and Susan H. Libby (eds), *Blacks and Blackness in European Art of the Long Nineteenth Century* (Farnham; Burlington/Vt.: Ashgate, 2014), pp. 19–45 (pp. 23–9).

99 Anon., *La vérité en riant ou les tableaux traités comme ils le méritent, en vaudevilles* (Paris: Marchand, n.d.) [Collection Deloynes, vol. 19, no. 529, pp. 648–9].

100 The proverb is listed identically but with slight shifts in its explanation, under the entry 'Noir', in all editions of the *Dictionnaire de l'Académie française* between 1694 and 1798.

101 Wheeler, *Complexion of Race*, pp. 1–4.

102 [Author unknown] *Le nouveau Arlequin, et son ami Gilles au museum* (Paris: Chez Lacroix), p. 9, no. 275 [Collection Deloynes, vol. 22, no. 624, p. 327]. See on this critique Reuter, *Benoist*, pp. 206–7, and Grimaldo Grigsby, *Extremities*, p. 59.

103 *Le nouveau Arlequin*, p. 9, no. 275 [Collection Deloynes, vol. 22, no. 624, p. 327].

104 This is discussed in more detail by Helen Weston, '"The cook, the thief, his wife and her lover": La Ville-Leroulx's *Portrait de Négresse* and the signs of misrecognition', in Valerie Mainz and Griselda Pollock (eds), *Work and the Image* (Aldershot: Ashgate, 2000), pp. 53–73; Grimaldo Grigsby, *Extremities*, pp. 57–8.

105 Most pronouncedly in Weston, '"The cook, the thief, his wife and her lover"', pp. 53–73; or Griselda Pollock, *Differencing the Canon: Feminist Desires and the Writing of Art's Histories* (London; New York: Routledge, 1999), pp. 297–300; James Smalls, 'Slavery is a woman: "race", gender and visuality in Marie Benoist's *Portrait d'une négresse* (1800)', *Nineteenth-Century Art Worldwide*, 3:1 (2004).

106 See in particular Tony Halliday, *Facing the Public: Portraiture in the Aftermath of*

the French Revolution (Manchester; New York: Manchester University Press, 1999), especially, pp. 195–7.

107 I am using the term 'subjection' following Judith Butler's reading of Foucault in *The Psychic Life of Power: Theories of Subjection* (Stanford/Cal.: Stanford University Press, 1997).

108 See Reuter, *Benoist*, pp. 25–52, 109–103; more generally on David's women students Mary Vidal, 'The "other atelier": Jacques-Louis David's female students', in Melissa Hyde and Jennifer Milam (eds), *Women, Art, and the Politics of Identity in Eighteenth-Century Europe* (Aldershot; Burlington/Vt.: Ashgate, 2003), pp. 237–61.

109 Mungo Park, *Travels in the Interior Districts of Africa: Performed Under ... the African Association, in the years 1795, 1796, and 1797* (London: printed by W. Bulmer and Co. for the author, 1800); see also Reuter, *Benoist*, pp. 198–9.

110 Smalls, 'Slavery is a woman'.

111 This is the generally accepted assumption, see in particular Reuter, *Benoist*, p. 198; Grimaldo Grigsby, *Extremities*, pp. 59–60.

112 Schmidt-Linsenhoff, *Ästhetik der Differenz*, vol. 1, p. 163; Viktoria Schmidt-Linsenhoff, 'Who is the subject? Marie-Guilhelmine Benoist's *Portrait d'une Négresse*', in Agnes Lugo-Ortiz and Angela Rosenthal (eds), *Slave Portraiture in the Atlantic World* (Cambridge: Cambridge University Press, 2013), pp. 315-43 (p. 322).

113 Baron Jean-Baptiste Boutard, 'Salon de l'an VIII: portraits peints par les femmes', *Journal des Débats* (6 brumaire l'an IX [1800]), pp. 1–2 [Collection Deloynes, vol. 22, no. 632, p. 2]. I largely followed Grimaldo Grigsby's translation, in *Extremities*, p. 42

114 Charles-Paul Landon, 'Peinture: Exposition du Salon au Musée', *Journal des arts, des sciences et de littérature*, 94 (20 Brumaire l'an IX [1800]), pp. 339–41 [Collection Deloynes, vol. 23, no. 635, p. 399].

115 Margaret A. Oppenheimer, 'Three newly identified paintings by Marie-Guillemine Benoist', *Metropolitan Museum Journal*, 31 (1996), 143–50.

116 Reuter, *Benoist*, pp. 212–14; Schmidt-Linsenhoff, *Ästhetik der Differenz*, vol. 1, p. 169; Schmidt-Linsenhoff, 'Who is the subject?', p. 329.

117 Schmidt-Linsenhoff, *Ästhetik der Differenz*, vol. 1, p. 166; Schmidt-Linsenhoff, 'Who is the subject?, p. 325.

118 Smalls, 'Slavery is a woman'.

119 Dorlin, *Matrice de la race*, pp. 156–9.

120 Ibid., pp. 203–9, Dorlin refers in particular to Landais, *Dissertation sur les avantages de l'allaitement des enfans par leurs mères* (Genève; Paris: Méquignon, l'ainé 1781).

121 See among others Renato Mazzolini, 'Las castas: interracial crossing and social structure, 1770–1835', in Staffan Müller-Wille and Hans-Jörg Rheinberger (eds), *Heredity Produced: At the Crossroads of Biology, Politics, and Culture, 1500–1870* (Cambridge/Mass.; London: MIT Press, 2007), pp. 349–73; Claude Blanckaert, 'Of monstrous Métis? Hybridity, fear of misrecognition, and patriotism from Buffon to Paul Broca', in Peabody and Stovall (eds), *The Color of Liberty*, pp. 42–65.

122 I would not go as far as suggesting the hand looks like a claw, as have done Schmidt-Linsenhoff, *Ästhetik der Differenz*, vol. 1, p. 177, or Weston, '"The cook, the thief, his wife and her lover"'; also Schmidt-Linsenhoff, 'Who is the subject?', p. 336.

123 Schmidt-Linsenhoff, *Ästhetik der Differenz*, vol. 1, p. 177; Schmidt-Linsenhoff, 'Who is the subject?', p. 336.

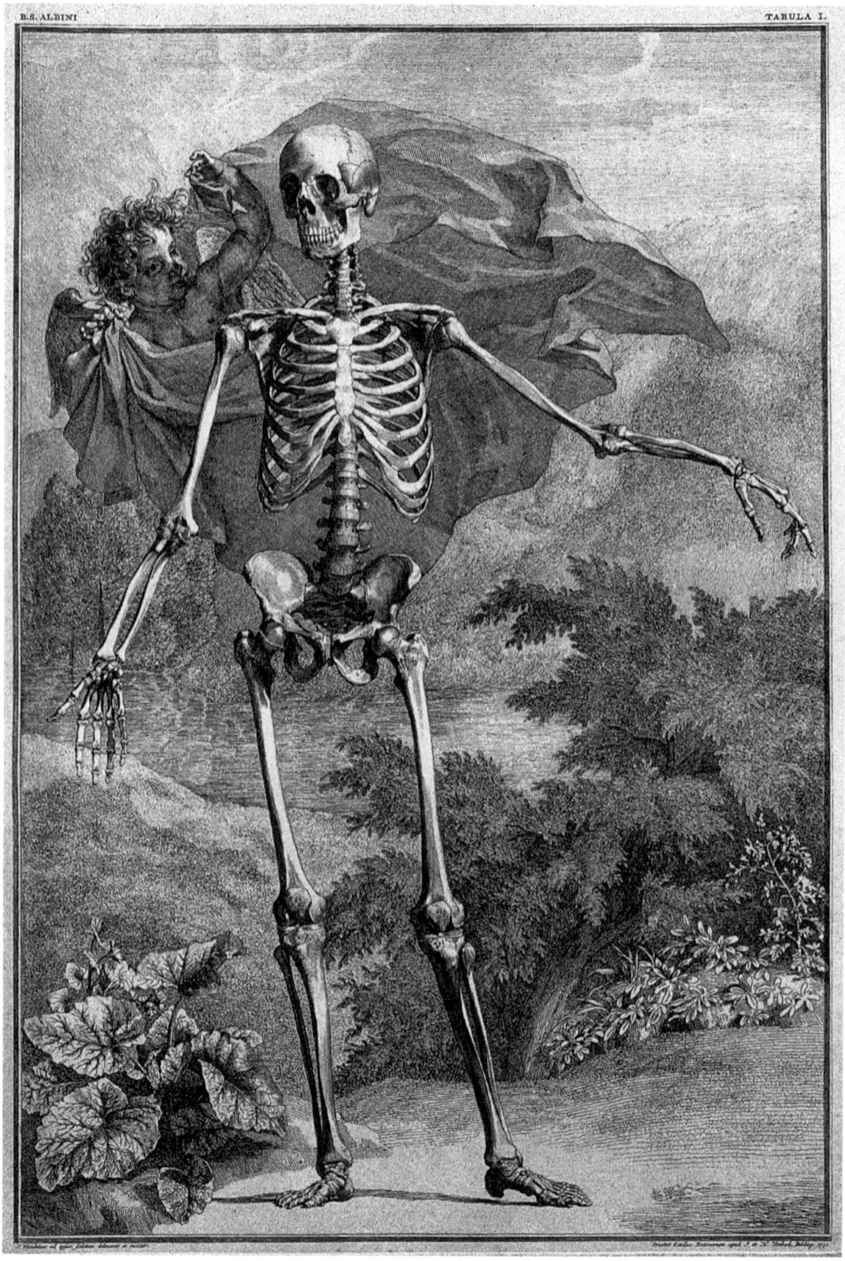

6.1 Jan Wandelaar, Putto unveiling a skeleton, from Siegfried Albinus, *Tabulae sceleti et musculorum corporis humani*, 1747, frontispiece, engraving, 56 x 39.8 cm (platemark).

Seeing through the skin 6

'If you wish to succeed in drawing, it is essential to study the body even to a great level of detail', stated Jean-Joseph Sue the younger in his 1788 *Élémens d'anatomie, à l'usage des peintres, des sculpteurs et des amateurs.* Then still working as assistant to his eponymous father, professor of anatomy at the Académie royale de peinture et de sculpture, Sue stressed the significance of anatomical study for artists and continued that they should 'curiously and observantly eye all the parts of the body, both internal and external, that compete [concours] to form the subject'.[1] The choice of the verb *concourir* prompts some ambivalence here, as it might indicate that inner and outer parts work together harmoniously to 'form the subject' or that they are in competition with each other. In its latter sense it points towards a potential tension between the inner and outer parts of the body, a conflict brought out by the practices of observation. While typically studying and representing the human body as it appears from the outside, covered by the skin, artists were expected to be aware of the bones and muscles that give the body its proportions and shape.

Indirectly, Sue's text also addresses a dilemma at the heart of anatomical knowledge production, whether pursued by artists or medics: in order to understand the structure and working of the living human one has to go through the corpse. Indeed, Sue insisted that artists should pursue the messy business of dissection, that they should

> have carried the scalpel through the labyrinth of this beautiful machine, gone through, visited and interrogated all its routes; have contracted and relaxed all its muscles; have confirmed via the sense of touch, all its forms and minute protruberances; have dismounted and mounted again the different pieces of the edifice of bones; have disjoined and rejoined the articulations … hence know the entire interior mechanism in order to better grasp the changes it can cause on the exterior.[2]

In the end though, all this hands-on exercise with the human marionette is aimed at the eye and a fantasy of translucency: 'one renders nature much more

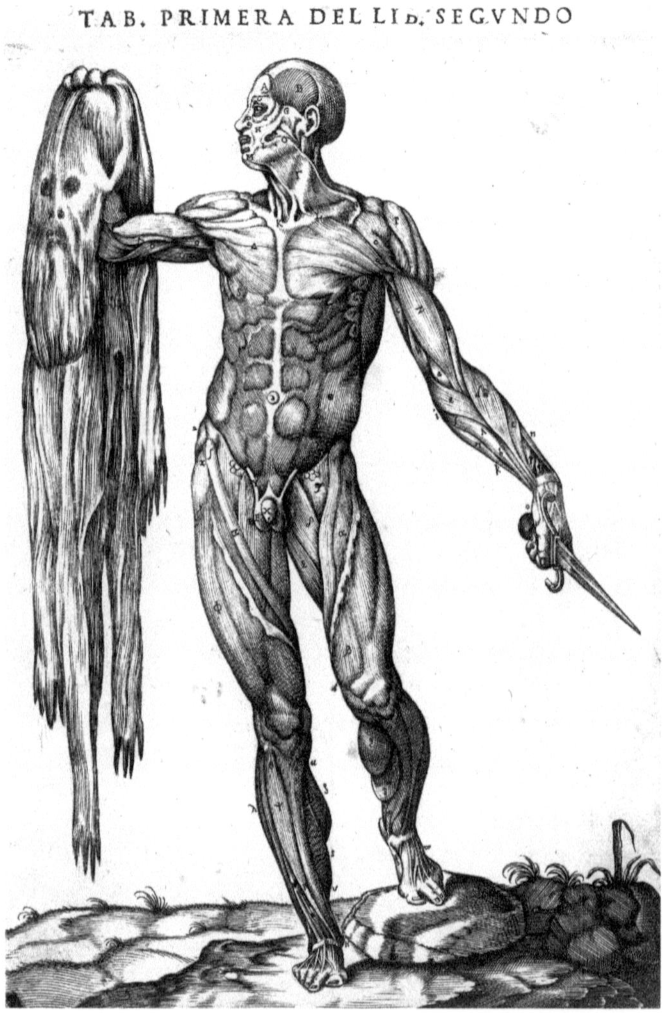

6.2 Gasparo Beccera (attributed to), Male figure with flayed skin, from Juan Valverde de Amusco, *Historia de la composition del cuerpo humano*, 1556, engraving.

faithfully if one sees it act through the veil in which it is covered. The more an artist is instructed on anatomy, the more this veil will be transparent for him.'[3]

Stressing the significance of expert guidance, Sue justified his own position and underlined the significance of artistic anatomy. In doing so, he heavily drew on the rhetoric of transparency that was highly prominent during the Enlightenment and which gained political urgency during the pre-revolutionary period. At the same time, Sue mobilised well-known tropes of anatomical parlance and imagery and used the metaphor of the veil that has to be lifted or rendered transparent in order to retrieve 'nature'. A similar symbolism is at stake in Jan Wandelaar's frontispiece for Albinus's prominent 1747 *Tabulae sceleti et musculorum* in which a flying putto lifts a cloth from a skeleton, thus theatrically staging anatomy and the anatomical atlas it preludes as instruments of revelation (Figure 6.1). In the context of anatomical knowledge production the veil, which has the potential to hide and disclose, has a bodily equivalent – the skin – which has to be removed in order to gain access to what is often understood and privileged as the inner truth of the human body. As Bohde has pointed out in relation to images of flaying, anatomy had been shaped since the sixteenth century by a metaphysics of interiority which was accompanied with a hierarchy of inside and outside, body and soul. The artist's acquaintance with anatomy was regarded as more than just a knowledge of bones and muscles, but as an insight into nature's compositional plan, itself associated with the conceptual aspect of *disegno*.[4] The skeleton and, to a lesser degree, the muscles were regarded as the essence of the body while skin was merely an envelope, an opposition that could still be conflated with the art theoretical notion of drawing versus colour during the nineteenth century.

However, there were also significant transformations in the theories and practices of artistic anatomy, and skin was at the very heart of them. As a veil and cover, skin itself frequently became a metaphor for the challenges in the artistic interpretation of the body. This chapter will discuss the ways in which the organic and metaphoric function of skin is played out in nineteenth-century medical discourse, and more specifically in the discourse, practices and imagery of artistic anatomy. Traditionally, skin had to be physically or symbolically removed to give way to insights into the body's interior. In contrast, nineteenth-century artistic anatomy directs the eye increasingly on to the body's surface and makes the artist look at a veil that remains physically intact. Artistic anatomy stresses the aesthetic role of skin and its contribution to the shaping of the human form. As much as the emerging life sciences of the time, the discipline is obsessed with the body as living entity. And in continuation of a process which started in eighteenth-century medicine, and vitalist medicine in particular (as discussed in chapters 3 and 4), skin is increasingly perceived as an active organ. This acknowledgement further challenges the desire to gain access to the body's inner secrets, and I will raise the question how this obstacle is dealt with in the discourses of artistic anatomy and the practices of artistic observation.

Looking at the body via a living tegument which wraps and shapes it, but which is also rendered semi-transparent via the projection of medical knowledge on to it, artistic anatomy develops methods of teaching that could – in theory – make dissection obsolete. Yet, one of the paradoxes of nineteenth-century artistic anatomy in France is that it focused on the exterior forms of the body, while the professors of artistic anatomy at the École des beaux-arts in Paris dissected and demonstrated on the cadaver more than ever before.[5] Leaving this latter aspect aside though, this chapter will concentrate on a new kind of artistic anatomy, called anatomy of exterior forms. New illustrated publications stressed the significance of the body's surface and developed iconographies that put a new regime of visual observation into place. I will discuss this shift in focus, from looking into a skinless body to looking on to the surface, and argue that this transformation goes along with a re-distribution of inside-outside relations during which skin becomes a potential hermeneutic barrier, as well as a metaphor for the transmission of knowledge and a medium for its communication.

Anatomy without skin

As a discipline predominantly concerned with the interior formation of the body, anatomy tended to pay little attention to the human skin as an organ. Since the sixteenth century anatomy produced its knowledge first and foremost via the practice of cutting into the dead body. In its etymology and early modern understanding, anatomy was more or less synonymous with dissection, and Denis Diderot and anatomist Pierre Tarin writing in the *Encyclopédie* followed a well-established tradition when referring to it as 'the art of dissection'.[6] The medical dismantling of the body typically begins with a cut through the human tegument, and many anatomical illustrations stage the opening of the body as a process of unpeeling that starts with the skin.[7] Along with the actual material practice of opening the body, the removing of its physical envelope also became a symbol of the unveiling of the body's secrets, and thus associated with anatomical knowledge production as such.[8] The well-known illustration showing a flayed man standing in *contrapposto* and triumphantly holding his skin for Juan Valverde de Amusco's 1556 *Historia de la composition del cuerpo humano* is a self-conscious representation of anatomy as a discipline that looks beyond the skin (Figure 6.2). This anatomical body is formed and held together by well-defined muscles, apparently without the need for an exterior envelope. The figure is reminiscent of iconographies of flaying, as in scenes of the flaying of the martyr Bartholomew or the mythological satyr Marsyas, but, with a knife in its own hand, suggests an act of heroic self-peeling.[9] This 'rhetoric of self-dissection' was widespread in anatomical images of the sixteenth century.[10] In a period when anatomy also became, as Katharine Park has suggested, 'an invitation to reflect on what it meant to be human – to be not only mortal, fragile, and prone to illness but also part of a divine plan', the images allowed viewers to envisage this reflection as an act of self-dissection.[11] While scenes of self-dissection became less frequent in subsequent centuries, peeled off and hanging or folded back skin

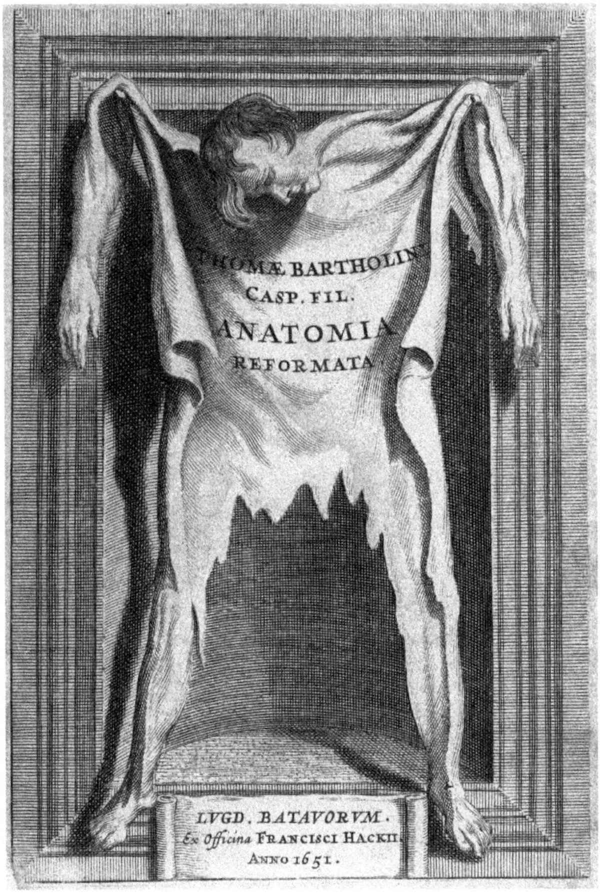

Human skin hanging from a frame, from Thomas Bartholin, *Anatomia reformata*, 1651, frontispiece, engraving, 15.5 x 10.5 cm (platemark). 6.3

remain recurrent motifs in anatomical imagery, for example in the illustration for Riolan's *Encheiridium* of a male figure with opened abdomen (Figure 5.2, discussed in the previous chapter), or in one of Gérard de Lairesse's illustrations for Bidloo's 1685 *Anatomia humani corporis* where skin hangs off bodies like rags with a pelt-like interior (Figure 2.10). A skin entirely removed from the human body featured frequently on the title pages of seventeenth-century anatomical tracts printed in the Netherlands, such as Thomas Bartholin's 1651 *Anatomia reformata* (Figure 6.3). The removal of the tegument stands here for anatomical knowledge production, and the opening of the book at this skin-page is aligned with the opening of the corpse for dissection, turning the anatomical book as a whole into a corpus.[12] In these front pages the letters of the title are printed on the skin thus recalling the usage of skin as parchment,

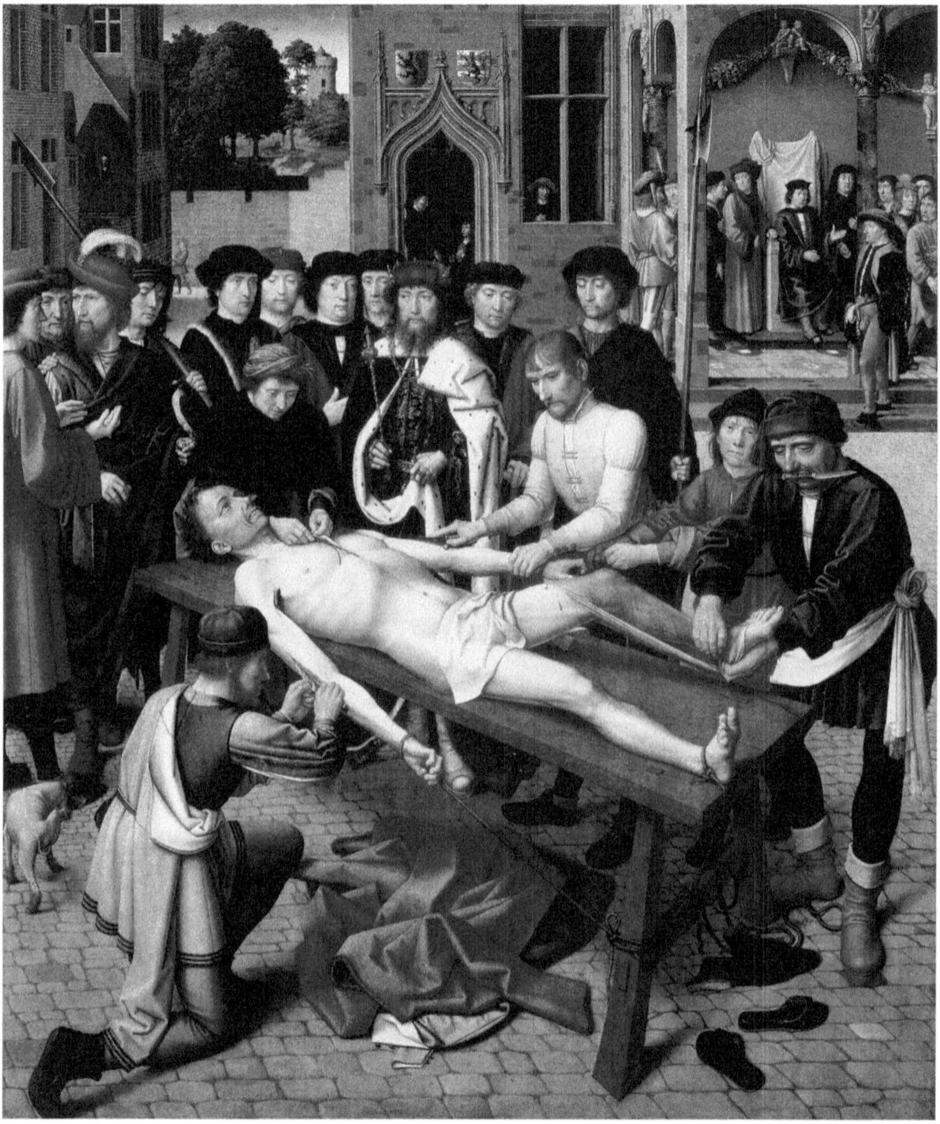

6.4 Gerard David, *The Flaying of Sisamnes*, 1498, oil on canvas, 182.2 x 159.2 cm.

in which the skin is the medium carrying the words or illuminations. But in the anatomical title pages, skin is more than just a medium and material support aligned with the pages of the anatomy book; it also hints at the violent aspect of anatomical knowledge production. The motif is, as Bohde has argued, related to the iconography and story of the judge Sisamnes, known especially from Gerard David's late fifteenth-century diptych (Figure 6.4). Sisamnes' punishment for corrupting the law was to be flayed alive with his skin serving thereafter as a moral warning as it was displayed above or served as a lining for the chair of future judges. On the title pages of anatomies the skin is equally evocative of guilt and punishment, and emphasises the ties between anatomy and jurisdiction.[13]

While images of *écorchés* displaying their bare muscles were prominent in anatomical illustrations, actual bodies were probably seldom flayed entirely in medical dissections. It was a different matter when artists started dissecting in the late fifteenth century (and Leonardo and Michelangelo were famed for having done so). Artists were more specifically concerned with the layers just underneath the skin, the configuration of the exterior muscles mainly responsible for the outer appearance of the body. With the formation of art academies, beginning with the Florentine Accademia del disegno and the Accademia di San Luca in Rome, anatomy was institutionalised as part of art training, and the study of the external and internal form of the human body as practised in life drawing and dissection became a core element of *disegno*.[14] It is unlikely that many art students actually carried out dissections themselves or even followed dissections, but the ideal art academy as envisaged in many early modern drawings and prints includes dissection and often specifically flaying. A late sixteenth-century drawing of an academy scene by Jan van der Straet (or Giovanni Stradano) for example, which circulated in print, prominently shows the flaying of a body hanged from a scaffold: an elderly, bearded person (looking like a scholar rather than a student) is in the final stages of removing a male corpse's skin, and his thick spectacles emphasise minute observation along with the manual skills in handling the knife (Figure 6.5). The écorché is prepared for study, and a young artist with his drawing utensils in hand looks attentively at the écorché's leg, the eyes directed towards a further operator's fingers grabbing the dead body and seemingly removing some last pieces of skin. The print makes an issue of the studious and violent aspects of artistic anatomy simultaneously.

The French Académie, following the example of the Italian art academies, included anatomy in its curriculum from its foundation in 1648. The actual teaching, however, remained rather patchy for more than a century. The surgeon François Quatroulx, in charge of the training in anatomy from the outset, started proper courses only in 1666 and, according to the limited existing sources, used among other things a skeleton, plaster casts of body parts taken from a flayed male corpse and anatomical prints from atlases such as Vesalius's *Fabrica*.[15] In addition, interested artists had the opportunity to follow dissections and demonstrations offered once a year in the Jardin du Roi. These anatomical performances enjoyed royal patronage, were public and free of charge and proved, depending on the anatomist and demonstrator concerned, very popular.[16] Whether a knowledge of anatomy was useful for

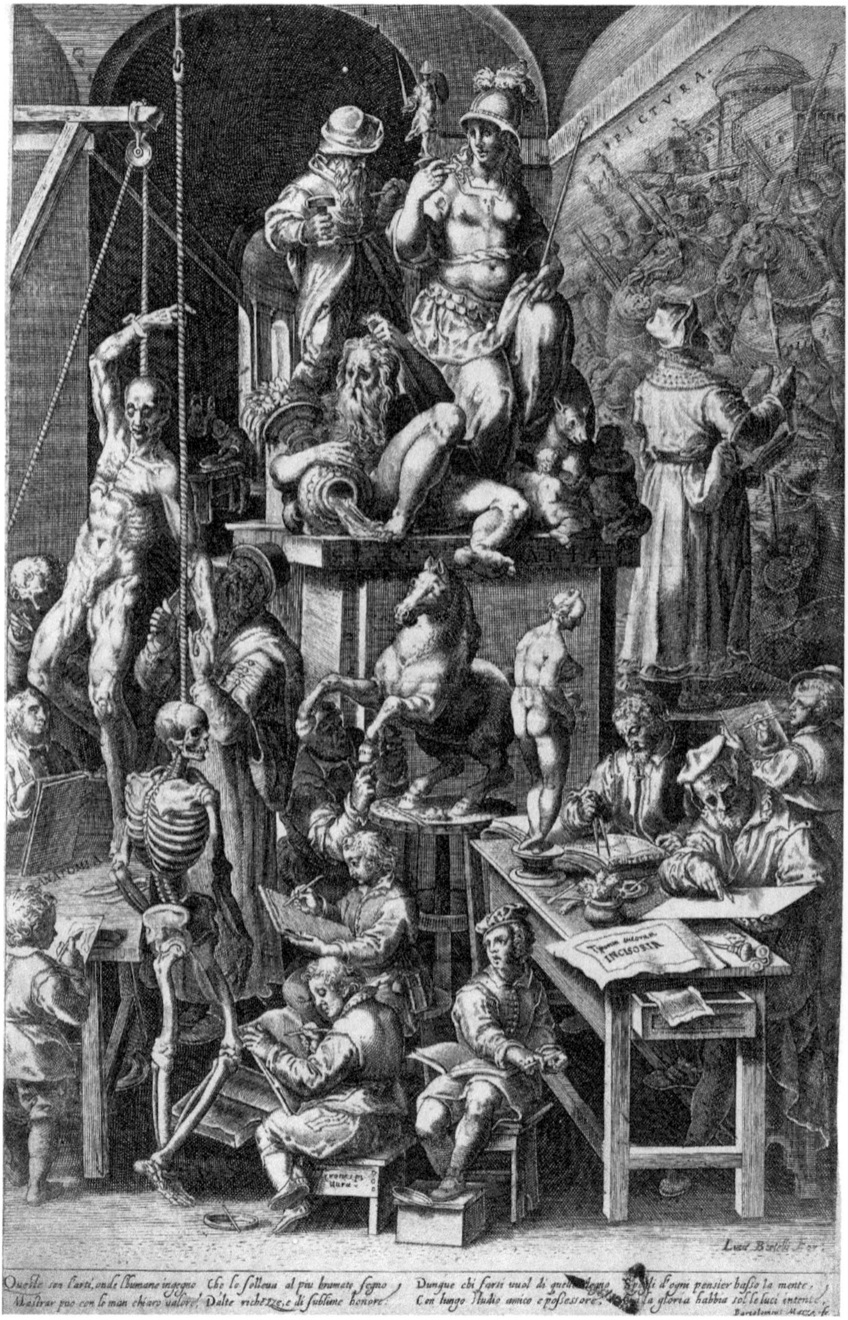

6.5 Bartolomeo Mazza after Jan van der Straet, *Art Academy*, ca 1580, engraving, 45.4 x 29.5 cm.

artists was, however, always a subject to debate. In mid-eighteenth-century France there was a lively critical debate as to what degree artists needed this kind of specialist knowledge, and art critics such as La Font de Saint-Yenne favoured invention and mastery of colour over scrupulous observation and technical skills that can hardly be acknowledged and assessed by a non-specialist audience of amateurs. With characteristic polemical verve, Diderot considered it even dangerous to look underneath the skin.[17]

The Académie royale pursued, around the same period, a different policy and the teaching of anatomy for artists was taken more and more seriously. During the second half of the eighteenth century, after Sue (the father) had been promoted to professor of anatomy at this institution, a more rigorous and sustained teaching was provided, and from 1772 onwards Sue offered an anatomy course to art students with demonstrations alongside the dissected body in the lecture theatre of the Charité hospital in Paris. This strengthening of artistic anatomy coincided in 1774 with the appointment of the Comte d'Angiviller as director of the Bâtiments du Roi, in charge of royal art commissions and the Académie. D'Angiviller himself initiated academy reforms, demanding respect for the *règlement* and the routines of life drawing. A promoter of a new classicism, he reiterated the significance of history painting and its pivotal element: the male nude.[18] The *nouveau règlement* of the Academy threatened students not attending the anatomy course with sanctions. In addition, following a proposition by the *conseiller* of the academy, Maurice Quentin de La Tour, a Prix de la demi-figure peinte (also known as Prix du torse) was instituted in 1776. For this competition, students were asked to work towards a painted, life-size study of a male torso, taking the following steps: to first draw from the academy's écorché – at this time probably a version of the écorché by the sculptor Houdon – to then work from the life model from different angles, and finally to take these up again to render the figure as if 'flayed' and to indicate the muscles' names.[19] Thus art students were being asked to use observational techniques in combination with anatomical knowledge in order to simultaneously look on to and through the skin, to visually and manually (by drawing and painting) de-flesh and re-flesh the body. This enterprise was aided by a new course running in parallel to the dissections at the Charité and taught in one of the academy's drawing rooms, where Sue demonstrated anatomy alongside the life model.[20] As his son proudly mentioned in his *Élémens d'anatomie* he thus adopted a method that William Hunter had already practised in his courses at the Royal Academy in London.[21] In the aftermath of the French Revolution anatomy moved even further into the heart of the Parisian art institutions. The anatomy theatre installed at the Louvre (parts of which had been transformed into a public museum in 1793) was close to the premises of the former Académie royale, provisionally re-named École de dessin and to become the École des beaux-arts. In 1804 the anatomy theatre moved with the institution to the Collège des Quatre-Nations, just across the Seine.[22]

Among the tools used for teaching artists the composition of the human body, anatomical illustrations played a major role; and until the nineteenth century artists would more or less study the same images as anatomists and medical students, and just focus on plates with particular interest for the purposes of the visual arts, usually the skeletons and muscle-figures. The first French anatomical atlas explicitly addressing artists was the 1667 *Abrégé d'anatomie, accommodé aux arts de peinture et de sculpture* published under the name of the painter and member of the Académie François Tortebat.[23] The successful volume, re-edited several times during the eighteenth century, has

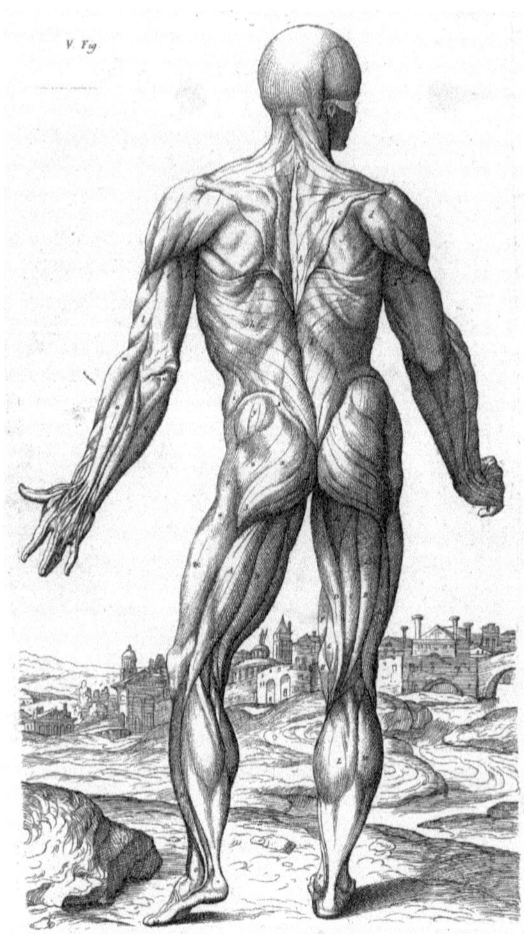

6.6 Muscle figure after Vesalius from François Tortebat, *Abrégé d'anatomie*, 1667, figure 5, engraving, 42.3 x 25.5 cm.

twelve pages of illustrations drawn and engraved by Tortebat after Vesalius's *Fabrica* and its accompanying book, the *Epitome* (also 1543). The adaptation to artistic purposes lies mainly in the condensation of the textual explanations provided and in the reduction of plates to three skeletons and seven écorchés displaying the outer and inner layers of muscles in various views, and the addition of two nudes (Figure 6.6).

The introduction discusses the necessity of a special anatomy treatise for artists. While anatomical knowledge is considered 'absolutely necessary for the perfection of art' given that the human body is 'the most noble object for painting', it concedes that a certain economy is appropriate and that tracts written for physicians have more detailed information than is required by artists.[24] Consequently, the medical explanations provided are in the abridged and clearly laid out form of tables, indicating the medical terms for each of the human muscles and their position in relation to other body parts as well as their function. For the bones a brief general description of their location and function, and a legend referring to the images of the skeleton is provided.

The introduction, moving between addressing artists, draughtsmen and more specifically painters, interestingly challenges the more traditional association of anatomy and drawing, in making a claim for the anatomical expertise of a famous colourist: Titian. It is thus likely that Roger de Piles, who soon claimed authorship for the introduction, was indeed involved in the production of the *Abrégé*'s text or at least its preliminaries.[25] The text first anticipates objections to the artistic study of anatomy by referencing the then familiar critique of Michelangelo, an artist particularly associated with his anatomical knowledge and his expertise in muscular nudes, according to which excessive study of bones and muscles puts the artist at risk of falling into a 'crude and dry manner'.[26] These doubts are immediately dispelled, in order to emphasise the relevance of the tract's endeavour by stressing that the life model cannot be adequately seen and understood without a knowledge of the muscles and their functions. The challenge is thus – as still expressed in Sue's artistic anatomy – the integration of surface observation and anatomical knowledge in order to turn the individual, imperfect body of the (in the academic context always male) model into that of the functional and aesthetically pleasing universal human it stands in for.

The inclusion of the familiar concern about excessive anatomical study and the mentioning of Michelangelo, serve finally to bring in Titian as the model artist who not only had anatomical knowledge but also knew how to conceal it. As generally in the seventeenth century, the Venetian painter is assumed to be the draughtsman of 'the beautiful anatomical figures' for Vesalius's works.[27] This attribution serves in this case not so much to prove the artistic quality of the plates (as in some twentieth-century art historical texts) as to attest Titian's anatomical knowledge and to single him out as an artist who perfectly balanced his understanding of internal structures and external forms. He 'possessed anatomy' but did 'nevertheless paint flesh with great delicacy and tenderness'. The general warning of the *Abrégé* is to 'not forget that the muscles are covered by the skin which softens them, and renders them more or less perceptible depending on the age and sex'.[28] Skin is thus considered as the natural covering for a vital but unsightly interior. Moving swiftly from this point to Titian's painterly practice, the text suggests that this smoothing function is taken over in painting by the making of flesh with paint – the production of *carnations* lending the bodies *morbidezza*.

As generally in early modern art theory, flesh is emphatically associated with life and lifelikeness, while skin can have both aesthetic and softening functions but is often evoked as a removable cloth, something to be removed to gain anatomical insight. The description of the figure demonstrating the external muscles states: 'This figure is denuded of the skin, the fat, the fleshy membrane, the nerves, veins and arteries that are on the surface of the body.'[29] It went on to suggest that the écorché had been deliberately drawn for artists by Titian. Yet, this didn't fully tackle the conflict of insight and aspect. Only the construction of Titian as both anatomically aware and expert in the rendering of lifelike flesh solved this problem for the *Abrégé*.

A few anatomical illustrations of that period more specifically designed for artists tried to address the conundrum of integrating the dead and live body with a particular pictorial solution. The first among them were images by Chrysostome Martinez, a Spanish anatomist and draughtsman who, apparently with the intention of producing an anatomical atlas directed at both physicians and artists, made a set of eighteen original anatomical etchings. Of these, only two became well known as they were re-issued by Martinez as engravings in 1689 in Paris, and reprinted there in 1740 and in 1780 for the Académie (Figure 6.7).[30] As later drawings inspired by them suggest, they were used for artistic study and teaching.[31] The distinctive feature of Martinez's images is that they show several views of the human body simultaneously. One print, predominantly concerned with proportions, features a male figure in back, side and front view showing alternately bones, muscles – and especially in the face – the body covered by skin. They invite one to see the body as a space made up of various partly intertwined layers, something the user of atlases such as Vesalius's *Fabrica* and versions of it could only do mentally, by flipping through the illustrated pages of the book and combining the insights of distinct images of bones, and internal and external musculature. The second print focuses on different views of human bones. In a lower zone, on what seems to be the plinth of a tomb, bones are represented for their own sake, as they are lined up individually and often cut up to display the marrow in some detail. On top of the architectural platform beyond, bones are articulated to form animated skeletons in a variety of 'as-if-alive' poses; such representations

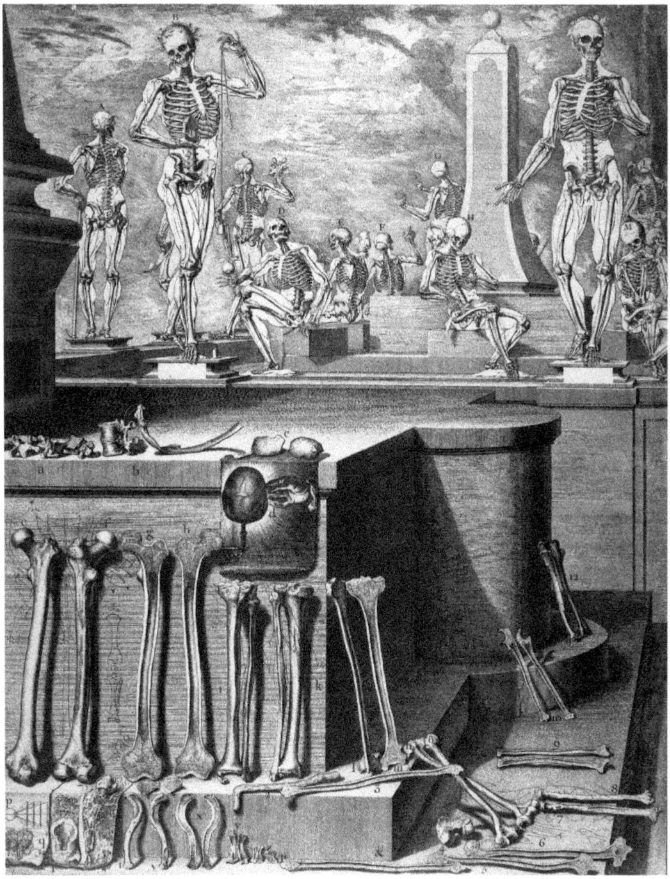

Chrysostome Martinez, *Skeletons in monumental architecture*, 1689, engraving, 68.5 x 53.5 cm. 6.7

frequently occur in early modern anatomical atlases. Each skeleton is underlain, though, by a white form in the shape of a human figure, and all are set against a background of weather phenomena in various shades of grey. This produces an effect of transparency, as if the skeleton could be seen through flesh made of glass. Given the graveyard setting, they can simultaneously be seen as resurrected, held together by their virtual shape rather than reincarnated in flesh.

Later in the second half of the eighteenth century, this attempt to provide images that render the skin transparent was taken up in the artistic anatomies by the sculptor Edme Bouchardon and the physician Johann Heinrich Lavater (the physigonomist's son).[32] The three osteological engravings by Gabriel Huquier were initially drawn by Bouchardon, according to the editor's preface, after the skeleton in the Académie. They show the bones surrounded by flowing lines forming the outer shape of the figure and not restricting it to a two-dimensional outline. This results in an interlacing of lines, an image of flowing features, rather than the illusion of a firm but transparent masculine body, and might be one of the reasons why later historiographers of anatomical illustrations such as Ludwig Choulant had little positive to say about Bouchardon's images.[33] Possibly in an attempt to bring more clarity into this mode of anatomical visualisation, Lavater introduced the use of two colours – a sanguine red besides the usual black ink – into his illustrations (Figure 6.8). They indicate the bone structure in relatively bold black lines while the shapes of exterior forms are subtly alluded to by reddish lines. Fading into the background though, they don't quite hold the pieces of the partial skeleton together.

These figures seem, in one way or another, to take issue with the curious liveliness of articulated skeletons prevalent in anatomical illustrations of the sixteenth to eighteenth centuries without ever being able to resolve its paradoxes. The skeleton is, of course, never a natural entity whether as a three-dimensional object made of prepared bones or when represented in a two-dimensional image. It is a re-assemblage of the durable parts of a human or animal body and as such, as anthropologist Elizabeth Hallam has suggested,

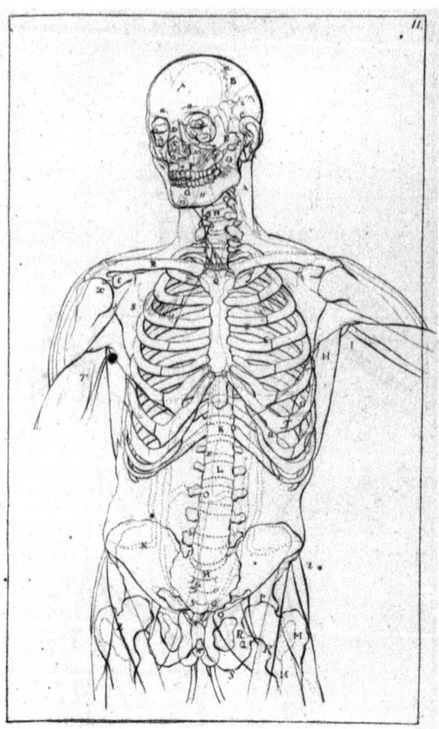

6.8 Muscles and skeleton of the human torso, from Johann Heinrich Lavater, *Élémens anatomiques*, 1797, plate 11, engraving, 21 x 12.5 cm (platemark).

an articulation in the double sense of the term 'as a properly joined body, and articulation of intelligible speech or language'.[34] The many skeletons moving through anatomical prints as if alive articulate medical knowledge about the body's bony structure and resurrect the dead body on which anatomy as 'art of dissection' is based. Often staged as animate emblems of mortality themselves, they can simultaneously recall and defy death. This way of dealing with anatomy's conundrum and the discipline's limited ability to access the vital body became increasingly problematic with the gradual development of modern medicine and associated imagery which understood itself as scientific and objective and took an ever more fervent interest in the physiological operations of the body and the understanding of life itself. Yet the conflict between the desire to comprehend life and the means of achieving knowledge about it were certainly not resolved by nineteenth-century medicine and physiology. On the contrary, revolutionary and post-revolutionary French medicine (as discussed in chapter 4), working under the shadow of the guillotine or with the guillotine as an experimental machine, only got closer to the cut between life and death.

Flaying ancient sculptures

An alternative visual strategy to engage with the deadness of the anatomical body was, as I will argue in what follows, the addition of an outline holding the skeleton together and turning it into a fully shaped figure. Even though introduced before, this device only became widespread during the nineteenth century and turned the animated skeleton into a living body imagined as transparent. It was particularly prevalent in artistic anatomy, a discipline that developed an independent genre of medical textbooks during the nineteenth century.[35] While the contour holding together the bones and defining the body's shape became increasingly diagrammatic, it was also more explicitly identified with the physical envelope of the body: the skin. This is most clearly the case in Jean-Galbert Salvage's *Anatomie du Gladiateur combattant* published in 1812 (Figure 6.9). The project systematically pursued a strategy of artistic anatomy that had occasionally been employed before, as it anatomises famous ancient sculptures, in this case the *Apollo Belvedere* and more prominently the statue of a fighting warrior known as *Borghese Gladiator*, by imagining the bone and muscle structure underneath the marble surface (Figure 6.10).[36]

Salvage's *Anatomie* is a patriotic and imperial enterprise through and through. The author of both text and plates was a graduate of the medical faculty of Montpellier who served as a surgeon for the republican army, and continued to work as a military surgeon in various Parisian hospitals after his return from the battlefields in 1796.[37] With the ambition of putting his anatomical knowledge into the service of the arts as well, he took drawing lessons, and in 1804 he submitted a prospectus, the manuscript and the drawings for

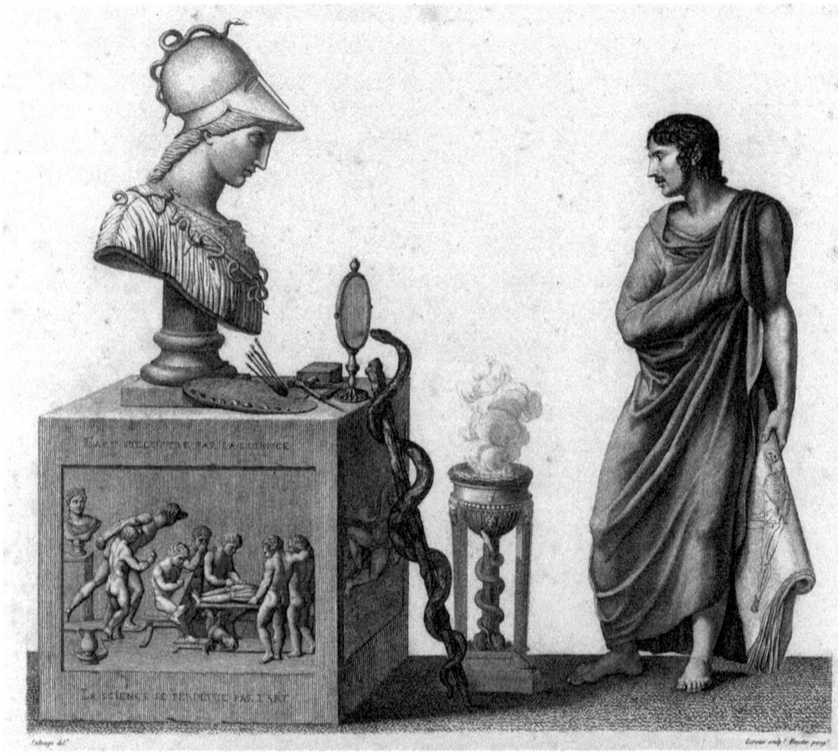

6.9 Lervoux after Jean-Galbert Salvage, frontispiece from *Anatomie du Gladiateur combattant*, 1812, engraving, 33.5 x 37.5 cm (platemark).

an atlas to the Classe des beaux-arts of the Institut de France (the institutional successor of the Académie royale). The relevant committee, of which Jacques-Louis David and Jean-Antoine Houdon were members, welcomed the *Anatomie du Gladiateur* without reservation, stating in their report that there had never been a comparable work of that quality.[38] Despite this official approval it took eight years until the atlas was finally printed, complete with engravings by Jean Bosq after Salvage's drawings. Purchased by the French State for its art schools in Paris and the provinces, it became the leading artistic anatomy in early nineteenth-century France.[39] Featuring anatomical insights into the *Borghese Gladiator* and the head of the *Apollo Belvedere*, it appropriated two ancient sculptures which had not only been models of artistic study and emulation ever since they were unearthed in the sixteenth and early seventeenth centuries; they had also ranked high in the neoclassical canon of ancient masterpieces and were as such targets of Napoleon's art appropriations in the aftermath of the 1796–97 Italian campaign and the later French occupation of parts of Italy.[40]

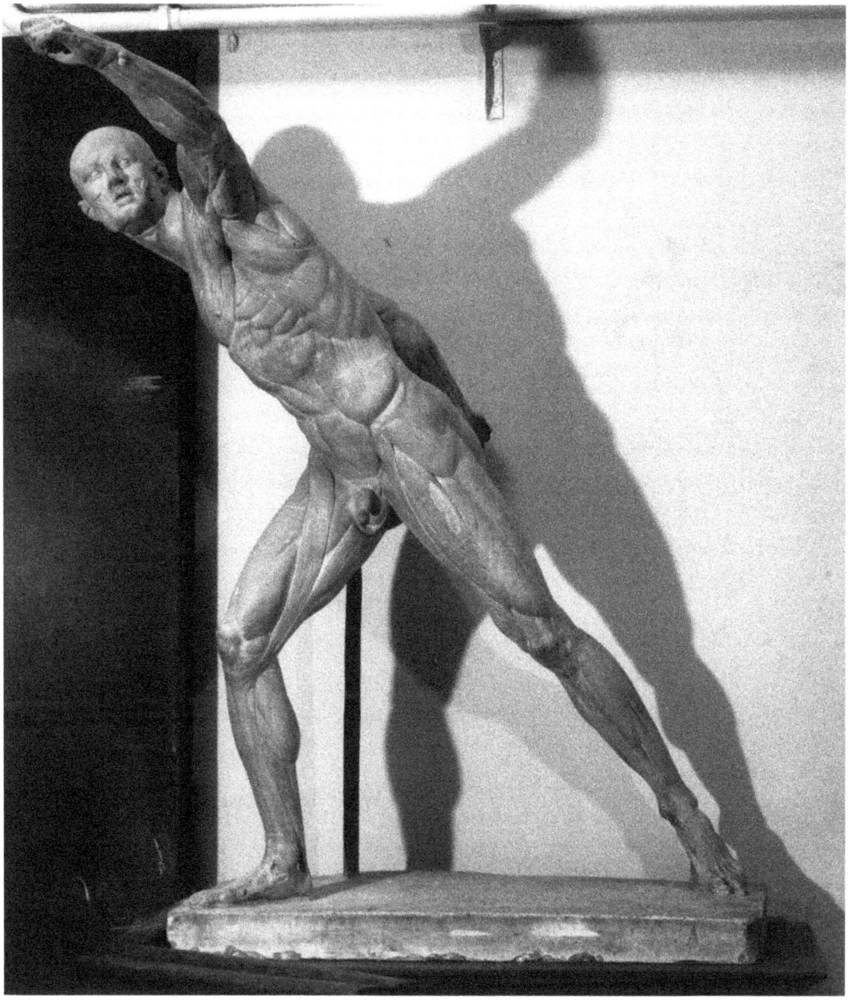

Jean-Galbert Salvage, Écorché copy of the *Borghese Gladiator*, 1804, plaster, 150 cm. 6.10

Even though Salvage would finally re-equip his drawn écorchés and skeletons with a contour serving as virtual skin, dissection and flaying were at the basis of his project. This is highlighted in the frontispiece for the work (Figure 6.9), which features a male figure – the author's idealised self-projection as a man in ancient gown and the straight lines of what was considered a Greek profile. With anatomical drawings in hand, he is worshipping a bust of Athena, goddess of wisdom and the arts, and surrounded by symbols of art, beauty and medicine. Athena's pedestal is decorated on the front side with an inscription celebrating the collaboration of art and sciences, which is visually emphasised by a relief that stages putti performing a dissection while another, to their left, chisels a sculpture in the shape of the *Borghese Gladiator*. One of the putti attending the dissection, or more precisely the flaying of a cadaver, is holding his nose, to indicate the smell such an enterprise entails. The frontispiece thus not only promotes the necessity of artistic anatomy but also affirms the self-heroisation of Salvage who stressed the hardships of the tasks he undertook to create the atlas and écorchés in his introduction.[41] The anatomist had easy access to corpses from healthy young men due to his post at the military hospital in Paris established at the former convent Val-de-Grâce, and he dissected numerous bodies to study the arrangement of muscles and bones when put in the pose of the *Borghese Gladiator*. He also produced three casts taken from bodies of young soldiers flayed in this position, soldiers whose bodies were relatively unharmed, as Salvage explained, since they had died in a duel.[42] In a close interaction of anatomical and artistic practices, the same procedures were applied to a cast of the ancient sculpture itself, when Salvage carved into the plaster to make an écorché figure displaying the virtual musculature of the *Gladiator*. Three casts taken from the flayed dead soldiers in the pose of the sculpture were purchased by the École des beaux-arts in 1811 and remained in the school's anatomy theatre until the early twentieth century.[43]

While the peeling of the actual skin of the cadaver or its plaster version (in the cast made from the sculpture) was crucial for Salvage's research into the formation of the *Gladiator*'s skeleton and musculature, in Salvage's drawings and the engravings for the atlas the bodies are resealed with a contour. If Salvage's studies were literally made over the dead bodies of the Napoleonic battlefields, the illustrations resurrect intact male bodies taking the ideal shapes of an ancient warrior and reanimate them via the *Gladiator*'s dynamic pose.

In the illustrations for the *Anatomie du Gladiateur* Salvage equipped the skeletons and écorchés with an outline indicating the outer confines of the ancient sculpture thus also reasserting a completeness the statue itself has never had in post-ancient times, given that it had – like most ancient marbles – only survived in fragmented form. While the plates engaging with the muscles and bones of the head and neck take another famous sculpture, the *Apollo Belvedere*, as a model for anatomical study, plates five to fifteen show the *Gladiator*, highlighting different anatomical elements: the skeleton, the interior musculature and the exterior musculature each seen from various angles. (Figure 6.11, plate 14a–b). The prints deploy a two-colour system to differentiate between elements of the body: bones are systematically printed in black, muscles in a sanguine red. The text of the legend referring to the respective parts of the body also uses this distinctive colouring in the letter print. In addition, the use of sanguine – with all its associations of blood – recalls the living (or dead) fleshiness of these parts, imbuing the abstracted contour with a residue of the *carnations*. Beyond this symbolism of sanguine however, the two-colour

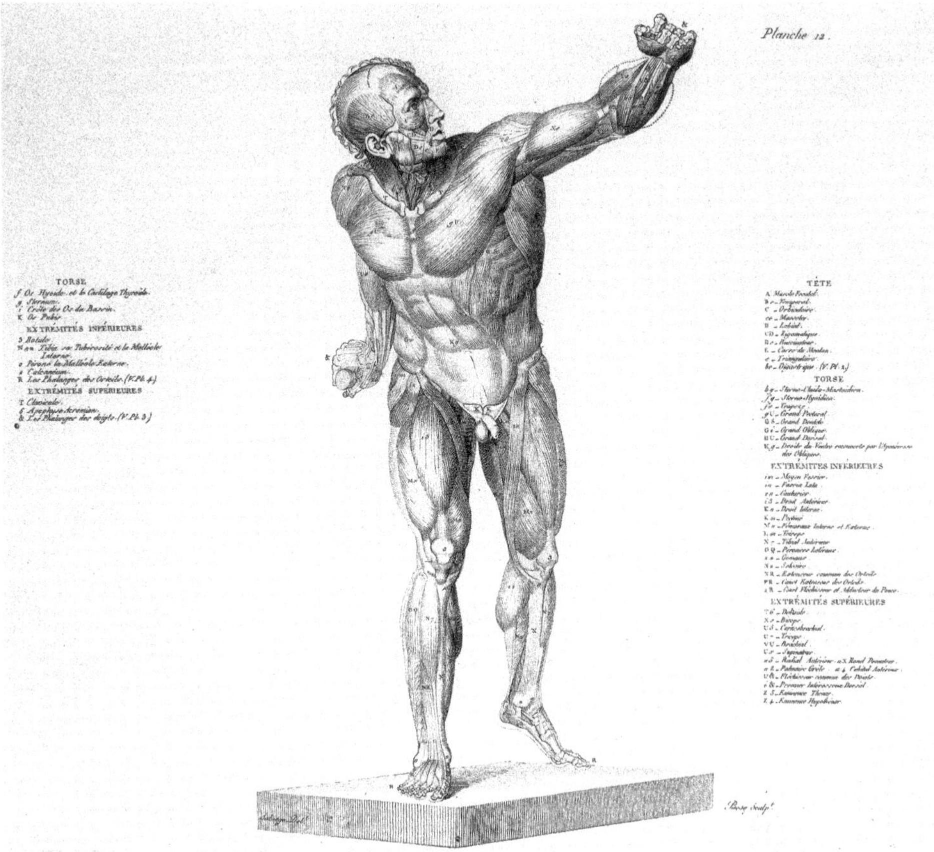

Bosq after Jean-Galbert Salvage, exterior muscles, drawn after the front view of the *Borghese Gladiator*, from *Anatomie du Gladiateur combattant*, 1812, plate 12, engraving in red and black ink, 32 x 36 cm (platemark). **6.11**

system has the more structural function of facilitating the discrimination of bones and musculature. In the plates engaging with the interior musculature, parts of the skeleton appear in black from behind the muscles or are laid bare in areas with fewer muscles, as in the shin bone. Red dominates in the plates focusing on the external muscles with only a few black bony parts showing through. An additional contour is just indicated in some areas, such as the feet, thus suggesting that the forms of the Greek athlete are predominantly determined by his impressive and well-defined muscles. In the plates staging the virtual skeleton of the *Gladiator* the outer shape of the sculpture becomes more prominent as it is indicated with a thick and continuously drawn outline which circumscribes (with the exception of the hands) almost the entire figure, producing more than the other plates the illusion of lucidity. The plates are thus an attempt to reconcile anatomy's look into the body and a surface view – and the athletic body facilitates this. The contour indicates the outer extent of the sculpture and corresponds almost entirely with the confines of the represented body. It can thus become a symbol or virtual double of the skin, the organ that shapes the body's outer appearance and serves – as it was understood in early nineteenth-century medicine – as its borderline.

Skin appears not only symbolically in the *Anatomie du Gladiateur*. As far as I see, the atlas is the first treatise on artistic anatomy that discusses the human skin, its structure and functions in detail. And, like Sue (the younger) before him, Salvage engaged with the question of human variety, skin colour and complexions. However, following Julien-Joseph Virey's polygenism and his hierarchical thinking about human races, Salvage took a far more rigid approach to human variety than Sue and, for that matter, later authors of artistic anatomies like Pierre-Nicolas Gerdy.[44] Salvage divided humankind into two main groups labelled 'white' and 'negro race', the differences between which he believed to be fixed by heredity.[45] In line with the explicitly racist readings of Enlightenment authors such as Camper by naturalists or anthropologists like Virey, Salvage saw a clear hierarchy in which 'la race blanche' is distinguished by their beauty and character. Positing black and white as extremes of a colour scale, encompassing a whole range of skin tones, allowed him nevertheless to draw a clear and unambiguous line between two fundamental races using this abstract contrast. Further attempts were made to categorise humans according to age group, with gender and temperament mixed in. Salvage maintained the distinction traditional humoral theory made between the phlegmatic, sanguine, choleric and melancholic temperaments and associated skin textures and tones with each of them. While the phlegmatic's tissue is spongy and their skin of a bland white, the sanguine features flourishing white skin and the choleric a velvet skin of olive tone.[46] These are explicitly referred to as skin colours and not as complexions. The latter term still occurs in the text but solely with reference to the temperaments as such. For Salvage skin colour is hereditary and a marker of race, and is now completely separated from the more flexible, non-hereditary notion of complexions (discussed in chapter 3). Variation in skin tone and temperament as well as the multi-coloured expressiveness of the face implicitly became for him a prerogative of the universal 'white'.

In the section specifically dedicated to the 'integument' Salvage pays particular attention to the organ's structure and physiology; and it is in relation to the skin's vital functions that its colouring comes into play as well. Elaborating on the organ's contribution to a body's shape as well as on its functions, he combined neoclassical aesthetics with vitalist medicine. He referred repeatedly to Bichat's considerations of the *système dermoïde* and *épidermoïde* in his 1801 *Anatomie générale* (discussed in detail in chapter 4), thus integrating, in abbreviated form, the then most up-to date medical knowledge into his artistic anatomy. Salvage generally stated that 'skin serves as envelope of the exterior parts of the body, it is perfectly moulded on them and attached by the means of cellular tissue'[47] and considered it as a lively contact zone thus echoing Bichat's understanding of skin as 'limite sensitive'. Again like Bichat, and most anatomists of the time, he distinguished between the thin and transparent epidermis and the dermis, which is itself divided into three topologically and functionally discrete but interconnected elements: the corium, the papillae and the reticular body.[48] He defined the corium as the thickest part of the skin, with a spongy consistence due to criss-crossing fibres, and as having the primary function of securing and protecting the body.[49] The reticular corpus is – and this again was by then a generally accepted medical fact – described as the location of the colouring matter in the skin (*couleur de la peau*). Following Bichat, who paid much attention to the fluids circulating through the skin but considered questions of 'the colouring matter of the reticular corpus'[50] of greater interest to the naturalist than to the physician, Salvage took, in this instance, a more vitalist than classificatory turn. He specially emphasised the vivacity of the facial skin, a site where the passions surface owing to a capillary system that channels the blood and thus makes the face blush (or pale).[51] Still, rather than the bodily fluids affecting the complexion, it is now on the contrary the skin colour that 'determines the fluids contained in the reticular body' and which is, Salvage continued, 'of a reddish white in most Europeans, paler in children and women, and generally more red in the face than elsewhere'.[52] This aspect of skin, the activity of fluids in the vessels of the reticular body, is treated only in the text and not illustrated in the *Anatomie du Gladiateur*. But one of the footnotes refers to a remarkable illustration for Moreau de la Sarthe's augmented French version of Johann Kaspar Lavater's essays on physiognomy, which was provided, along with illustrations of the facial muscles, by Salvage himself (Figure 6.12). It accompanies the section on the 'anatomy and natural history of the face' added by Moreau de la Sarthe to the translation of Lavater's original text. It shows an isolated, cut off face serving to represent, as the accompanying text explains,

> the reticular corpus seen under the skin, and developed by an injection. The more one looks at it, the more one will be surprised by the distribution and this communication of vessels. And yet, these distributions, these communications are even more considerable in nature; and if the injection had penetrated into the whole extension of the vascular network that this plate represents, it would appear red in all points of the surface.
>
> It was by skilfully letting well-coloured foreign liquids pass through the reticular body that the famous Ruysch gave cadavers of children all the sparkle and freshness of life.[53]

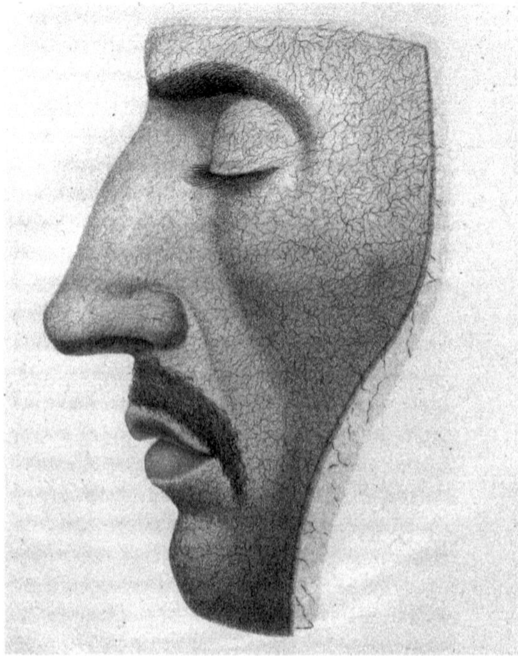

6.12 F. Kaiser after Jean-Galbert Salvage, blood vessels of the face, from Lavater (ed. Moreau de la Sarthe), *L'art de connaître les hommes*, 1820, vol. 4, plate 190, 23.3 x 15 cm.

The face curiously resembles (except for the shut eyes) the idealised self-portrait of Salvage on the frontispiece of the *Anatomie du Gladiateur*. However, whatever face was injected this way, it could have hardly been that of the draughtsmen himself. But this is not the only paradox of an image representing an experiment for which a face has to be cut off to demonstrate the liveliness of its skin. It shows the face as an isolated mask, with its skin criss-crossed by a multitude of red-coloured lines indicating the vessels filled with the red liquid that simulates the blood and the ability of the face to record and display changing physiological and emotional states. Fusing the discourses of art theory and medicine, Moreau de la Sarthe refers to this capillary network also as the site 'where nature has placed the *carnations*'. The injection in the physiological experiment and its fictional representation in Salvage's face and the flesh tones produced by painters conflate in a manner that had been characteristic of the parlance on flesh, its colours and their painterly representation – *chair* and *carnations* – for centuries. In the eyes of *médecin-philosophe* Moreau de la Sarthe, who strove to anchor psychology in the materiality of bodily processes, the *carnations* became a matter of physiology. In this account of skin and face, the *carnations*, rather than being fully embodied, have themselves withdrawn into the skin and become a psycho-physiological effect on the canvas of the face.[54] It is a view in which the facial skin is both a medium and a dense fleshy entity, and Salvage's image of the injected face-mask shows it as a surface in a flesh tone with a multitude of red vessels and as a thick layer in a buttery yellow.

Even though no image capturing the physiology and depth of skin was included in the *Anatomie du Gladiateur* itself, Salvage's textual account of the papillae and the sense of touch largely followed the vitalist notion of skin and is in line not only with Bichat but also with earlier Enlightenment views of the skin as an exquisitely sensible organ. The papillae are described like the emanations of an altogether neuronal body, whose nerves transgress the dermis and end in tactile buds just beneath the epidermis making 'sensibility … the exclusive property of skin'.[55]

The only area where Salvage significantly departed from Bichat is in his elaborations on the cellular tissue or what he also called 'adipose membrane'. This fatty layer, which had been described by earlier anatomists as a part of the skin,[56] became a kind of physiological no man's land between body and skin for some nineteenth-century physicians. For Salvage it has a significant aesthetic function because it:

> Fills the intervals between the muscles, lifts the skin and keeps it uniform. It contributes to the charm of the body parts by lending them gentle and rounded forms under which the muscles are softly drawn in men, and are, so to speak, completely hidden in women and children. When it is distributed in the right proportions over the whole body, it contributes to individual beauty by leaving the imprint of health and freshness that a body's well-nourished appearance has to offer.[57]

Combining medical and artistic vocabulary throughout, Salvage specifically referred to the *mollesse*, an aesthetic quality prominent in neoclassical art discourse when praising the softly drawn forms of a well-proportioned body. Akin to the Italian *morbidezza* the *mollesse* was traditionally associated with the softness of flesh and flesh tones; it receded into the outlines in neoclassicism but remained a trope of vivacity in the image of the body. Due to the choice of the *Borghese Gladiator* – a model of muscular athleticism – this aspect does not really play out in the illustrations for the *Anatomie du Gladiateur* where instead quickness is evoked via the dynamic movement of the figure and recalled through the use of sanguine in the colour version. The materiality of skin and flesh though gets lost in the interstice – an empty space between muscles and contour brought in to foster an imaginary transparency.

Ever since Susie Orbach's 1978 classic *Fat is a Feminist Issue* we have known that fat is never neutral material and it is certainly not in Salvage's treatise.[58] The author carefully distinguished between men, women and children, as the latter two groups ward off a piercing anatomical observation with a well-nourished adipose membrane. It is the soft and dense skin of women in particular that serves both as a chaste veil and as a hermeneutic barrier. It is the virile and muscular body whose anatomy is speaking.

Surface anatomy

The male body is not simply translucent, however. This becomes an issue in a group of anatomical texts published later in the nineteenth century that more explicitly guide the artist's attention towards the surface. Labelled or conceived of as 'Anatomies of exterior forms' they paradoxically engage with the internal structure of the body via its exterior.[59] The first treatise with such a title was Pierre-Nicolas Gerdy's 1829 *Anatomie des formes extérieures du corps humain, appliquée à la peinture, à la sculpture et à la chirurgie*. The author, who was among the more prominent physicians of the first half of the nineteenth century, taught in a variety of academic positions – anatomy, physiology, surgery as well as hygiene – and also published on sense physiology and the philosophy of the senses.[60]

In the late 1820s around the time of the death of the younger Sue, Gerdy offered an anatomy course for artists at the Académie de médecine.[61] After Sue's death he also applied for the position of anatomy professor at the École des beaux-arts, but the institution preferred to hire Édouard Émery, who continued teaching very much in the traditions of the Sue dynasty, putting particular weight on the practice of dissection.[62] In contrast, Gerdy, whose courses were very popular with art students, devised a method of teaching that centred around the life model and the idea of anatomy as visible via the surface. The treatise, which seems to be a direct outcome of this teaching, takes artistic concerns as its point of departure, as it looks at numerous art works from the collections of the Louvre to assess their anatomical precision – and does not shy away from critiquing even the most famous ancient sculptures – and focuses entirely on what is accessible to the eye when looking at the exterior forms of the body. What he provides is arguably the most extensive elaboration on the body's surface ever written: more than three hundred pages of minute description of physical forms. In the case of each bodily area, Gerdy first characterises the larger form, then the topography of the surface going from larger planes to small furrows and elevations. The introductory sentences regarding the arm and hand – a body part to which alone 60 pages are dedicated – states for example:

> The arm is a member that is rounded like a cylinder, but compressed from the outside to the inside. It is, on its exterior, hollowed out by some kind of longitudinal, not very deep furrow that starts at the deltoid muscle's dimple and fades before reaching the level of the crook of the arm. This furrow is produced by

> the recess of the skin caused by the projections that render sensible the margins of the neighbouring triceps and the biceps, situated at the back and the front of the arm respectively.[63]

In a related footnote Gerdy discussed (as for other characteristics of external anatomy) a number of ancient and modern art works where this feature is more or less exactly rendered. He particularly praised David and two of his mature male figures, Tacitus in the *Intervention of the Sabine Women* and the main figure in his *Leonidas at Thermopylae*, for the truthful imitation of this detail. Gerdy thus turned anatomy into a matter of attentive observation and exact imitation in image or words. If Gerdy's obsession with the details of the body's surface is unique, his use of extensive descriptions is not. Bichat, whose anatomical works were extremely comprehensive, developed in his *Anatomie descriptive* a complete ethics of medical description, in demanding a 'precise and rigorous style' in which every detail elaborated upon is scrupulously verified on the basis of dissection.[64] He believed in full co-ordination of the observing eye, dissecting hand and linguistic emanation. Bichat's trust in autopsy and the possibilities of language made him a fierce opponent of medical illustrations and models. Gerdy considered dissection dispensable for artists, but his book follows a similar ethics of dense description based on empirical knowledge through observation. In its quest for total comprehension, Gerdy's medical ekphrasis conforms to the 'ideal of an exhaustive description' that Foucault considers to be one of the characteristics of nineteenth-century clinical thought. This ideal envisions a 'correlation between the visible and the expressible, namely the continuous correlation of an entirely … faithful description … Thus language ... establishes a correlation between each sector of the visible and an expressible element that corresponds to it as accurately as possible'.[65]

The accurate verbal account thus relies on exact observation and fosters the desire for equally thorough visibility. In this exchange between seeing and describing, skin baffles the medical or artistic eye when looking at the intact body. Something always gets lost in translation as the skin forms a physical barrier that is in the way of full comprehension. Something has to remain obscure for the artist to keep the hierarchy of expertises in place, and the eyes see only like 'through a cloud what the mind can't understand'. To clear the mist, anatomy has to instruct the artist:

> Anatomy coming to the aid of the eye, gives transparency to the skin, and reveals to the artist's intelligence, the forms of the surface of the body, by recalling to him the hidden parts under the veil that covers them. It is thus to say that anatomy is like a magnifying glass that makes forms perceptible up to the tiniest detail, so that the artist enlightened by anatomy can see much better.[66]

Anatomical didactics makes the body's surface legible and renders distinct the 'subcutaneous forms despite the skin that veils them'. Skin thus acquires a paradoxical role as it simultaneously covers and educes the internal structure and becomes itself the material hinge for the complex relationship between knowing, speaking and seeing. This mediation is not an easy process; skin is more than just a veil as it makes an active contribution to the formation of the bodily forms.

> If the skin, precisely joined to the parts that it covers, did not fall into creases by virtue of its suppleness, if it did not modify forms in certain places through its thickness, it would merely faithfully translate the parts that it covers without contributing to their production; but it is not just that. Fortunately, it modifies the forms in certain places, it alters them in others, and above all, it veils them. These observations suffice to demonstrate that its study should inspire the interest of artists.[67]

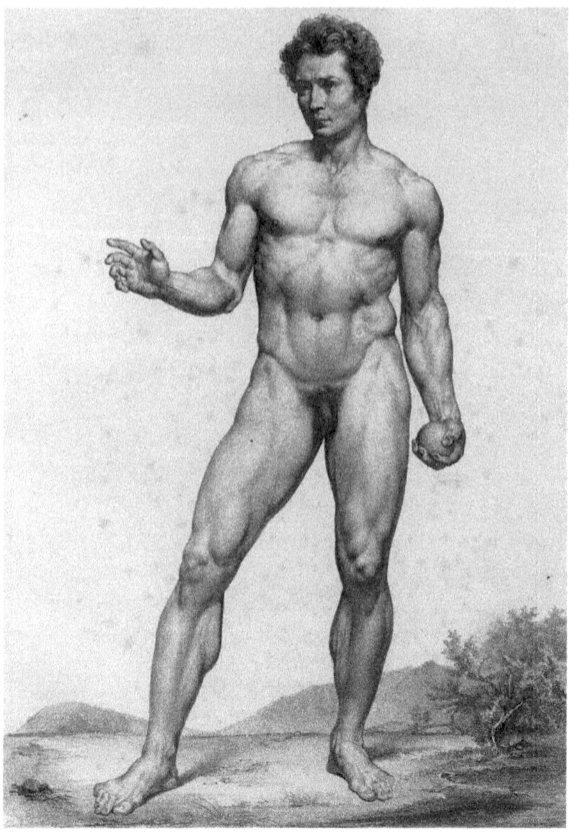

6.13 Langlumé after Demesse, male nude, from Pierre-Nicolas Gerdy, *Anatomie des peintres*, 1829, plate 1, lithograph.

Literally speaking of skin as a translator, Gerdy aligned the organ's role with his own function as an instructor who renders anatomical knowledge visible for artists without ever giving it all away.

Gerdy's project of a comprehensive artistic anatomy remained incomplete, and rather than complementing the *Anatomie des formes extérieures* with considerations on the inner formation of the body, he stopped with the surface. This might have been due to his misfortune in not securing the professorship at the École des beaux-arts, but it is emblematic of artistic anatomy's move towards morphology. Gerdy's publication also came with only a small number of illustrations: three academic nudes in a separate, larger format atlas and three matching schematic figures in the text volume itself (Figure 6.13 and 6.14). The latter indicate with lines the boundaries between muscles, and number the bodily regions listed in the legend, thus mapping the areas put into relief through shading in the lithograph. The three lithographs from the atlas stage a heroised male nude placed on to a comparatively small-scale

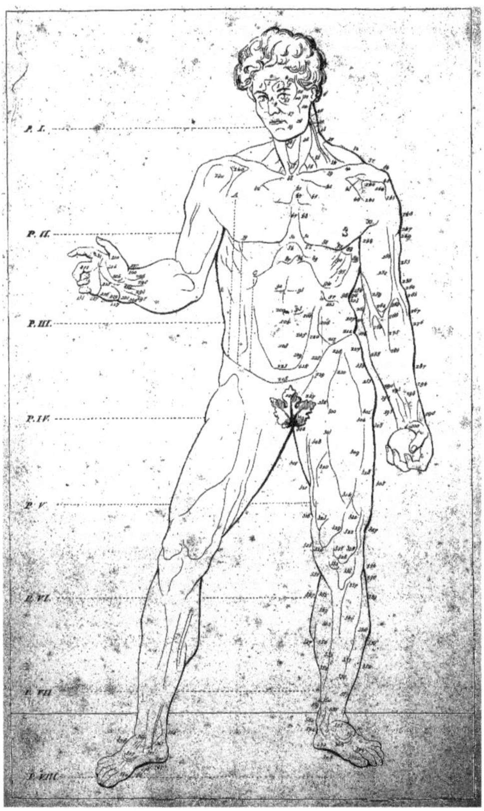

Fourquemin after Demesse, schematic view of male nude, from Pierre-Nicolas Gerdy, *Anatomie des formes*, 1829, plate 1, lithograph, 20.4 x 12 cm. 6.14

landscape background and approximating the pose and physical features of an ancient sculpture, the *Discobolus* at rest, a Greek sculpture associated with the classical canon of Polyclitus. The figure is at rest, lacking the dynamism of the *Borghese Gladiator*; the two statues thus represented alternative models of ideal athletic masculinity. Marble versions of both sculptures had been purchased by Napoleon from the collections of his brother-in-law, Prince Camillo Borghese, and they entered the Louvre around the same time (ca 1808).[68]

In comparison with the ancient model, the lithograph emphasises and details the muscles of the discus thrower. In a short explanation of the plates, Gerdy admitted that he adopted the pose of the ancient figure, to ultimately represent 'man himself' and further elaborated that he had asked his draughtsman, Demesse,

> to conserve the grandiosity of ancient forms as much as nature allowed. For the same reason, I have asked him to reject all the little furrows and depressions, that are not necessarily tied to our organisation, and which are only miseries of nature and disturb the major lines of beautiful forms. However, I believed I had to make him draw the most minute details when they belong to the unchanging natural character of our structure.[69]

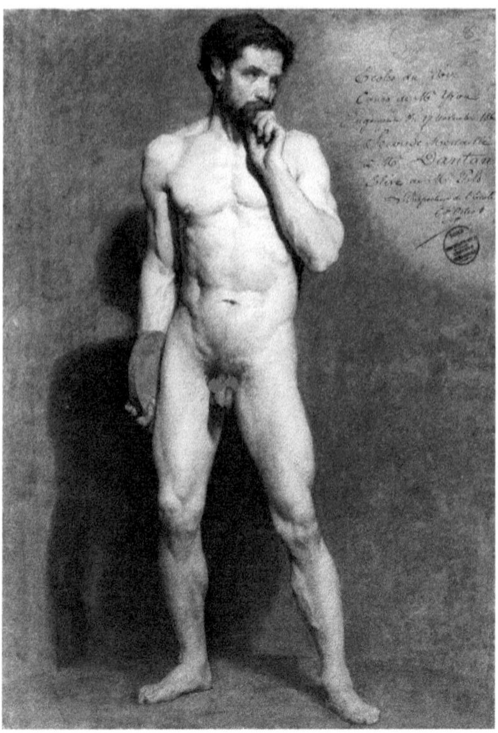

6.15 Edouard Dantan, *Male* académie, 1868, black chalk, charcoal and gouache on paper, 61.5 x 45.5 cm.

The nude thus combines emulation of ancient art, observation and idealisation. It complies with the neoclassical aesthetics of *académies* of that period and in particular those produced by David and his school. And rather than embodying Winckelmann's vision of ideal beauty, Demesse's muscular nude is in line with what Émeric-David had promoted as 'beau réel' in his 1805 *Recherches sur l'art statuaire*, one of the most significant art theoretical texts of the Napoleonic period.[70] Émeric-David had pleaded for a reconciliation of idealisation and truth to nature, an idea not very far from that of the early historian of medical illustration, Ludwig Choulant, who about half a century later promoted an 'ideal' kind of anatomical image. Choulant favoured this type of scientific image 'constructed from the constant mean proportion of several types'.[71] Demesse's male nude for the *Anatomie extérieure* is put in the pose of a man getting ready to launch a bowl, as Gerdy explains, an 'attitude, which, although simple, allows one to make the muscles more perceivable'.[72] It is a pose made for description and study with eye and pencil, and not at all a natural pose, as all muscles are active simultaneously. The lithograph renders the body smoothly, producing through subtle shading a pronounced and detailed relief. Without looking like an écorché, it indicates all the muscles via a modulated surface.

Demesse's nude seems to have been a productive model for artistic exercise, and many of the life drawings made at the École des beaux-arts later in the nineteenth century adopt a similar style – producing even surfaces and a pronounced variegated relief of muscles. Almost forty years after the publication of Gerdy's atlas at least one life model session took up the pose of the *Discobolus* and the resulting drawings closely echo the lithographs from the *Anatomie des formes* (Figure 6.15). While Gerdy's all-embracing descriptions were probably too detailed to be of lasting practical use for artists, his overall approach proved highly successful during the second half of the century, and later nineteenth-century artistic anatomies not only reference him prominently but also adopt the perspective of surface anatomy. Among them were most notably Julien Fau's 1845 *Anatomie des formes* and Paul Richer's 1890 *Anatomie artistique, ou description des formes extérieures du corps humain*, both of which came with less extensive text and a larger number of illustrations. In the enlarged 1865 second edition of his treatise, Fau covered the entire internal and external anatomy in a single volume, and included general remarks on the development of the human, and on human variety and temperaments (very much in the manner of Salvage). The work comprised 25 plates drawn and lithographed by Leveillé, an experienced anatomical draughtsmen who had previously worked under Nicolas-Henri Jacob for France's most comprehensive nineteenth-century anatomy atlas, Bourgery's *Traité complet de l'anatomie de l'homme*. From the start, Fau's *Anatomie des formes* was very popular, soon translated into English by the Scottish surgeon and anatomist Robert Knox, and re-edited several times both in England and France. Even though Fau also commissioned a new écorché for artists made by Eugène Caudron,[73] he seconded Gerdy in his emphasis on the surface: 'The whole object of artistic anatomy is completely misunderstood by those artists who represent living man, with the angular forms of the dead dissected body of anatomical schools; the cellular tissue and the integument play a part sufficiently important to merit also the attention of artists.'[74]

Skin, he argued, is what first meets the eye when looking at a body and has a considerable impact on the human form. It makes it look pleasant and is indirectly associated with *mollesse* and life. 'It invests the whole exterior, reproducing the internal forms; but the presence of the cellular tissue, and the thickness of the skin itself, modifies these forms, and, diminishing their asperities, bestow on them a peculiar grace. There is a wide difference between the écorché, and the body covered with the external integument.'[75]

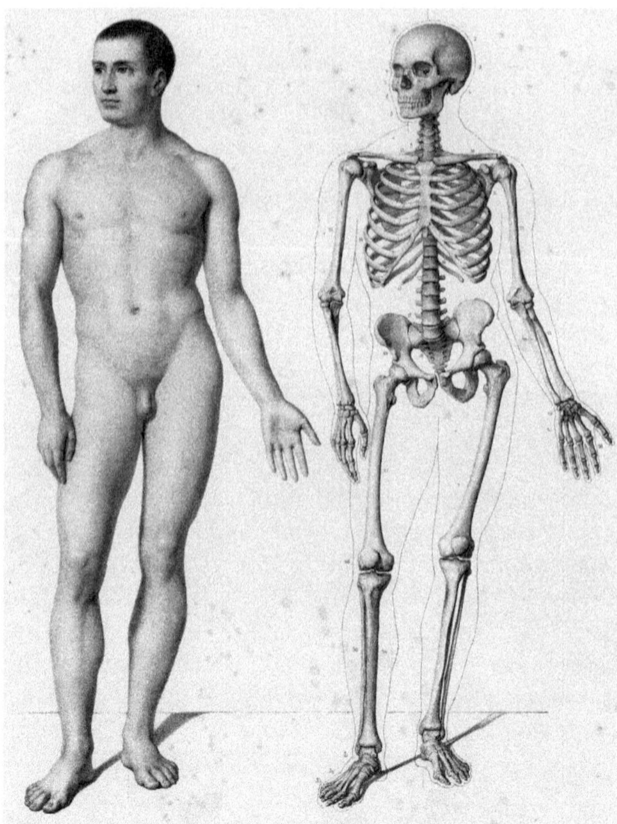

6.16 Leveillé, Male nude and skeleton, from Julien Fau, *Anatomy of the External Forms of Man*, 1849, plate 2, lithograph, 34.5 x 27.5 cm.

Explicitly referring to Bichat's notion of skin as 'sensitive limit', Fau also highlighted the organ's function as a communicative membrane perforated by minuscule openings connecting superficial and internal parts.[76] And, as in Gerdy, the organ does not only communicate bodily fluids and sensory information but also 'translates' and transposes anatomical knowledge.[77] The illustrations stress this latter function of the human tegument as most of them simultaneously present an external view of the body along with insights into the structure of muscles or bones. In plate 2 for example (Figure 6.16), a male nude representing here the universal anatomical human, is shown frontally in relaxed *contrapposto* position with one hand resting on the thigh while the other is opened and directed towards the viewer in order to expose different areas of the arm. In this pose, the figure is a hybrid of an emulation of an ancient sculpture and a more diagrammatic, standardised anatomical 'man' arranged for convenient anatomical demonstration. The body is highly idealised with a smoothly rendered surface showing much less musculature than the male figure from Gerdy's atlas. Muscular activity is however more prominent in illustrations focusing on individual body parts, especially the arm, in action. More than a change in the visual strategies of artistic anatomy as such, this to some degree contradictory imagery might be an indication of the ambivalent attitudes towards muscular masculinity at the time. As Andrew Shelton has shown, in the aftermath of the July Revolution, a strong, potentially violent working class, embodied by a muscular man, was frequently juxtaposed to a physically less potent middle class. These anxieties were played out, for example, in the reactions to Ingres' *Martyrdom of Saint Symphorien* exhibited at the Salon of 1834; the painting, featuring two brawny lictors, was accused by some critics for its '*musculomanie*'.[78]

The figure in Fau's anatomy atlas is much more restrained. Due to its muscular moderation, it is also much less telling as regards its internal structure, and requires additional images to become transparent. The figure is, in fact, shadowed by its skeleton, an assemblage of bones in the nude's pose and circumscribed by a contour. The skeleton and its – individual – bones rather than the mapped surface areas as in Gerdy's muscular nude are indexed and identified in the corresponding description of plates. The image of the skeletal structure thus needs to be aligned with that of the exterior formation and vice versa. Both the nude and the articulated skeleton with its contour stand in for the living body. In the nude figure skin works as a surface that forms the appearance of the body as well as rendering it aesthetically pleasing, and as a cover which hinders direct access to anatomical knowledge. In the skeletal figure it is simultaneously an indication of shape, and an abstract borderline recollecting an imaginary self. Only when mentally blending the two images – as if with a stereoscope, an instrument invented at the time – is it possible to form a view of a transparent body in three-dimensions.

The modelling function of skin in a more material rather than abstract sense is emphasised in a number of further plates showing the head and trunk for which the same generic male figure serves as a model. Some of them also use the system of the two shadowing figures. Plate 12 for instance (Figure 6.17), features two figures in profile cut at the level of the nose and thigh, with the one on the right displaying the external musculature. The muscles are rendered so as to suggest relief, while the skin is seen as a straight cross-section emphasising the varying density of the dermis which is thicker on buttocks and lower belly, and thinner around the breast, shoulders, neck and so forth. Through this representation of its distinctive structure it is clearly shown as an organ with its characteristic cellular tissue – as described by Bichat – and with its function of filling smaller depressions and thus modelling the exterior form in a way described by Fau in his text. The skin is displayed here as having an idealising effect on the outer appearance which the artist representing the body is meant to capture and enhance.

Nineteenth-century artistic anatomies particularly stress the modelling or aesthetic role of skin, but this function is also present in the general definitions of skin and in the illustrations for the leading anatomical atlases of the period, such as Jules Cloquet's 1821–31 *Anatomie de l'homme*, the first of its kind to have lithographic illustrations, or Jean-Baptiste-Marc Bourgery and Nicolas-Henri Jacob's multi-volume *Traité complet de l'anatomie de l'homme* issued between 1831 and 1854. In the main, they describe skin as an envelope of varying thickness moulded around the internal organs and serving as protective barrier, which engages in organic exchanges between the inner and superficial parts of the body, as well as between the body and its environment. They also consider it as the seat of the sense of touch, before elaborating on the details of its structure and physiology. They also each provide a set of detailed microscopic views of the organ.[79] But it is in illustrations regarding the musculature that the varying density of the organ is indicated in a manner Fau and Leveillé would adapt for the *Anatomie des formes extérieures*. In a lithograph for Cloquet's atlas showing the muscles of the male abdomen seen in profile, the anatomical cut into the body is emphasised, and explicitly thematised in the legend which points to the 'skin incised above the bend of the hip'.[80] Skin is rendered here as a thick layer of tissue seen from above and with a texture clearly distinct from that of the muscles and the smooth, undisturbed surface of the body (Figure 6.18). The then still relatively new medium of lithography, where the image is drawn on a stone, rather than incised into a copper plate, is particularly apt for rendering the different materialities of various tissues. Lines mimicking crayon drawing give a smoothness to the almost sculptural surface of the figures.

The image production for Bourgery's atlas was overseen by his co-author Nicolas-Henri Jacob, an artist who had studied with Jacques-Louis David and later became a professional anatomical draughtsman, producing the

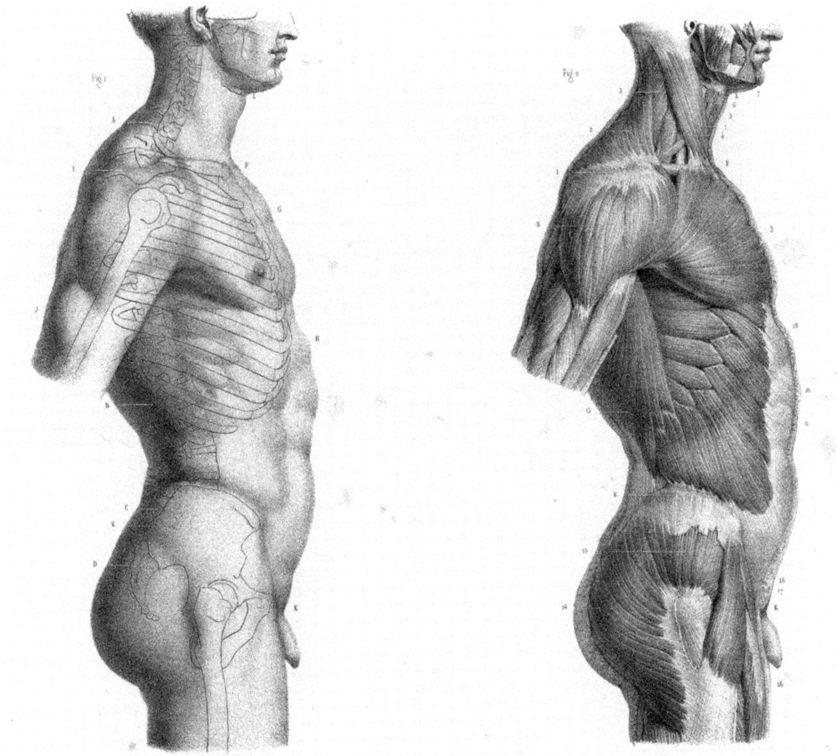

6.17 Leveillé, Exterior view with outlined skeleton and muscles of male trunk, from Julien Fau, *Anatomy of the External Forms of Man*, 1849, plate 12, lithograph, 27.5 x 35.8 cm.

majority of the illustrations for the *Traité complet*. If Leveillé's lithographs for Fau's artistic anatomy seem less sophisticated than the illustrations for these two medical atlases in terms of the amount of detail and the differentiation between different organic textures, this is not a result of the draughtsman's lack of skill. Given that he had contributed to Bourgery and Jacob's *Traité complet* and is indeed introduced as 'élève de M. Jacob' on the title page of Fau's atlas, it should be seen simply as an attempt to dispense with visual information deemed too specialised for the artist.[81] In addition, there are pictorial solutions which are specific to the *Anatomie des formes extérieures* as they especially address the artistic mode of looking at the body. Most important among them is the pairing of figures to demonstrate the body's external and internal formation. The illustrations of the external muscles of different body parts each include a cross-section through the skin and a drawing demonstrating the view from outside. Moreover, rather than adding the skeleton in a third view, the respective bones are inscribed on to the figure in their relative

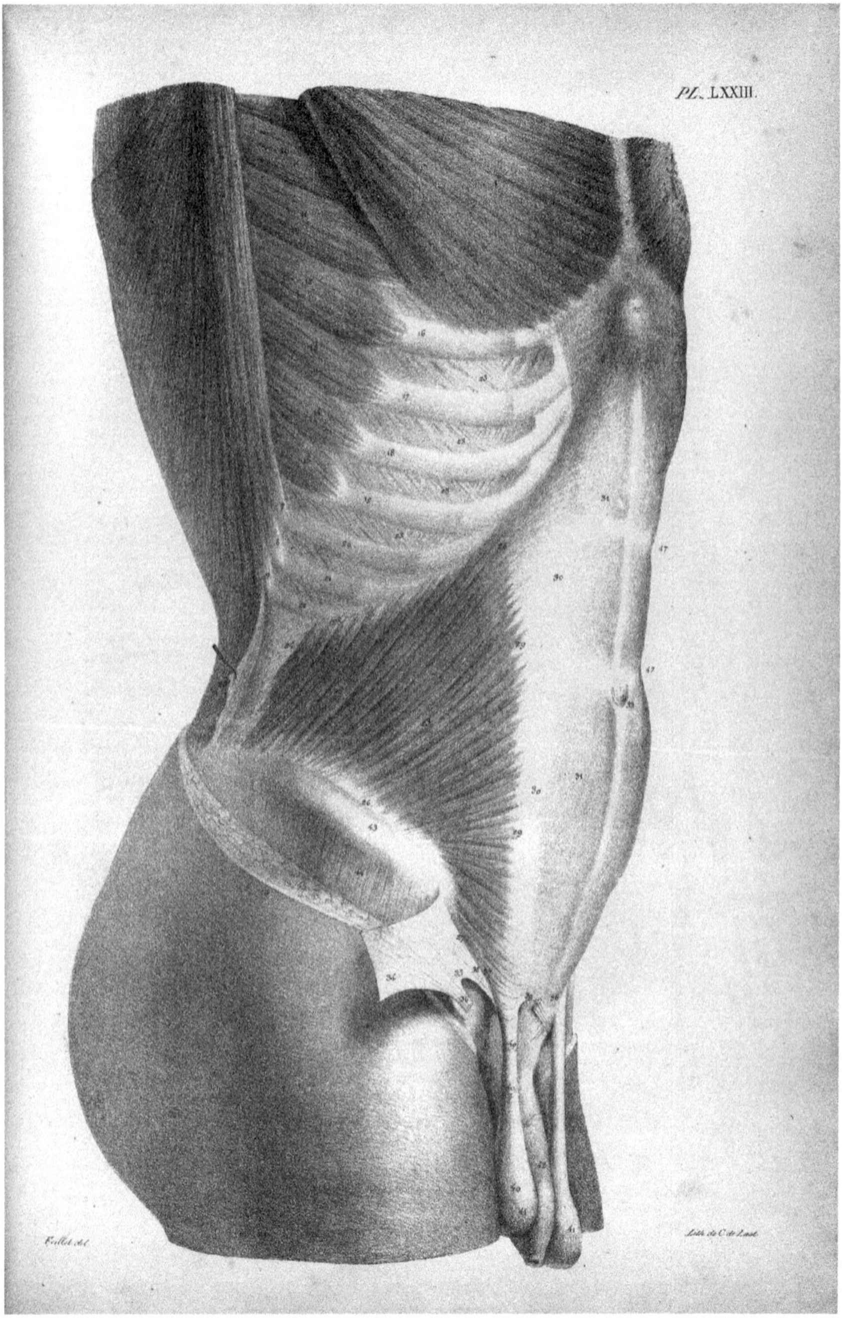

6.18 C. de Last. after Feillet, Muscles of the abdomen, from Jules Cloquet, *Anatomie de l'homme*, 1821–31, vol. 1, plate 73, lithograph, 50.5 x 23 cm

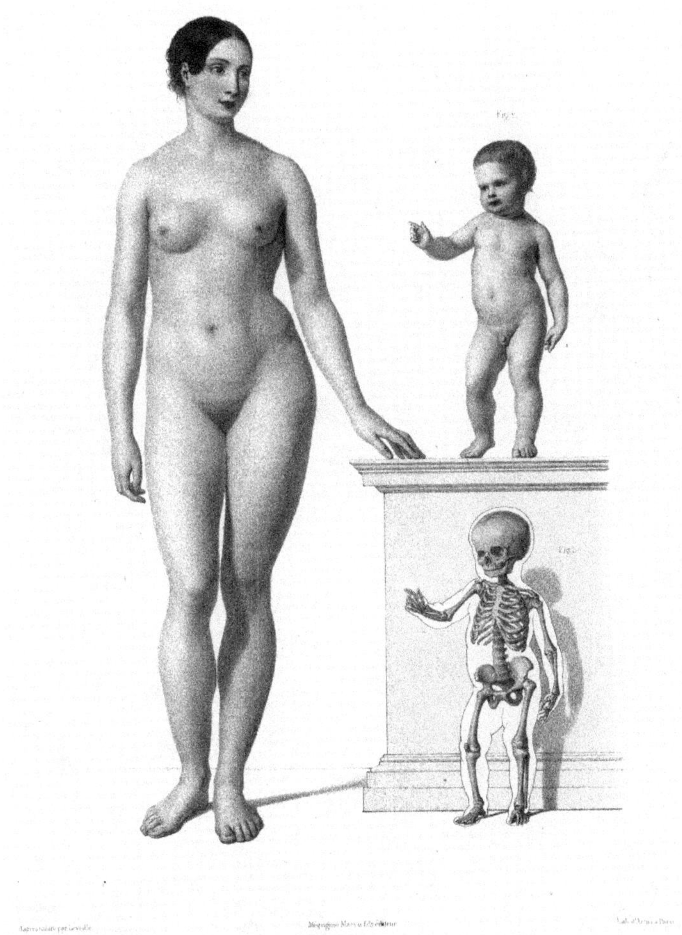

Leveillé, Female nude and child, lithograph from Julien Fau, *Anatomy of the External Forms of Man*, 1849, plate 5, lithograph, 35.5 x 27.5 cm. 6.19

positions, though with a certain ineptness at times, for example in the profile view of the trunk, where the upper ribs are printed on to the arm in the area where arm and thorax overlap. And, since the bones are actually printed on to the nude figure, it isn't quite clear whether we see them on or in the body. The purpose of the illustration and the associated anatomy lesson is, however, to make the artist see the body in layers and project anatomical knowledge on to the surface when working with the life model. It is like an x-ray view *avant la lettre*, able to render the body transparent and to see both soft and hard tissue. The surface of artistic anatomy's body becomes a projection screen for anatomical knowledge.

There is however no transparency for the female body and only two out of the 24 plates are at all dedicated to women (Figure 6.19). In line with the practice of general anatomy atlases, anatomy is exemplified via a universalised and idealised male body, a norm which constructs bodies of women and races other than 'white' as aberrations. Typically, the sections on female anatomy are restricted to the form of the reproductive organs. Fau's atlas goes further, however, as woman's interior is completely omitted. The relevant two plates stage a female nude frontally and from the back, in a setting which, unlike all the others, is slightly reminiscent of the early modern anatomy atlas in including a prop, a socle or part of a sarcophagus on which the woman's left hand rests. While the corresponding male nude is shadowed by its skeleton, the female nude is accompanied by a male toddler standing on the pedestal with his outlined skeleton underneath. The woman is thus reduced to her reproductive duties while her musculature and bone structure are left out. This turns the female interior into a taboo in a manner reminiscent of Diderot's discussion of the horrors of the écorché provided almost a century earlier in his *Notes on Painting*:

> Study of the écorché doubtless has its advantages; but is it not to be feared that this écorché might remain in the imagination forever; that this might encourage the artist to become enamoured of his knowledge and show it off; that his vision might be corrupted, precluding attentive scrutiny of surfaces; that despite the presence of skin and fat, he might come to perceive nothing but muscles, their beginnings, attachments, and insertions; that he might overemphasize them; that he might become hard and dry, and that I might encounter this accursed écorché even in his figures of women? Since only the exterior is exposed to view, I prefer to be trained to see it fully.[82]

While generally suggesting attention should be paid to the surface, and warning of the damaging effects of excessive anatomical knowledge for artists, Diderot is particularly revolted by imagining women's physical interior. Overall though, he was as ambivalent about the écorché as were the nineteenth-century teachers of artistic anatomy and authors of respective treatises. Himself an amateur anatomist, and co-author of the aforementioned article on anatomy for the *Encyclopédie*, he advised Catherine the Great to purchase a copy of Houdon's écorché sculpture for the art academy in St. Petersburg.[83] The École des beaux-arts in Paris continued to use écorchés throughout the nineteenth century. The artistic anatomies of the nineteenth century can be seen as an attempt – whether successful or not – to control artists' anatomical knowledge by containing it. Rather than an over-productive imagination haunted by the écorché, the nineteenth-century artist was meant to project a rationalised medical image on to the body's surface. In nineteenth-century artistic anatomy as a discourse, a didactic strategy and a disciplined observational technique exercised by artists in the life room, skin acquires a multiple role: it is seen as an envelope with the aesthetic function of lending the body – as if by means of artistic idealisation – a unified shape. As a consequence it also becomes an obstruction, a hermeneutic barrier to anatomical enquiry. And yet, to the trained medical or artistic eye, it can refer to the body's interior formation, and is thus understood as a translating membrane. Generally described in nineteenth-century anatomical discourse as a communicative organ, a transmitter between the body and its environment, skin is perceived as a medium. This can be viewed as part of a tendency of the nineteenth century to see the body as a fully legible 'screen body', a development that Charles Grivel has discussed in relation to late nineteenth-century French novels and associated with the emergence of new technologies such as photography.[84] But, looking at artistic anatomy and the medical discourse on skin more generally speaking, these notions of the body and skin already emerge towards the end of the eighteenth century, built on a long tradition of using and perceiving skin as medium or canvas, and they never manage to result in a fully formed fantasy of a transparent human tegument.

Be that as it may, the complexity of skin as both a communicative membrane and sealed envelope – both a surface inviting projections and pleasing cover haunted by images of the interior that are never fully controlled by the observational practices of artistic anatomy – is particularly relevant to the female portraits and nudes by Jean-Auguste-Dominique Ingres discussed in the next chapter.

Notes

1 Jean-Joseph Sue (the younger), *Élémens d'anatomie, à l'usage des peintres, des sculpteurs et des amateurs* (Paris: Méquignon, l'ainé 1788), p. 2.
2 Ibid.
3 Ibid.
4 Daniela Bohde, 'Skin and the search for the interior: the representation of flaying in the art and anatomy of the cinquecento', in Florike Egmond and Robert Zwijnenberg (eds), *Bodily Extremities: Preoccupations with the Human Body in Early Modern European Culture* (Aldershot: Ashgate, 2003), pp. 10–47 (pp. 20–1).
5 Philippe Comar (ed.), *Figures du corps: une leçon d'anatomie à l'École des beaux-arts* (Paris: Beaux-arts de Paris, 2008), pp. 42–7.
6 Diderot and Tarin in the article 'Anatomy' of the *Encyclopédie ou dictionnaire raisonné des sciences, des arts et des métiers*, ed. Denis Diderot and Jean le Rond d'Alembert (accessed via University of Chicago: ARTFL Encyclopédie Projet (winter 2008 edn), ed. Robert Morrissey, http://encyclopedie.uchicago.edu/), vol. 1, 1751, p. 409. For a definition of early modern anatomy see Andrew Cunningham, *The Anatomist Anatomis'd: An Experimental Discipline in Enlightenment Europe* (Farnham; Burlington/Vt.: Ashgate, 2010), pp. 20–1.

7 On the sequence of actual dissections see Cunningham, *The Anatomist Anatomis'd*, pp. 26, 69.

8 Daniela Bohde, *Haut, Fleisch und Farbe: Körperlichkeit und Materialität in den Gemälden Tizians* (Emstetten: Edition Imorde, 2002), p. 310; Claudia Benthien, *Skin: On the Cultural Border Between Self and the World* [1999], trans. Thomas Dunlap (New York; Chichester: Columbia University Press, 2002), pp. 63–94.

9 See in more detail on the connection between religious or mythological scenes of flaying and anatomical practice in sixteenth-century Italy Bohde, *Haut, Fleisch und Farbe*, pp. 297–342, and Bohde, 'Skin and the search for the interior'.

10 On the 'rhetoric of self-dissection' Jonathan Sawday, *The Body Emblazoned: Dissection and the Human Body in Renaissance Culture* (London; New York: Routledge, 1995), pp. 110–29.

11 Katharine Park, *Secrets of Women: Gender, Generation, and the Origins of Human Dissection* (New York: Zone Books, 2006), p. 264.

12 For a media-archeology of the anatomy atlas which considers these questions more broadly see Markus Buschhaus, *Über den Körper im Bilde sein: eine Medienarchäologie anatomischen Wissens* (Bielefeld: transcript Verlag, 2005).

13 Daniela Bohde, 'Pellis Memoriae Peccatorum: die Moralisierung der Haut in Frontispizen und Anatomietheatern der Niederlande im 17. Jahrhundert: ein blinder Flecken in der Medizingeschichte nach 1945', in Albert Schirrmeister (ed.), *Zergliederungen: Anatomie und Wahrnehmung in der Frühen Neuzeit* (Frankfurt a. M.: Vittorio Klostermann, 2005), pp. 327–58, with critical reference to Benthien, *Skin*.

14 Bohde, *Haut, Fleisch und Farbe*, pp. 309–12.

15 Comar (ed.), *Figures du corps*, pp. 19–20; Martial Guédron, *De chair et de marbre: imiter et exprimer le nu en France (1745–1815)* (Paris: Éditions Champion, 2003), pp. 68–73.

16 Cunningham, *The Anatomist Anatomis'd*, pp. 98–104.

17 On this debate see Morvenna Joly, 'L'obsession du "dessous": Diderot et l'image anatomique', *Recherches sur Diderot et sur l'Encyclopédie*, 43 (2008), 57–70.

18 Thomas E. Crow, *Emulation: Making Artists for Revolutionary France* (New Haven; London: Yale University Press, 1994); Abigail Solomon-Godeau, *Male Trouble: A Crisis in Representation* (London: Thames & Hudson, 1997).

19 Guédron, *De chair et de marbre*, pp. 85–6; Gudrun Valerius, *Académie Royale de Peinture et de Sculpture 1648–1793: Geschichte. Organisation. Mitglieder* (Norderstedt: Books on Demand, 2010), pp. 246–7; *Procès-verbaux de l'Académie royale de peinture et de sculpture, 1648–1793*, ed. Anatole de Montaiglon, 10 vols (Paris: Société de l'histoire de l'art Français, 1875–92), 25 April 1776, vol. 8, pp. 217–18.

20 Comar (ed.), *Figures du corps*, pp. 25–6; *Procès verbaux de l'Académie royale*, ed. de Montaglon, 1 June 1776, vol. 8, p. 224.

21 Sue, *Élémens d'anatomie*, p. v.

22 Comar (ed.), *Figures du corps*, pp. 28–39; Margaret A. Oppenheimer, '"The charming spectacle of a cadaver": anatomical and life study by women artists in Paris, 1775–1815', *Nineteenth-Century Art Worldwide*, 6 (2007), www.19thc-artworldwide.org/spring07/46-spring07/spring07article/142-qthe-charming-spectacle-of-a-cadaverq-anqthe-charming-spectacle-of-a-cadaverq-anatomical-and-life-study-

by-women-artists-in-paris-17751815atomical-and-life-study-by-women-artists-in-paris-17751815.

23 The publication date is sometimes indicated as 1668 (as the privilège on the last page states 'Achevé d'imprimer pour la première fois le douzième janvier 1668') but most copies (such as the ones in the British Library and the Wellcome Library that I have been using) say 1667 on the frontispiece.

24 François Tortebat [and Roger de Piles], *Abrégé d'anatomie accommodé aux arts de peinture et de sculpture* (Paris: chez ledit Tortebat, 1667–68) (unpaginated).

25 Roger de Piles, *L'art de peinture de C. A. Du Fresnoy. Enrichie de Remarques, & augmenté d'un Dialogue sur le coloris* (Paris: Nicolas Langlois, 1668), p. 91. From the 1733 edition of the *Abrégé* onwards both de Piles and Tortebat are listed as authors. See also Morwena Joly's catalogue entry in Comar (ed.), *Figures du corps*, p. 178.

26 Tortebat [and de Piles], *Abrégé d'anatomie* (unpaginated). This reproach was common in Venetian art theory and addressed to Michelangelo among others by Ludovico Dolce in his 1557 *Dialogo della pittura intitolato l'Aretino*, and taken up by Gian Paolo Lomazzo in his 1584 *Trattato dell'arte de la pittura*. See Daniela Bohde, '"Le tinte delle carni": zur Begrifflichkeit von Haut und Fleisch in italienischen Kunsttraktaten des 15.–17. Jahrhunderts', in Daniela Bohde and Mechthild Fend (eds), *Weder Haut noch Fleisch: das Inkarnat in der Kunstgeschichte*, pp. 41–63 (p. 47).

27 Bohde, *Haut, Fleisch und Farbe*, pp. 302–3.

28 Tortebat [and de Piles], *Abrégé d'anatomie* (unpaginated).

29 Ibid.

30 Comar (ed.), *Figures du corps*, p. 178.

31 See for example the 1773 drawing by Lambert-Sigisbert Adam reproduced in Comar (ed.), *Figures du corps*, pp. 180–1.

32 Edme Bouchardon, *L'anatomie nécessaire pour l'usage du dessein* (Paris, chez Chereau et Joubert, 1741); Johann Heinrich Lavater, *Élémens anatomiques d'ostéologie et de myologie à l'usage des peintres et des sculpteurs*, trans. Gauthier de la Peyronie (Paris: Ziegler, 1797).

33 Ludwig Choulant and Mortimer Frank, *History and Bibliography of Anatomic Illustration* [1852] (New York: Hafner, 1945), p. 275.

34 Elizabeth Hallam, 'Articulating bones: an epilogue', *Journal of Material Culture*, 15 (2010), 465–92 (p. 467).

35 Édouard Cuyer and Mathias Duval, *Histoire de l'anatomie plastique; les maîtres, les livres et les écorchés* (Paris: Picard & Kaan, 1898), pp. xi and 253.

36 Earlier examples include Errard's anatomical drawings for the Académie de France à Rome. See Comar and Joly in Comar (ed.), *Figures du corps*, pp. 226–9.

37 On Salvage's biography see Raymond Lifchez, 'Jean-Galbert Salvage and his *Anatomie du gladiateur combattant*: art and patronage in post-revolutionary France', *Metropolitan Museum Journal*, 44 (2009), 163–84.

38 *Procès-verbaux de l'Académie des beaux-arts, publiés pour la Societé de l'Histoire de l'Art Français*, ed. Marcel Bonnaire, vol. 2 (Paris: A. Colin, 1940), 4e séance du 5 Brumaire an XIII [27 October 1804], pp. 287–8. The prospectus was published in the *Nouvelles des Arts*, vol. 4, 1804, pp. 76–80. Jean-Galbert Salvage also quotes it in his *Anatomie du Gladiateur combattant, applicable aux beaux-arts, ou, traité des*

os, des muscles, du mécanisme des mouvemens, des proportions et des caractères du corps humain (Paris: chez l'auteur, 1812), p. ij. See also Dorothy Johnson, *Jacques-Louis David: Art in Metamorphosis* (Princeton/N.J.; Chichester: Princeton University Press, 1993), pp. 156–9; and Dorothy Johnson, *David to Delacroix: The Rise of Romantic Mythology* (Chapel Hill/N.C.: University of North Carolina Press, 2011), pp. 102–3; Guédron, *De chair et de marbre*, p. 84; and in most detail on the making of Salvage's atlas Lifchez, 'Jean-Galbert Salvage'.

39 Choulant, *History of Anatomic Illustration*, p. 332.

40 See on the two sculptures and their reception Francis Haskell and Nicholas Penny, *Taste and the Antique: The Lure of Classical Sculpture, 1500–1900* (New Haven; London: Yale University Press, 1981), pp. 148–51, 221–4.

41 Salvage, *Anatomie du Gladiateur*, first two pages of introduction.

42 Ibid., p. ij.

43 Comar (ed.), *Figures du corps*, p. 230; Lifchez, 'Jean-Galbert Salvage', pp. 174–8.

44 Pierre-Nicolas Gerdy, *Physiologie médicale didactique et critique* (Paris: Crochard, 1832); and on Gerdy, Claude Blanckaert, 'Of monstrous Métis? Hybridity, fear of misrecognition, and patriotism from Buffon to Paul Broca', in Sue Peabody and Tyler Edward Stovall (eds), *The Color of Liberty: Histories of Race in France* (Durham/N.C.; London: Duke University Press, 2003), pp. 42–65 (pp. 53–4).

45 Salvage, *Anatomie du Gladiateur*, pp. 28–9.

46 Ibid., p. 30.

47 Ibid., p. 35.

48 Ibid.; Xavier Bichat, *Anatomie générale, appliquée à la physiologie et à la médecine*, 4 vols (Paris: Brosson, Gabon et Cie, 1801), part 2, vol. 4, pp. 646–68; and for a definition that summarises the early nineteenth-century medical knowledge on skin the article by Chaussier and Nicolas-Philibert Adelon in the *Dictionnaire des sciences médicales*, vol. 39 (Paris: Panckoucke, 1819), pp. 565–609, here in particular pp. 565–6.

49 Salvage, *Anatomie du Gladiateur*, p. 35; see for comparison the relevant section in Bichat, *Anatomie générale*, part 2, vol. 4, pp. 646–56.

50 Bichat, *Anatomie générale*, part 2, vol. 4, p. 659.

51 Salvage, *Anatomie du Gladiateur*, p. 3; Bichat, *Anatomie générale*, part 2, vol. 4, pp. 655–65.

52 Salvage, *Anatomie du Gladiateur*, p. 35.

53 Moreau de la Sarthe in Johann Kaspar Lavater, *L'art de connaître les hommes par la physionomie*, trans., ed. and augmented by Jacques-Louis Moreau de la Sarthe, vol. 4 (Paris: L. Prudhomme 1806), p. 305.

54 Moreau de la Sarthe in Lavater, *L'art de connaître les hommes*, vol. 4, pp. 299–300.

55 Salvage, *Anatomie du Gladiateur*, p. 35.

56 See for example Riolan, discussed in chapter 5, p. 147.

57 Salvage, *Anatomie du Gladiateur*, p. 37.

58 Susie Orbach, *Fat is a Feminist Issue: The Anti-Diet Guide to Permanent Weight Loss* (New York: Paddington Press, 1978).

59 The earliest usage of the term I found was in Bouchardon's *Anatomie nécessaire*, which is referred to as 'Livre d'Anatomie extérieure' by its editor in the directions to the reader, but it is only during the nineteenth century that books carry this title.

60 On the biography of Gerdy see Jules-Auguste Béclard, *Notices et portraits: éloges lus à l'Académie de médecine* (Paris: Masson, 1878), pp. 107–36.
61 Gerdy published an announcement *Cours d'anatomie appliquée à la peinture et à la sculpture* according to which the course, covering the entire human anatomy and finishing with 'promenades anatomiques dans les jardins et les musées publics', would be held from 22 January 1827 onwards and take place every evening with the exception of Thursdays and Sundays.
62 Comar (ed.), *Figures du corps*, p. 42. See also Anthea Callen, 'The body and difference: anatomy training at the École des beaux-arts in Paris in the later nineteenth century', *Art History*, 20 (1997), 23–60; Jean-François Debord, 'De l'anatomie artistique à la morphologie', in Jean Clair (ed.), *L'âme au corps: art et sciences (1793–1993)*, exh. cat. (Paris: Réunion des musées nationaux, Gallimard, 1993/94), pp. 102–17.
63 Pierre-Nicolas Gerdy, *Anatomie des formes extérieures du corps humain, appliquée à la peinture, à la sculpture et à la chirurgie* (Paris: Bechet jeune, 1829), pp. 174–5.
64 Xavier Bichat, *Traité d'anatomie descriptive*, new edn, revised and corrected, vol. 1 (Paris: Gabon, 1829), p. xxvi.
65 Michel Foucault, *The Birth of the Clinic: An Archaeology of Medical Perception* [1963], trans. A. M. Sheridan Smith (London: Tavistock, 1973), p. 113.
66 Gerdy, *Anatomie des formes*, p. xiii.
67 Ibid., p. xiv.
68 At the Louvre the sculpture is now referred to as 'Athlète au disque dit "le Discophore"'. See the entry on the work by Marie-Bénédicte Astier at the Louvre website: www.louvre.fr/oeuvre-notices/athlete-au-disque-dit-le-discophore, last accessed 15 July 2016.
69 Gerdy, *Anatomie des formes*, p. 327.
70 Johnson, *Jacques-Louis David*, pp. 160–2; and Mechthild Fend, *Grenzen der Männlichkeit: der Androgyn in der französischen Kunst und Kunsttheorie zwischen Aufklärung und Restauration* (Berlin: Reimer, 2003), pp. 107–8.
71 Choulant, *History of Anatomic Illustration*, p. 22; Lorraine Daston and Peter Galison, *Objectivity* (New York: Zone Books, 2007), pp. 70–5 and p. 428, fn. 27, who adapt and comment on Choulant's categories.
72 Gerdy, *Anatomie des formes*, p. 327.
73 Julien Fau commented on the figure in his *Explication d'un nouvel écorché à l'usage des artistes* (Paris: Méquignon-Marvis, 1844).
74 Fau here quoted from *The Anatomy of the External Forms of Man, intended for the use of artists, painters and sculptors*, trans. Robert Knox (London: Bailliere, 1849), pp. 101–2. Knox skipped parts of Fau's text, while adding some considerations of his own.
75 Fau, *Anatomy of the external forms*, p. 18.
76 Julien Fau, *Anatomie des formes extérieures du corps humain a l'usage des peintres et des sculpteurs* (Paris: Méquignon-Marvis, 1845), pp. 18–19. The paragraph referring to Bichat is omitted in Knox's translation.
77 See for example Fau, *Anatomie des formes extérieures*, p. 197.
78 Andrew Carrington Shelton, *Ingres and His Critics* (Cambridge: Cambridge University Press, 2005), pp. 15–53.

79 Jules Cloquet, *Anatomie de l'homme, ou Description et figures lithographiées de toutes les parties du corps humaine*, 8 vols (Paris: Impr. de C. de Lasteyrie, 1821–31), vol. 3 pp. 329–31; Jean-Baptiste Marc Bourgery and Nicolas-Henri Jacob, *Traité complet de l'anatomie de l'homme, comprenant la médecine opératoire*, 8 vols (Paris: C. A. Delaunay, 1831–54), vol. 3, pp. 303–11. See more generally on both atlases and the use of lithography for the illustrations K. B. Roberts and J. D. W. Thomlinson, *The Fabric of the Body: European Traditions of Anatomical Illustrations* (Oxford; New York: Clarendon Press, 1992), pp. 535–46; and Benjamin A. Rifkin, *Human Anatomy: From the Renaissance to the Digital Age* (New York: Abrams, 2006), pp. 254–79.

80 Cloquet, *Anatomie de l'homme*, vol. 1, p. 200.

81 Choulant, *History of Anatomic Illustration*, p. 347, is full of praise for the plates and also highlights 'the contours drawn around' the skeletons.

82 *Diderot on Art*, trans. John Goodman, introd. Thomas Crow, 2 vols (New Haven; London: Yale University Press, 1995), vol. 1, p. 193. See on this passage by Diderot, Joly, 'L'obsession du "dessous"'; and especially with regards to the échorché's gender also Benthien, *Skin*, pp. 87–9.

83 Joly, 'L'obsession du "dessous"', pp. 61–70; Zofia Ameisenowa, *The Problem of the Écorché and Three Anatomical Models in the Jagiellonian Library*, trans. Andrzej Potocki (Wroclaw: Zaklad Narodowy im Ossolinskich, 1963), p. 71; Maurice Tourneux, *Diderot et Catherine II* (Paris: C. Lévy, 1899), pp. 428–9.

84 Charles Grivel, 'Der siderale Körper: zum Prinzip des Kommunikation', in J. Hörisch and M. Wenzel (eds), *Armaturen der Sinne: literarische und technische Medien 1870 bis 1920* (München: Fink, 1990), pp. 177–99.

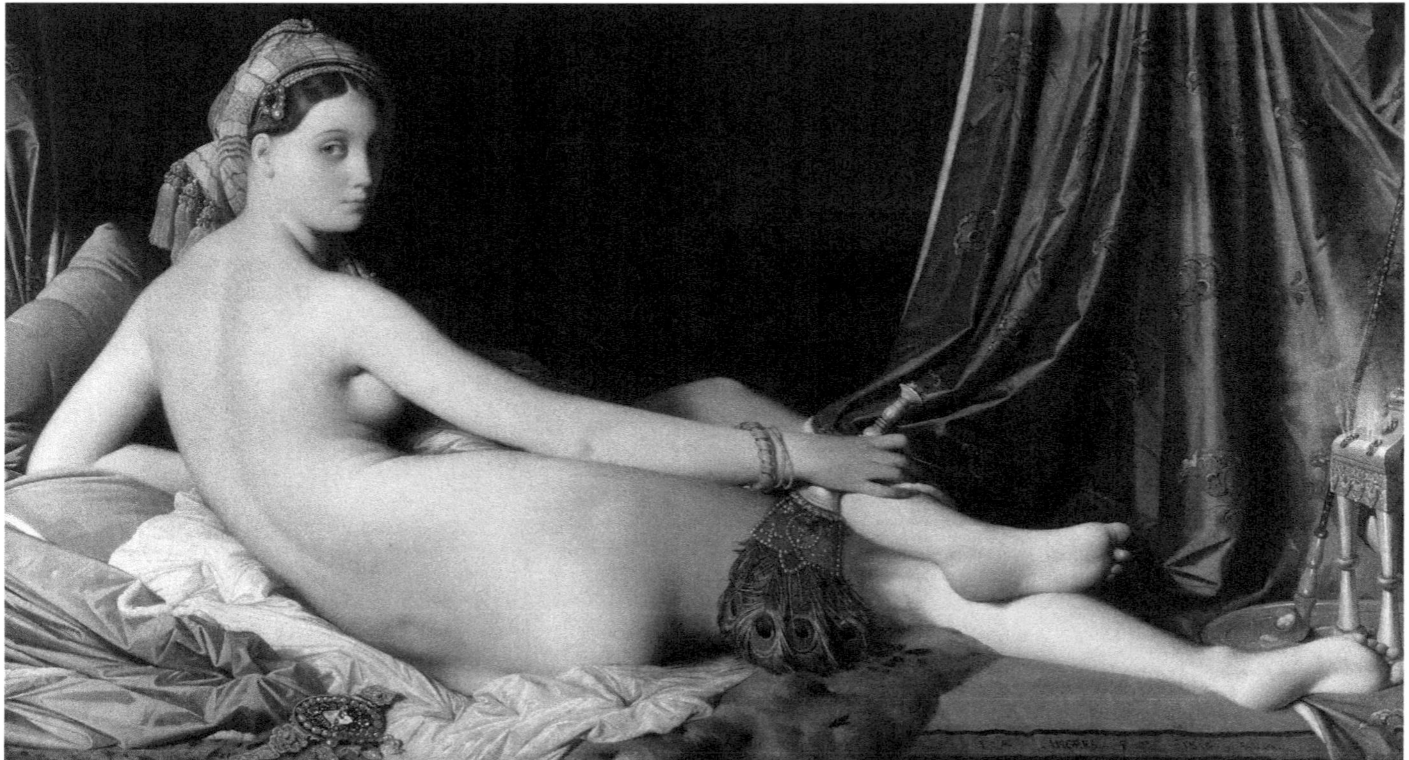

7.1 Jean-Auguste-Dominique Ingres, *Grande Odalisque*, 1814, oil on canvas, 91 x 162 cm.

Hermetic borderline 7

'In this figure there are neither bones nor muscles, blood, life or relief, nothing finally that constitutes an imitation. The flesh tone is greyish [*la carnation est bise*] and monotonous ... It is obvious that the artist sinned consciously, that he wanted to do badly, or that he believed he was resuscitating the pure and primitive manner of the masters of antiquity.'[1] With these words Charles-Paul Landon commented upon Jean-Auguste-Dominque Ingres' *Grande Odalisque* exhibited at the Salon of 1819 (Figure 7.1). According to Landon, as correspondent and member of the Institut de France the official voice of art criticism, Ingres failed to make use of appropriate painterly techniques to breathe life into his female nude. Evidently, the critic did not wish to see a flat surface in a painting, but the illusion of a three-dimensional body of blood and flesh. Assuming the procedures of artistic anatomy would be applied, Landon expected the artist to allude to the interior structure of the body, using light and shade to produce a sense of relief. Ingres made no such attempts, yet the painted body still prompted Landon, apparently accustomed to this way of seeing and assessing the human figure in representation, to recall muscles and bones. At the same time, the critic made it perfectly clear that Ingres had consciously refused, against his own capabilities, to use and demonstrate his knowledge of artistic anatomy. This is why Landon associated Ingres' aesthetic choice with a purified classicism, a style and attitude promoted with particular vigour during the years Ingres was a student of David by a group of rebellious students known as *barbues* or *primitives*, who wished for a return to the simple forms of early antiquity.

The artist's antipathy for anatomy is proverbial; it was recorded, for example, in his pupil's memoirs of the Parisian studio Ingres opened in 1825. According to Amaury-Duval, Ingres advised his pupils to draw or paint only what they saw. This plea for naivety was far from new, and especially topical at a time when artists, including the *barbues* and David himself, questioned what they considered to be the now obsolete 'science' of the pre-revolutionary Académie.[3] In Ingres' case, it was a quest to do away with preconceived knowledge which must have included anatomy, given that the artist called this discipline, 'a dreadful science, a horrible thing', which he could only think of with 'disgust'.[4] However, as I will argue, the relationship between Ingres' approach to the body in his nudes and portraits and contemporary anatomy was more complex than Amaury-Duval's recollections suggest. This chapter will engage with the artist's attention to the body's surface – which he shared with contemporary artistic anatomy – and the reduction of modelling of physical forms based on study of their interiors, especially in his female nudes and portraits. At the same time, Ingres changed the terms of the fabrication of *carnations*, as his painting of flesh and skin became deliberately non-physiological, prompting questions about the kind of materiality the painted body is meant to have or refer to. Critics registered Ingres' peculiar handling of skin and flesh as one of the artist's idiosyncrasies and their writings manifest a gradual shift in the understanding of the body in paint. In this process, certain traditional art historical terms the first chapters of this book sought to explore – in particular the term *carnation* – partly lost their validity. In Ingres' paintings themselves the established association of flesh and paint was replaced by the alignment, on the one hand, of the skin with the images' ground, be it canvas or paper, and, on the other, of the depicted skin and the polished painterly surface.

Ingres, anatomy and the male nude

Ingres was, as Landon pointed out, familiar with the principles of artistic anatomy. He had undertaken a course of study in which the practice of life drawing was central and the study of anatomy was difficult to completely avoid. After early initiation by his father, a painter and sculptor working in Montauban, the eleven-year-old boy entered, in 1791 and in the midst of the revolutionary period, the Académie royale des beaux-arts in Toulouse, the only academy in the provinces directly affiliated with the Académie royale in Paris, and with a very similar curriculum.[5] The training was centred around the study of the human figure, and, according to the regulations, divided into four consecutive stages, in which pupils first drew body parts, then whole figures, before, in their third year, continuing with studies after reliefs and three-dimensional objects as well as copies from paintings, to finally study the life model until they were considered able to make their own compositions.[6] The painter Jacques Gamelin, known today mainly as the author of an artistic anatomy, the *Nouveau recueil d'ostéologie et de myologie*, printed in Toulouse in 1779, had long left the Académie by the time Ingres studied there. But it is quite possible that the bizarre illustrations – osteological and myological plates mixed with battle scenes which were as gory as they were imaginative – still circulated at the school and made a lasting impression on the young Ingres (Figure 7.2).

In 1797, after finishing his studies in Toulouse, Ingres continued his education in Paris where he soon joined the studio of David. Ingres thus entered

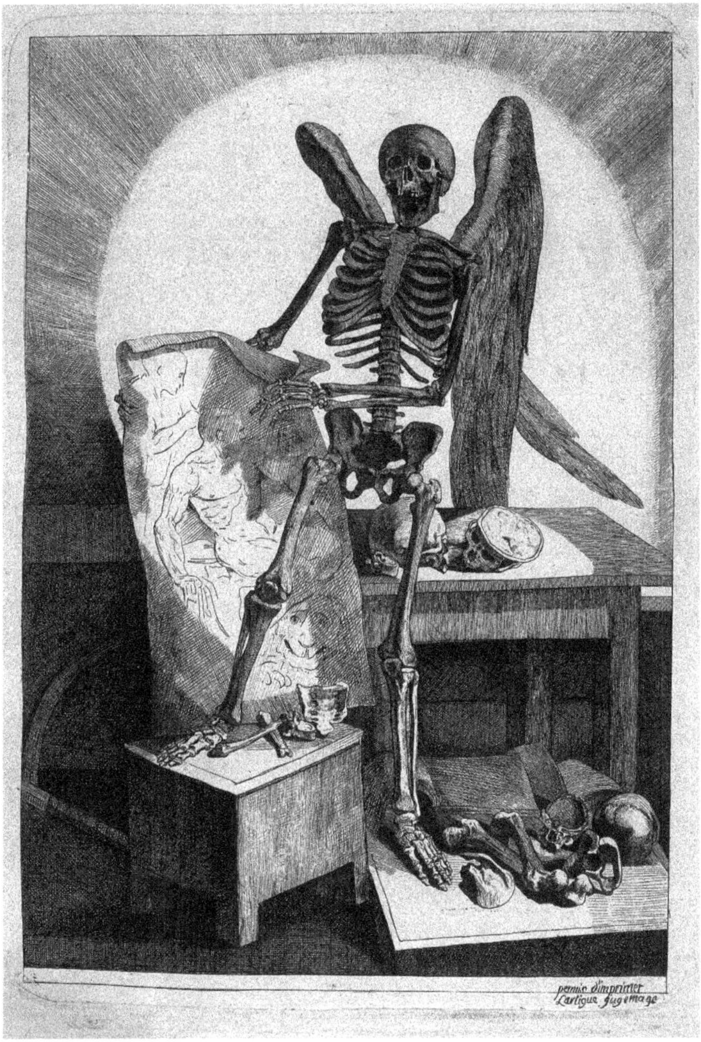

Jacques Gamelin, skeleton with drawing, from *Nouveau recueil d'ostéologie*, etching, 35.2 x 25.1 cm (platemark). 7.2

a setting where particular emphasis was placed on life drawing and on the rendering of muscular male nudes that could be developed into the heroic bodies of history painting.[7] Judging from the visual and verbal accounts of David's studio no anatomical aids such as skeletons or écorchés were employed. But Ingres' time at the École des beaux-arts and in David's studio, itself located at the Louvre, coincided with the period during which Sue (the younger) gave his public lessons in artistic anatomy at the amphitheatre set up in the building (discussed in chapter 4). There is no specific record of Ingres attending these lessons, but they were part of the curriculum and certainly hard to ignore given the proximity of the anatomy hall, the art school, studios and the Gallery of Antiquities installed in 1798 and officially inaugurated in 1800. Ingres frequented the latter galleries at the time to work on drawings for the illustrated catalogue of the French national art collections kept at the Louvre, since 1793 a public museum.[8] It might well be that Ingres' oft-reported distaste for anatomy resulted from his early exposure to the macabre anatomical images by Gamelin, and later to the dissections and animal-beheadings performed by Sue as part of his teaching in artistic anatomy and his studies into the physiology of life and death.

The École des beaux-arts, which Ingres attended, as was customary, while assisting at David's studio, paid equal attention to life drawing, and the production of painted *académies* as preparations for the major competition, the Prix de Rome, was a requirement. There are four male nudes still in existence that Ingres produced in this context.[9] Dating from 1800–1 they all suggest the intensive study of male anatomy, as far as is possible from the observation of the exterior forms within the setting of a life drawing class. One of the more or less life-sized torsos was certainly made in December 1800 for the contest for the best *demi-figure peinte* (as explained in the previous chapter, generally called Prix du torse) and won Ingres admission to the Rome prize competition

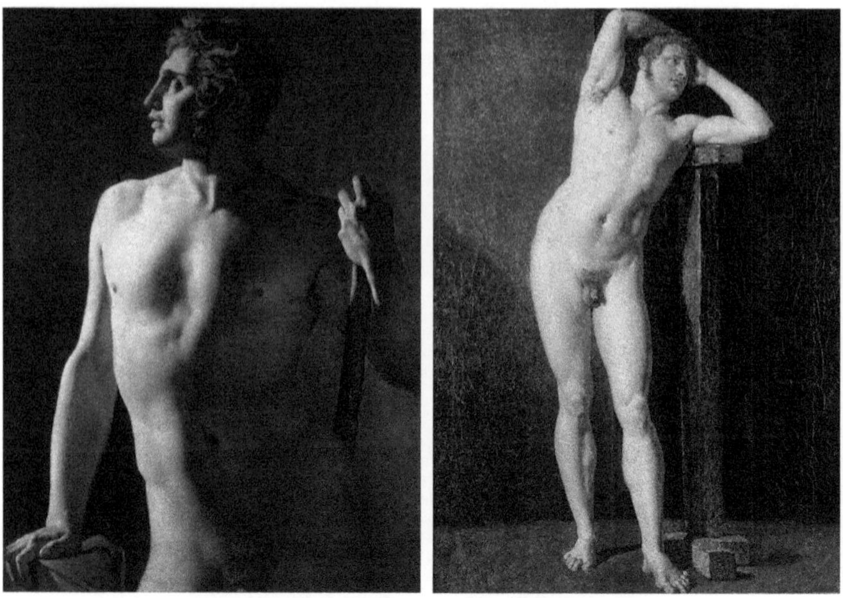

7.3–4 [*left*] Jean-Auguste-Dominique Ingres, *Male* académie (torso), 1800–1, oil on canvas, 102 x 80 cm. [*right*] Jean-Auguste-Dominique Ingres, *Male* académie, 1801, oil on canvas, 79 x 56 cm.

(Figure 7.3). This nude is softly modelled, with brightly lit areas while the zones in the shade are rendered in an earthy greyish brown. This mixture of glow with matt earthy pigments makes it similar to David's 1794 *Death of Bara*, a painting that the artist kept in his studio after Thermidor, as well as to Jean Broc's contemporary *Death of Hyacinthus* (1801). In comparison with the two languid nudes by this fellow student and member of the *barbues*, Ingres, adhering to the exercise, went less far in the reduction of detail and shows his mastery of the male physique by emphasising the life-imbued fleshiness of the model. Two further, rather small format, male nudes were probably also produced as studies required for the admission to the Prix de Rome contest.[10] These standing nudes leaning on wooden supports show many of the characteristics of the school of David: the direction of the incidental light is clearly indicated and the gradations of light and shade are used to lend the body relief and to emphasise the muscles (Figure 7.4). The flesh tones are predominantly rendered in a bright yellowish tone while the shades are kept in grey. Here and there a reddish hue produces a glow, an anatomically unspecific indicator of life and vitality.

Ingres took up these studies for his *Ambassadors of Agamemnon*, the composition which earned him the Prix de Rome in 1801. He used the task to demonstrate his mastery of the male nude, interpreting the prescribed topic as a frieze of men of various ages, from the young supple Patroclus, via the sinewy Achilles and the forceful mature Ajax to the frail old man further in the background. Ingres subtly nuanced the degree of muscularity, intimating the muscles of the ephebes and modelling them fully in the adult men. However, he surprisingly renounced another traditional element for the differentiation: the skin tone of all men is uniformly that of a light beige while the shades are rendered in gradations of bluish grey. The merging of observation of the life model with an idealised version of nature represented by ancient sculpture is particularly apparent in the figure of Patroclus. Ingres developed the pose with the crossed legs from one of his standing nudes.[11] The elegance of the figure with the swaying hip owes much to the *Apollo Sauroctonos*, although Ingres exaggerated the movement, resulting in a further eroticisation of Achilles' beloved friend at the expense of a more flowing outline.

Sufficiently experienced in the techniques of rendering a nude anatomically plausible and in the balance of idealisation and observation to get the academic blessing of the Rome prize, Ingres went on to reduce the relief of his nudes. In the known *académies* he produced while a stipendiary in Rome, *Oedipus and the Sphinx* and a *Woman in a Bath* (better known as the *Valpinçon Bather*), he departed in several respects from this institutionalised and accepted neoclassical version of the body in paint (Figure 7.5 and 7.6; plate 15). Even though he won the prize in 1801, Ingres' departure was delayed until October 1806. By the time the artist arrived at the Villa Medici, the new

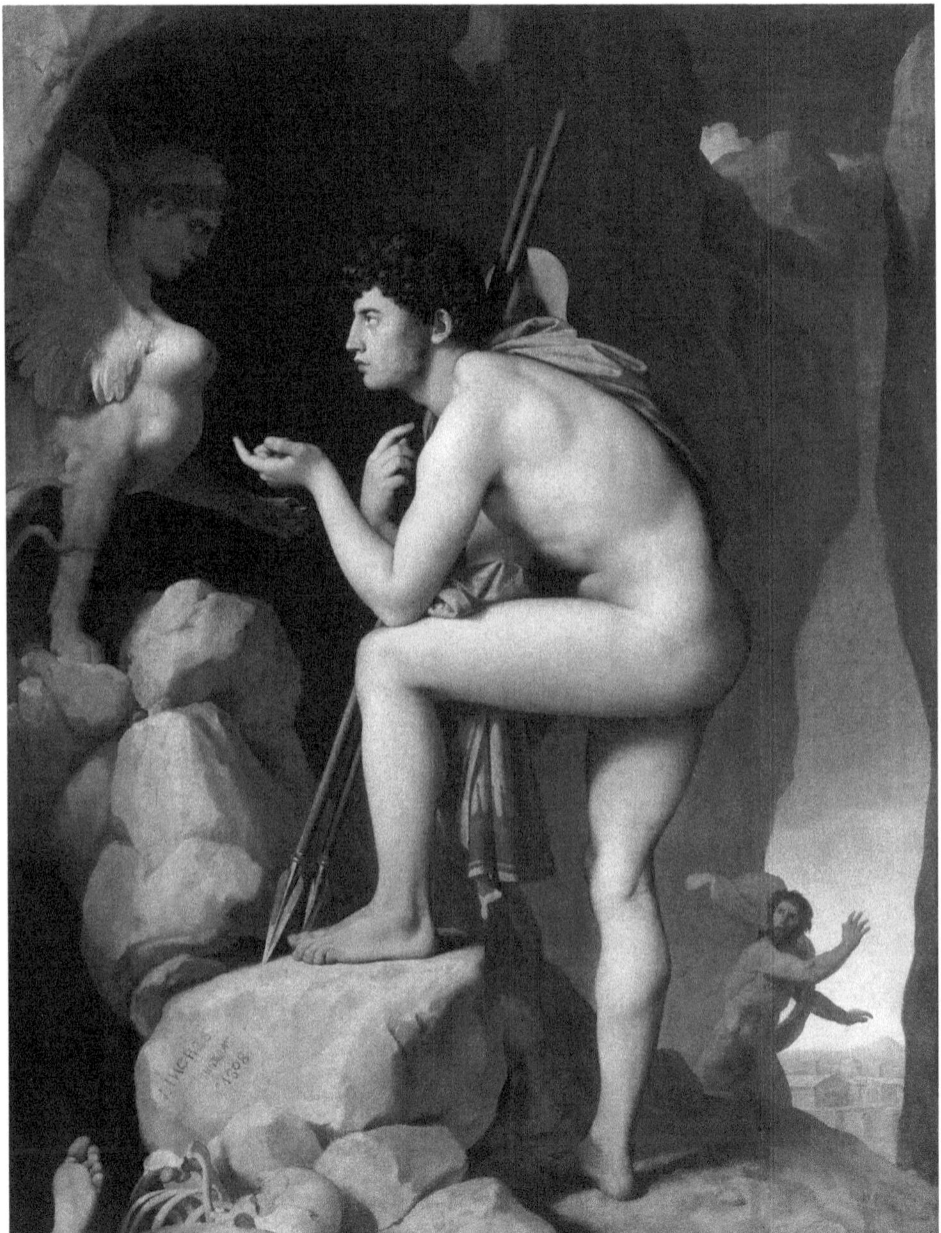

7.5 Jean-Auguste-Dominique Ingres, *Oedipus and the Sphinx*, 1808, oil on canvas, 189 x 144 cm.

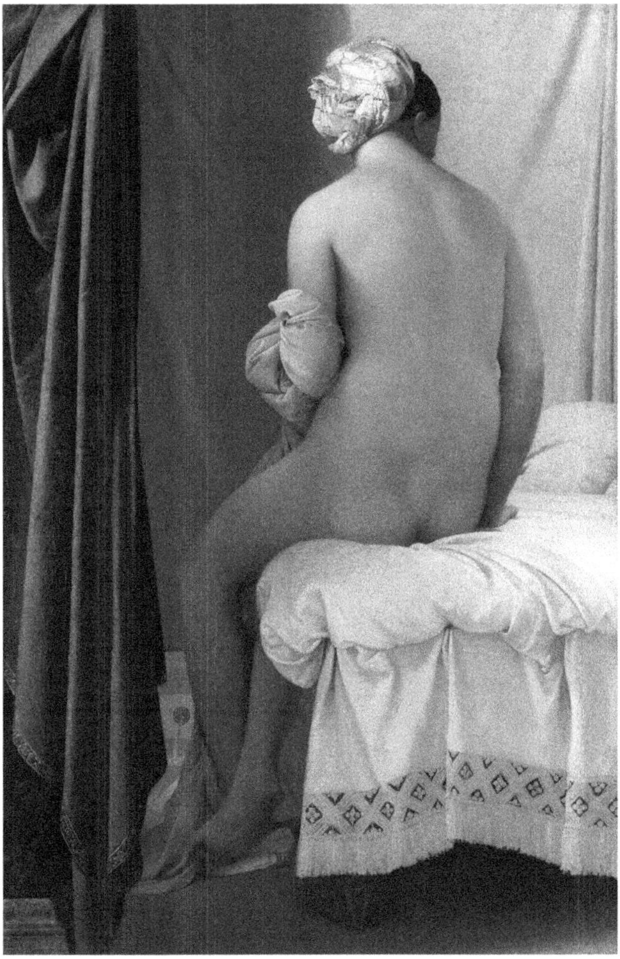

Jean-Auguste-Dominique Ingres, *Baigneuse de Valpinçon*, 1808, oil on canvas, 146 x 97 cm. 7.6

location of the Académie de France à Rome, he had already started a professional career in Paris: he had received several private commissions, among them the portraits of the Rivière family (discussed later on) and two highly prestigious commissions for Napoleon showing him as Premier consul (1804) and on his imperial throne (1806); and he had displayed works in the Salons of 1802 and 1806. It was probably in acknowledgement of these achievements that Ingres was granted, only a couple of weeks after his arrival in Rome, a house with studio of his own, the pavillion San Gaetano, separate from the other students yet in the grounds of the Villa. This allowed for a certain degree of independence, which is revealed, I believe, in the way the artist approached the institutional requirements. While the separate studio enabled Ingres to hire his own models (including female ones), it can be assumed that Ingres took part in the students' prescribed activities, which included daily life drawing exercises from 6 a.m. to 8 a.m. in the summer months and 6 p.m. to 8 p.m. during the winter season.[12] In any case, Ingres accomplished one of the major tasks set for the *pensionnaires*, that is, the production of painted nudes to be sent back to Paris in order to demonstrate the work and progress made in Italy. According to a report by Guillon-Lethière, director of the French Academy in Rome after the death of Joseph-Benoît Suvée, Ingres completed two male and two female *académies* between his arrival in 1806 and 1808, two of which were dispatched to Paris.[13] Other students submitted female nudes too: Joseph-Denis Odevaere, another former student of David, sent a nude that was referred to as 'Une femme au bain', while Ingres' *Baigneuse* was labelled 'Une femme assise'; among the sculptures there was likewise a female nude.[14] While not unprecedented, it remains astonishing in so far as life drawing in the academy (both in Paris and Rome) remained during most of the nineteenth century uniquely concerned with the male nude, with the *académie* being the most literal embodiment of the institution.[15] According to what is known from the *Correspondance des directeurs* and the regulations of the re-established Académie de France à Rome the models employed during the time that Ingres had his stipend were male. It is unlikely that an explicit point about this was ever made, and it seems that it simply went without saying. On the other hand, the fact that some of the figure study requirements of 1806 were actually female nudes was equally not worth a special mention by either the director of the Academy in Rome or members of the Classe des beaux-arts of the Institut de France who assessed the works upon reception. Their concern was far more with the overall quality of the works, which they found to be rather weak.

Looking at Ingres' two *envois de Rome* together, it can be argued that the painter did more than just fulfil his duties as a *pensionnaire*: he challenged the format by reflecting upon it. Granted, with his *Oedipus and the Sphinx* he placed himself in the tradition of the school of David, whose members had been particularly ambitious with their *envois de Rome*. As Thomas Crow has shown in much detail, David and students like Drouais, Fabre and Girodet had revalued the academic exercise and had turned the products of the life room almost into history paintings, either by dramatising the body as such and/or by adding props, landscape and further figures to open up a narrative dimension in this way.[16] Similarly, Ingres' *Oedipus and the Sphinx* has a theme beyond the academic exercise, and although focusing on one male nude, only makes sense through the inclusion of a second figure: the Sphinx situated at the margins and cropped by the picture frame. Ingres thus added a figure that was at least partially female to a setting that was typically all-male.[17] The hero is represented just at the moment when he solves the famous riddle posed by the hybrid creature. Despite his future destiny, which will prove futile all attempts to act wisely and rationally, in this very moment he is a figure that acts with his intellect and argues fearlessly with the monster, gesturing simultaneously to the Sphinx who had asked the riddle: which creature is first four-footed, then two-footed and finally three-footed?[18] Pointing to himself, Oedipus does not only speak the answer – 'man' – but also embodies it. The academic male nude is thus staged as what it is and used to be, the ideal embodiment of universal manhood. However, the body is seen from an unconventional angle, in the rather distanced mode of the profile. The figure has almost the character of a silhouette as Ingres emphasised the contour and neglected interior differentiation, thus downplaying the traditional task of a painted academy: displaying the integration of anatomical study and life drawing by suggesting a relief of muscles. While not entirely undisturbed by muscles, as was the case in Girodet's 1793 *envoi de Rome*, entitled *The Sleep of Endymion*, the surface is fairly smooth and homogeneous in tone, and makes no particular attempt to emphasise the musculature. This corresponds to some extent with the subject matter. Almost ironically Ingres chooses an intellectual rather than martial hero, shown in a moment of reflexion and suspended action,[19] and reversed the efforts made by David (in particular in his so-called *Patroclus*) and, following him, Jean-GermainDrouais (in the *Wounded Warrior*) during the pre-revolutionary period to narrativise the body through dramatic staging of the muscles. Despite the fraught moment, Oedipus' muscles do not translate as interior tension; the hero's force lies in his solid posture, firm gaze and in the gestures of his hands. Self-contained and concentrated, Oedipus seems oblivious to the remains of the victims of the Sphinx placed in the lower foreground and partially descending into an undefined black hole. With one foot still in the flesh, and a sand-coloured skull and bones that almost blend into the surrounding rocks, these human remains add a temporal dimension as they hint at victims who fell prey to the Sphinx in the more or less distant past. But the juxtaposition of bones and nude also recalls the ways in which the exercise of life drawing in academic training is built up from the study of bones and skeletons and thus always haunted by death and dead body parts. Ingres' *Oedipus and the Sphinx* can thus be aligned with one of the prints from Gamelin's aforementioned 1779 *Nouveau recueil d'ostéologie et de myologie* (Figure 7.2), in which a winged skeleton, surrounded by further still lifes of bones and skulls, holds up a drawing of a male nude, thus making a point about the interconnection of flesh and bones, of life drawing and anatomy personified in a symbol of death. With Oedipus figuring as the male nude, death and anatomy are remembered as something to be left behind.

The judgement on Ingres' *académies* made by the members of the Classe des beaux-arts of the Institut de France upon reception of the *envois de Rome* in 1809 does not explicitly mention a lack of anatomical skills, but it grasps aspects of the painting that work to downplay them:

> One can find in the figure of Oedipus by Ingres parts that are correctly drawn, well painted and rendered with truth; however one would wish that the figure as a whole had more gradation of light and of colour. The head is of a pale tone that has nothing to do with the rest of the figure, and it lacks nobility … The thigh and the right leg are well painted and their design is true. The rock should have been more coloured and more solid, this would have given more value to the flesh tones [*chairs*] that do not stand out enough against the surrounding objects.[20]

For the committee there were two major issues. In their view, the painting was too monochrome as Ingres failed to distinguish between the colour of the body and its environment. The flesh, one might deduce, looks like sand and stone, thus lacking the liveliness usually associated with the *carnations*. In addition, they remark a lack of gradation and hence of shading, a technique normally used to create relief and thus to suggest muscles underneath the skin. This seems to have been the effect Ingres was actively seeking. He was able to push this even more in his female nudes. Turning to the female nude was a means 'to eliminate narrative' as Susan Siegfried has convincingly suggested.[21] This is an issue not only of topic but also of anatomy, as the female body allowed for a reduction of the appearance of muscles, the physical agents of movement and gestural expression. Ingres left anatomy further behind by, somewhat ironically, adopting a view of the female body he shared with nineteenth-century physicians. Most anatomists and art theorists agreed that women's skin and what they called 'adipose membrane' served to hide their anatomy to a large extent. This is why the critic Landon considered the female model inapt for the academic study of the nude, the main purpose of which was, in his eyes, to 'make the science of anatomy shine'.[22] Discussing a later *envoi de Rome* shown at the Salon of 1822, Léon Cogniet's *Jeune Chasseresse*, he generally bemoaned the relaxation of the requirements for the *pensionnaires* in Rome, and stated that female nudes are not appropriate for this kind of academic exercise. The younger generation of artists obviously did not agree with this assessment, and for Ingres the female nude was of interest for precisely the same reasons that she was unsuitable for Landon.

Skin and canvas: the *Baigneuse de Valpinçon*

Unlike Landon, the committee of the Classe des beaux-arts did not take issue with the fact that the *pensionnaires* sent female nudes, at least they made no comment of that kind. Their assessment of Ingres' *Baigneuse* resembles in many respects that of the *Œdipus*, as they praise the drawing but notice a want of variation in colour and shading:

> In the figure of a woman dressed with some kind of turban, we noticed parts which are finely drawn, well painted and rendered with truth. But one would have wished that the painting had more decided effects; it is hard to guess where the light comes from, the reflections of the body permeate among the tones of the linen in the half tones, and the figure does not cast any shadow on the plane where it rests. The curtain that forms a straight and dark line on the foreground of the painting is not successfully placed. Considering the talent that Ingres demonstrates in his works, one would desire that he rather engaged with the beautiful character of antiquity, and the grand and noble style that must have inspired the beautiful productions of the old masters of the good times of the Roman school.[23]

What is interesting about this appraisal is not so much what it says, but what it omits. There is no indication that the artist changed the gender of the nude and shifted its potential cultural connotations. The latter could be seen as hidden in the admonition that the artist should have taken his inspiration from 'the beautiful character of antiquity'. While the academic male nudes of the period generally followed bodily models of antiquity and made allusions to classical themes, Ingres situated his female nude in a vaguely defined environment. A curtain to the left introduces the space behind as a separate reality, all the more so as it ends on a base with no other function than carrying the artist's signature, thus assigning it as the artificial space of the painting, a vision materialised by the artist. The eye is both directed to and arrested by the woman's naked back – a large surface of immaculate skin stretched out like a projection screen. It is doubled in the canvas in the background that closes the shallow pictorial space. As I will argue, Ingres' painting very actively engages with this interaction of closure and visibility, and the immaculate skin as much as the painted fabrics plays an important role in this.

In the shallow space opened through the curtain, we get a glimpse of a basin and fountain, locating the nude in a bath and affording, in conjunction with the turban, an interpretation of the site as a Turkish bath or harem, and thus an association with the imaginary rather than geographical space that has tended to be called 'the Orient'.[24] This is certainly a direction in which Ingres took the topic himself in later revivals of his earlier nude, such as the 1828 *Interior of a Harem* or the late *Turkish Bath*. However, in the *Valpinçon Bather* Ingres did not employ local décor, for example, to evoke reality. His nude is situated in a generic bath, and the lack of shadows – criticised by the Classe des beaux-arts – suggests the site as a fantasy space. Moreover, there is more than just one 'Orient' at stake. The Orient as a concept and France's relation to the actual spaces and people associated with it were in considerable transformation between the period of Ancien Régime France, with its largely friendly diplomatic relationships with the Ottoman Empire via the rule of Napoleon in the aftermath of the Egyptian campaign to the later colonial engagement of France in North Africa. Ingres must have witnessed the impact that some of these developments, notably the Egyptian campaign, had on the artistic scene in Paris during the period before he left for Rome as he had a studio in the Couvent des Capucines, a former convent secularised during the Revolution and later allocated to artists.[25] Among the artists who had their studios in the convent during the first decade of the nineteenth century were Girodet and Antoine-Jean Gros, former students of David. Both artists were facing the challenges Jean-Joseph Sue had described in his 1797 *Essai sur la physiognomonie* (discussed in my chapter on skin colour) as they were engaging in paint with a multitude of complexions. Girodet produced his portraits of Mamelucks at the convent, while Gros was working on battle paintings commemorating Napoleon's Egyptian campaign. These large format canvases transformed history painting as they turned towards more or less contemporary events, however much mystified. This transformation went along with a shift in the significance of the male nude, once the linchpin of history painting. The modern French hero could – unlike the ancient Greek and Roman precursors which still populated many neoclassical history paintings – no longer convincingly be represented unclothed. Nudity was instead transferred to the enemies, and along with it orientalised, sexualised and frequently feminised.[26]

Given his time spent in the community of artists at the Couvent des Capucines, Ingres was certainly not unaware of the prevalence of oriental subject matter when he left for Rome and is likely to have been aware of the consequences these new topics had for the male nude and the relevance of its institutional incarnation, the *académie*. But Ingres' pictorial engagement with the Orient remained second hand. Unlike painters such as Eugène Delacroix or, later, Jean-Léon Gérôme, he never travelled to Turkey or North Africa, and took all the detail of decorative elements for later works such as the *Grande Odalisque* or the *Turkish Bath* (1852–59) from images, such as paintings or sixteenth- to eighteenth-century illustrated travel accounts.[27] In his *Baigneuse* he evoked what could be understood as oriental with very few attributes, which present themselves quite obviously as citations from other art works and remain culturally rather unspecific. The striped fabric wound around the woman's head is a hair-do often found in Italian Renaissance painting, and is thus taken from the type of source the *pensionnaire*s were meant to study and emulate. One well-known example is the so-called *Fornarina* by Raphael (Figure 5.11), a painter highly fashionable at the time and a particularly important artistic model for Ingres and certainly included in what the Classe des beaux-arts canonised as 'old masters of the good times of the Roman school'. What is more, the water basin in the background might well have been inspired by a painting such as David's *Paris and Helen* of 1789, and is thus a fitment that could evoke both antiquity and the Orient. This latter painting and its narrative – relating to the Trojan war – can also serve as a reminder that French relations with Asia Minor, the geographical location it refers to, were all but settled around 1800, since it could be associated both with antiquity and with the Ottoman Empire. While French neoclassical culture, especially during the Revolution, embraced and appropriated the ancients as their own ancestors, Turkey and Persia were rather associated with the strange, exotic and foreign.

The sparse *Baigneuse de Valpinçon* opens up an imaginary space, and if it evokes a bath or seraglio setting, this is mainly via the closure of both the represented and the pictorial space, the invitation into which is uncertain. This space is both inviting and impassable: the nude seen from the back allows the eye to linger on the body's surface while simultaneously blocking the view into the depth. The painted back is kept flat, with just enough gradation of tone to still be legible as a body. Faceless it remains non-descript, not showing any obvious signs of gender difference.[28] The pale, immaculate skin that works so well as a projection screen, was not, however, culturally neutral; it was simultaneously an element of ideal beauty and of racial distinction. In narratives of the harem, the white and spotless skin served as a marker of beauty and distinction, supported by the assumption that the most beautiful odalisques were light-skinned slaves imported from the Caucasus region. This was already the view in the late seventeenth century as seen in François Bernier's 1684 'New Division of the Earth' (discussed in chapter 5), but it gained new significance in the light of late eighteenth-century racial anthropologies, notably Johann Friedrich Blumenbach's theory that Caucasia was the home of the world's most beautiful people and the cradle of humankind.[29]

The best-known travel report providing an account of a harem and Turkish bath, as well as of its inhabitants' immaculate skin, was Lady Mary Wortley Montagu's letters published posthumously in 1762, and immediately translated into French.[30] Being a noble woman and an ambassador's wife, Lady Montagu had the privilege of travelling and the advantage of being granted access to spaces restricted to women. Staging herself as a foreigner who encounters a strange world with curiosity and wonder, she expressed surprise about the politeness and cultivation of women in a state of 'stark nakedness' so uncommon to the eyes of a British lady, and admires the women as 'well proportioned and white skinned; all of them smooth and polished by the frequent use of bathing'.[31] In an earlier letter she had already pointed out the 'shiningly white' skin and remarks that in a space where everybody is naked, 'the face would be hardly observed. I perceived that the ladies with the finest skins and most delicate shapes had the greatest share of my admiration'.[32] Montagu associated the unclothed women in the bath with art works, as she evoked drawings by Guido and Titian and suggested that the women in the *bagnio* could perfectly represent 'the figures of the Graces'. She thus not only made the women imaginable for her European readers,[33] but also framed them as images.

The *Baigneuse de Valpinçon* certainly allows, and allowed at the time of its production, associations of the harem or the Turkish bath and of the pristine women inhabiting it. These associations are however brought to the painting by those looking at it. The nude and the space it is framed by remain unspecific, offering themselves as projection screen rather than being explicitly 'oriental'. What aligns Ingres' painting and Lady Montagu's *bagnio* is their construction as closed space, whose inhabitants are brought to visibility as art. In the painting this is addressed via the painted white fabric that spans the entire background, without actually seeming very far removed, thus giving no real sense of the extent of this fictive room, but just making a point about its closure. It emphasises the flatness of the painting, by barring the depth and pushing the image to the foreground. And if a harem can be associated with this painted space, then potentially as a meta-pictorial metaphor of the closure of the pictorial space itself.

Flattened and situated nearly in line with the picture plane itself, the broad surface of the body is paralleled with the fabric. And some *trompe l'œil* folds were needed, to indicate that this is not just the painting's ground or background. It is only by showing itself as such that the cloth opens the possibility of being seen as an echo of the canvas on which the nude has been painted. It is thus not through unveiling but through a veil that Ingres' *Baigneuse* can be said to be staged as paint on canvas. Turning its back, the body is drawn into the flattened pictorial space and, with the drapery around its arm, wound into the white and greyish fabrics by which it is almost entirely surrounded.[34] Skin is clearly not the vibrant 'nervous canvas' that it had been evoked as by eighteenth-century physicians, artists and art theorists, nor a communicative membrane, but a mute surface which is nevertheless aligned with the medium of painting itself: a surface made of paint on canvas. The *Bather* exposes skin as an immaculate surface that looks untouched and untouchable both as an object represented and as a representation, since the painting as a whole looks – like most works by Ingres – as if it was barely touched by the artist's brush.

The nude, still legible as a body after all, is however not entirely flat nor completely sealed. The almost hermetic surface of the back hints at an orifice through the slight indication of a cleavage at the buttocks. The eyes are drawn to it, as the folds of the sheet on the bed bundle at the body's centre of gravity. Just below, the drapery pads in such a way as to echo the bottom that sits on it. This technique of echoing bodily forms in drapery and upholstery was often used in eighteenth-century erotic art, in paintings by Fragonard or, for example, Boucher's 1745 *Odalisque* where the forms of the reclining nude seen from the back (but looking at the viewer) are multiplied in the plush fabrics. But rather than amplifying sensual plenitude, the puffed up sheets which have more volume than the body itself in Ingres' painting are a deferral of bodily forms and openings. They reflect upon the body's flatness and provide a further link between skin and canvas while remaining erotically charged.

In Ingres' *Valpinçon Bather* closure and deferred openings co-exist, and a sense of untouchability is combined with the haptic appeal of the nude. This creates a strange feeling of ambivalence, and I use the terms 'touch' or 'tactile' versus 'haptic' to approach the different ways in which the sense of touch can be mobilised via two-dimensional images and the relationship between seeing and touching can work. Ingres' paintings produce their haptic effects and evoke the materiality of the different stuffs and forms precisely by almost entirely effacing the traces of the brush. The painted skin, especially, prompts a slippery ambivalence of smooth flatness and volume, a *noli me tangere* – a desire to touch and the inhibition of it at the same time.[35]

This ambivalence of haptic appeal and untouchability also characterises the body of a young woman in one of Ingres' early portraits, a work which also addresses tactility: the portrait of Caroline Rivière finished before the artist's departure to Rome (Plate 16). Painted along with those of her parents between 1805 and 1806 before being shown at the Salon in autumn 1806, the portrait sets the girl (born in 1793, she was about thirteen years old when portrayed) against a landscape background. With the body in semi-profile and the face turned towards the picture plane, neck, head and shoulder are neatly circumscribed like a silhouette. Through the eyes turned towards the viewer, and the rosy cheeks and red lips matched with earrings of the same colour, there is a certain freshness and open address despite the absence of an explicit facial expression. The portrait has a number of similarities with the back view of the bather: the ivory skin tone is brought out by being put next to the white fabrics, and the skin texture is concealed through the smooth finish of the painterly surface. But little of Caroline Rivière's skin is actually disclosed; besides the face and moderate décolleté, the garments only reveal fragments of her arms and hands. While the Empire dress is short-sleeved, the arms are covered by gloves reaching from the palms to the upper arm near the dress and disclosing just a slit of naked skin. Oversized and of somewhat chunky brazen brown leather, these gloves are like a badly fitted second skin, displaying all the folds Ingres usually avoids detailing in human skin. Even though the gloves allow the fingers – these fine instruments of touch – some freedom, they seem to prohibit the touching of the skin and of the most sensory item evoked in the canvas: a very soft looking white shawl around Mademoiselle Rivière's arms, which has been convincingly identified by Aileen Ribeiro as a *fichu de cygne*, a swansdown scarf.[36] The very thought of it prompts sensual feelings, and given that this was a very fashionable item at the time, it is likely to have been identified by contemporary viewers, possibly imagining the girl as a modern Leda. Interestingly, the critic Castagnary who, not always sympathetic to Ingres, was quite taken by this portrait, compared it to the works of Correggio known for his *sfumato* (otherwise so different from Ingres' polished surfaces) and a *Leda with the Swan* (ca 1532). While the arms of the painted adolescent would feel the lining of the leather gloves, they can't sense the softness of the feathers. Only a finger at each hand is painted on top of the shawl – whether they are meant to touch, in the imaginary space of the painting it is impossible to make out. Evenly painted, the skin of Caroline Rivière is as perfectly sealed as that of the *Valpinçon Bather*, and is visibly kept from the enjoyment of too intense and pleasant sensory perceptions. And yet, there are some apertures elsewhere. The glove leaves a gap at one of the arms, allowing a glimpse at the lining and into the space between the human and animal skin. And, one lower end of the scarf is turned inside out, showing instead of the rounded body of downs a suture with some black spots evoking an undefined inside. Remarkably, it is at this seam, which would most obviously be the work of the person who fabricated the swansdown garment, that Ingres left the trace of a brushstroke performing as such. Ingres generally worked with very thin layers of paint producing seamless surfaces and is reported to have renounced *la touche* as an 'abuse of painterly execution',[37] but rarely and selectively the handling is exposed. In the portrait of Caroline Rivière, the trace left is in a highly significant spot: placed on the suture of the shawl it surrounds an undefined opening and marks a point where both the painting and the piece of dress give an insight into their making.

The flattening and sealing of the body is thus never entirely complete, and it is not, as scholars like Robert Rosenblum and Uwe Fleckner, arguing from a modernist perspective, have suggested, merely a form of abstraction.[38] Instead, it is an engagement with the relationship between the flat and the haptic, the untouchable and the evocation of touch, between body and image, between canvas, skin and painted surface. These issues, along with the possibilities of embodiment by pictorial means, are, I will argue, further investigated in two remarkable drawings around the theme of *Venus Anadyomene*.

Skin and paper: a navel

In parallel to preparing his *envois de Rome* Ingres started working on a number of other female nudes. The genre gained currency during the Napoleonic period, and notably the *Grande Odalisque* and similar works were commissions by Joachim Murat, king of Naples and Sicily between 1808 and 1815, and his wife, Napoleon's sister Caroline.[39] As already discussed, Ingres' interest in the female nude went beyond the genre itself. Work on the topic of Venus Anadyomene started with drawings around 1807 and, like the oriental nude, it would preoccupy the artist for decades. Several drawings, even though related to the painting, seem independently to explore the emergence of bodily forms from the paper ground, and the relations between paper and skin. The reworked painted *Venus Anadyomene* was finally finished in 1848

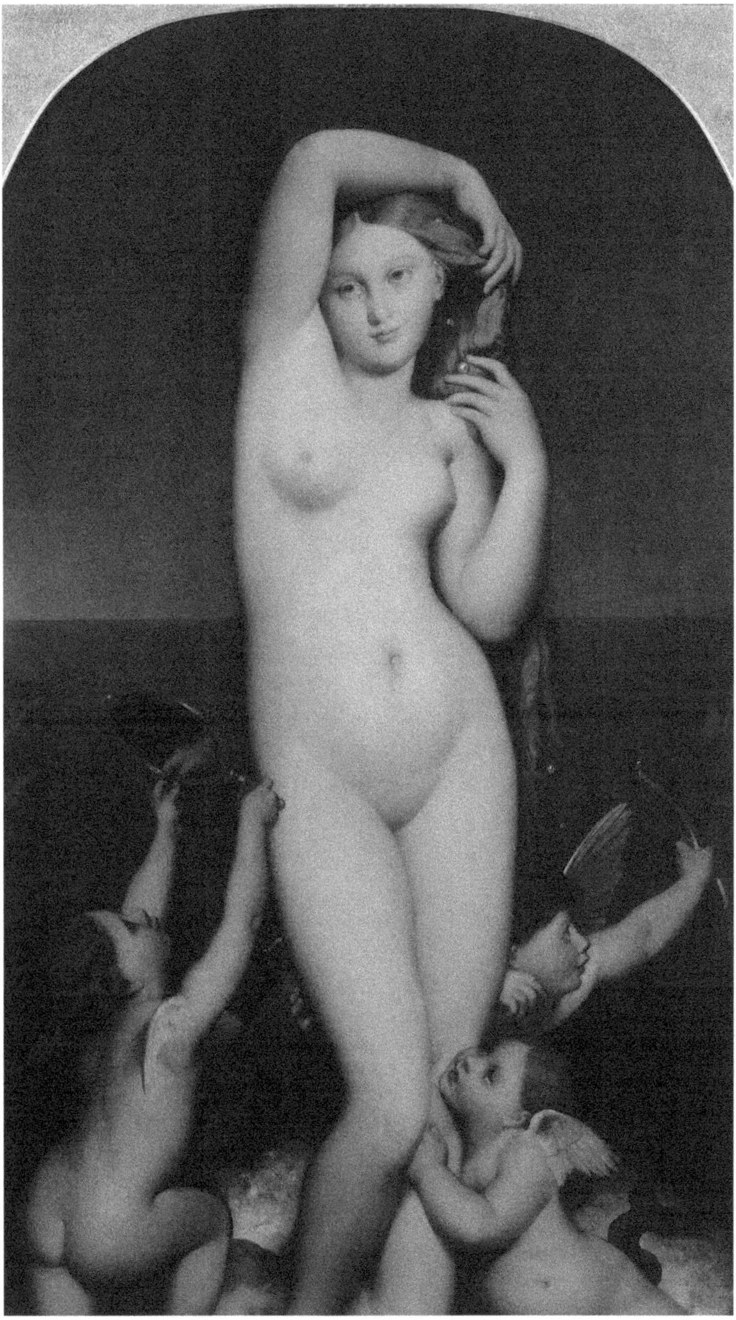

Jean-Auguste-Dominique Ingres, *Venus Anadyomene*, 1808/48, oil on canvas, 163 x 92 cm. 7.7

(Figure 7.7) and became, along with Ingres' *La Source*, the epitome of the idealised nineteenth-century female nude: almost entirely stripped of a narrative context, the paintings expose the female body frontally and represent it in a smooth cover of uniformly coloured flesh and skin.

Since antiquity the art literature had been aware of the fact that the ideal body is a construction built from parts, an insight that has been conceived in more psychoanalytical terms since the twentieth century: the flip side of the ideal and complete image of the self is the fragmented body, the 'corps morcélé'.[40] The body in pieces does not seem to have been a repressed fantasy in the case of Ingres. In an early pencil drawing for *Venus Anadyomene* (1807), he referenced Zeuxis, and the well-known story according to which the ancient painter constructed a painting of Helen – the embodiment of perfect beauty whom he lacked as a model – by fusing beautiful parts of five different women. The figure is surrounded by a plethora of written notes. With frequent repetitions, Ingres jotted down the parts of Venus to be painted – feet, breast, neck – and was obsessed with the question of their materiality. Equating Venus's body with precious materials like ivory and alabaster, he took up well-known literary tropes of praise of female beauty. He was particularly occupied with the question of its colouring, testing a multitude of words for shades of white culminating in the otherworldly 'alabaster breast that is equal to the argentine splendour of the moon'.[41]

The artist is also quite explicitly engaged with body parts in drawings on the theme of Venus Anadyomene produced from 1807 onwards.[42] One of the drawings singles out the head of Venus and is quite unique due to its cropping, or rather the way in which the arm and head are fitted on to the sheet (Figure 7.8). Unlike in the more traditional *Venus pudica* pose used in other (possibly earlier) drawings, such as the one just mentioned, but similar to the later painting the arm is laid around the head. The move away from gestures covering the body and expressing chastity, to a full disclosure of the naked front, can be seen as a way of turning skin itself into what was considered as women's natural veil and cover. For example, the art critic and theorist Charles Blanc later stated in his *Grammaire des arts du dessin*: 'A female body, even if it is naked, stays thus veiled under a transparent skin covering large draperies of muscles, that are the *pudeur* of the skeleton'.[43] As in the illustrations for Fau's anatomy for artists or Diderot's dread of a female écorché (both discussed at the end of the previous chapter), women's physical interior is made taboo, in this case in suggesting that nature had to veil the skeleton under a double layer of muscles and skin. In Ingres's drawing, the change of pose also results in the arm becoming a frame for the head. The arm's outer borderlines are not indicated; the drawn flesh ends sharply with the angular margins of the paper, thus aligning pictorial and bodily frame as well as the represented body with the sheet. What can be read as an arm, especially in view of the later painting and similar contemporary drawings that leave more space for the body, actually oscillates between the illusion of a three-dimensional volume and a flat shape that cuts out the face. The body thus merges into the support on to which it is drawn, and at the same time the image is not just a representation of a head but also a drawing about the emergence of a form on paper.

This can also be said about another unusual drawing, which, even though fragmenting the body, is a well-composed picture in its own right rather than just a preparatory sketch (Figure 7.9).[44] It is a more or less life-sized drawing of a navel placed in the upper half of a small piece of paper (5.3 x 6.3 cm). It has been suggested that the drawing dates from around 1808 and was made as one of the studies for Venus Anadyomene,[45] and it makes sense to consider it as such, as it can be interpreted as a reflection on processes of generation and separation. The navel is drawn as a circle and defines, along with a bit of shadow above it, the surrounding area as a belly. It is thus through this

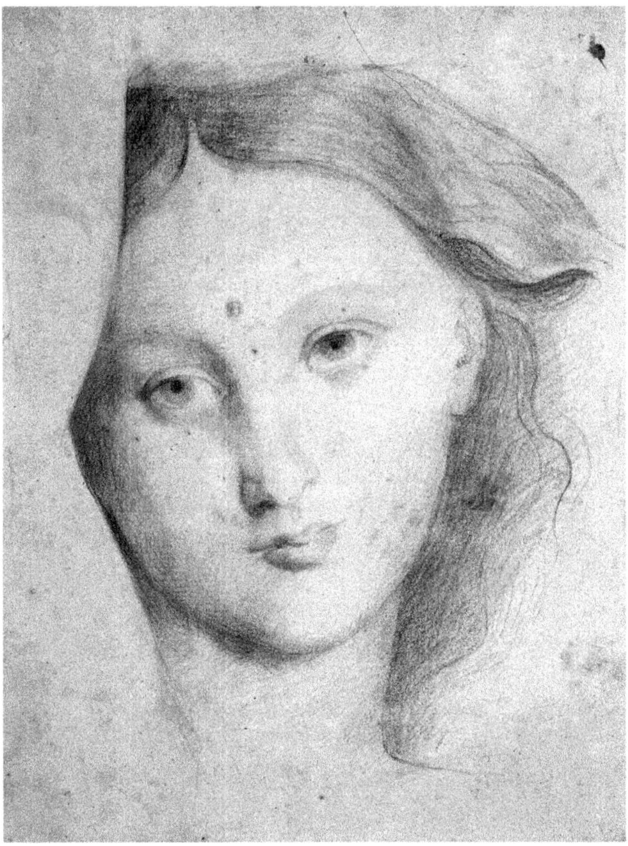

Jean-Auguste-Dominique Ingres, *Head of Venus*, ca 1808, graphite on paper, 27.7 x 20.8 cm. 7.8

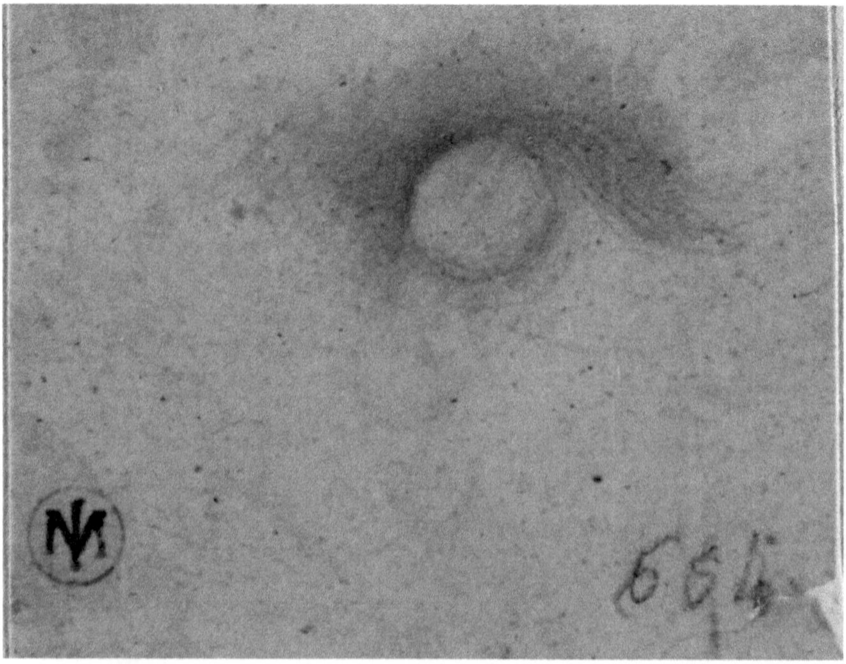

7.9 Jean-Auguste-Dominique Ingres, *Navel*, ca 1808, graphite on paper, 5.3 x 6.3 cm.

minimal sketch of a circle and a shadow that the viewer sees a curving out of the picture plane, the relief of a body. No line circumscribes the belly or trunk as such; it is marked by the navel and the illusion of a convexity limited by the edges of the paper. Due to this cropping the image oscillates between the flatness of the piece of paper and the volume evoked by the shading. Since the beige colour of the paper works convincingly enough as a light flesh tone, skin and paper collude here even more explicitly than skin and canvas in the *Baigneuse de Valpinçon*. A minimalist indication of a curved volume on a piece of paper, this drawing is, I suggest, as much a way of thinking about processes of embodiment through the means of visual representation as it is about a navel. Yet, the navel is not just any body part. It is a reminder of a former connection and the scar of a separation. But why this attention to the navel of a mythological figure, which, if logic works with deities incarnate, should not have one? As is well known, this particular manifestation of Venus rose from the spume as a fully fleshed adult. The goddess had never been in a womb and hence should carry no scar from the cutting of the umbilical cord. In the drawing, Venus does not rise from the sea but a highly significant body part rises from the paper, emerging as a somewhat rudimentary fantasy of autonomous male generative power (one for which the ancient gods had a high price to pay though).[46] The drawing of Venus' navel can thus be seen as a reflection about the production of an image as an act of separation or externalisation. The image of the navel stands in for the process of separation initiated by drawing a line and turning paper into skin.

The navel drawn by Ingres looks not so much like a 'piece of knotted skin', as Elisabeth Bronfen has called it, a folded entity that blurs any clear 'demarcation between the intimate and the external', but like a belly button. It is a neat seal hardly recalling a stoma, a very well disguised 'simulation of an erotogenic orifice'.[47] Rather than a marker of sexual difference, the belly button is a marker of separation which is, just like the orifice in the *Valpinçon Bather*, not specifically gendered.[48] Together with the belly button, the entire skin is the outcome of a separation. Formed by the pencil it merges with the paper and coincides with the image's surface making the drawing and body part a separate entity. As such, this particular belly button points to the closure of skin in Ingres' works more generally.

The concealment of the female body and a highly ambivalent relationship to bodily orifices have often been characterised by feminist scholarship as a quintessential aspect of the simultaneously eroticised and desexualised female nude. The idealisation of the female body in representation has been assessed as a classic instance of fetishism in the Freudian sense: the ideal female nude is understood as a fetish that manages anxieties about the female body imagined as castrated.[49] Fetishism thus works to deal with the castration complex and assuage the potential threat to masculine narcissism. However, the consistency with which Ingres renounced physiological or morphological realities in paintings such as the *Baigneuse de Valpinçon* or the *Grande Odalisque* does not provide the reassuring effect of the fetish.[50] On the contrary, Ingres pushed idealisation so far that it produced an inverse reaction. As scholars like Carol Ockman have pointed out, the artist's quest for perfection in form was taken to such an extreme that it often resulted in bizarre anatomical distortion, and the sensuous, undulating contours with which nudes like the *Grande Odalisque* are circumscribed can simultaneously please and trouble.[51] The body is sealed by a uniform skin made of a seamless layer of glossy paint, taking away any porosity as well as leaving the knowledge and procedures of artistic anatomy as far behind as possible. Ironically though, this foreclosure of any reference to the body's physiology and anatomical interior only brings the paradox of artistic anatomy to the fore. Critics like Landon, quoted at the outset, so accustomed to scrutinising the painted or chiselled surface for anatomical correctness, saw seamless skin, but thought of bones and muscles. Similarly, the art critic Auguste-Hilarion de Kératry famously deduced an extra lumbar vertebra in the Odalisque's spine to explain its unusual length.[52] Looking at this female nude, they exercised the techniques of mental dissection that artistic anatomy almost exclusively probed with male figures, from ancient sculpture to the life model.

Yet, Ingres was in line with some aspects of contemporary artistic anatomy, namely the discipline's increasing attention to the body's surface. He only went half way though, as he largely refused to model the painted skin as a surface legible with regard to its internal formation. The female nude was a means of renouncing this aspect of artistic anatomy more radically; this, again, was in keeping with a general understanding of female forms as disclosing less anatomical detail. This was notably argued by authors of artistic anatomies who wrote the female interior out of their treatises by ascribing to the women's body a higher degree of concealment, because it was more fleshy and rounded than that of the male. Sue (the younger), for example, suggested that 'in a well formed women … the arms are more chubby, … ; the muscles much less apparent, the members more rounded, their outlines more pleasant, the traits of the face finer, finally the skin more white and more delicate'.[53] Similar to Blanc's later remarks, Salvage's *Anatomie du Gladiateur* reinforced this view in claiming that women's muscles are 'completely hidden' by the subcutaneous fatty layer.[54]

Monochrome flesh tones

Ingres' early critics were apparently not willing to accept the consequential translation of this anatomical view of women's physical appearance into a female nude. They perceived a lack of' 'interior modelling' and hence detailing of parts of the body. In addition, there was also an issue with the flesh tones as such; early nineteenth-century art criticism lacked the suitable vocabulary to appreciate Ingres' particular way of making *carnations*. The artist did indeed only partially comply with what was understood as a successful rendering of flesh tones. The dominant contemporary practice still, was to employ all the primary colours in addition to the basic flesh tone typically consisting of, depending on the hue to be achieved, varying amounts of white, yellow (usually ochres) and red. The artist and art theorist Paillot de Montabert, a former student of David, suggested this kind of approach to *carnations* in his multi-volume *Traité complet de la peinture* (1829–51), a monumental summary of neoclassical doctrines mixed with insights from medical discourse:

> As far as the chromatic character of flesh is concerned, it consists of the transparency and the variation of tints (*teintes*). The finer the skin, the more these variations shine through. The light that penetrates the skin takes on the bluish tints of the veins, the red tints of the arterial vessels and also the colour of the fat and the tendons [white, as he explains elsewhere]. In consequence, all colours are as if they were confused and half-hidden though the skin, the epidermis of which refracts the rays that cross it via its texture. The skin, independent of its polish or roughness in certain areas, also offers, in particular on the cheeks, a certain

> velvety quality that the cold smoothness of the brush is unable to express. The shine of sanguine and golden colours, tempered by the tender and bluish tints showing through, can only be expressed by an artist with a very delicate eye.[55]

In a manner that had been characteristic of the art discourse on flesh tones for centuries, matters of artistic imitation and of physiological processes are entangled here. It is typical of neoclassical art theory, however, that the site in which the processes mimicked are located is designated as skin rather than flesh. In many portraits of David, skin is, as I have shown, rendered as a semi-transparent membrane via the use of thin strokes of blue to mimic veins underneath the epidermis and areas of red to signal the presence of blood and suggest vivacity. Ingres, in contrast, does not use these means to give a sense of the skin's translucency but turns the human envelope into a homogeneous opaque surface. In both portraits and nudes he works with one single skin tone gradually modified in its intensity to indicate a certain degree of shading and to produce some sense of bodily form. The effect looks almost like a grisaille in flesh tone, emphasising the haptic quality as the shading makes up for the lack of colour; and it seems logical that Ingres made a painted variant of his *Grande Odalisque* in grisaille (New York, Metropolitan Museum).

However, the soft ivory or honey tone is crucial for the appeal of Ingres' nudes, and in the *Baigneuse de Valpinçon* the very light hue of the skin is emphasised against the white fabrics with their greyish shades. The committee of the Classe des beaux-arts could only see this as a lack of variation, and with regard to the female nudes Ingres showed at the Salon of 1819, critics were generally in agreement with Landon (quoted above) that the flesh tones were too monochrome. Kératry, looking at the *Grande Odalisque*, spoke of 'teintes monotones' resulting in a kind of coolness, 'giving indication of no sentiment at all' – on the part of the painter as much as the painted nude. Critics could not accept this way of treating flesh tones, missing the customary variation of colour to produce vivacity. All the more surprising then, that Kératry added to his observations: 'and yet, I don't know how, but there is something of Titian'.[56] He thus evoked the artist who remained in the nineteenth century the exemplary master of flesh tones, still appraised in terms very similar to those of the sixteenth century as a painter in whose '*carnations* circulated blood'.[57] But blood was exactly what Ingres' painted bodies lacked in the eyes of most critics. His painting is decisively non-physiological and the artist did not use fine strokes of blue to indicate subcutaneous veins, nor reddish zones in the skin to signal blood circulation. And yet, it seems that Kératry saw a sensuality in Ingres' flesh tones without quite knowing the terms in which to appreciate it.

Among those who praised Titian's mastery of flesh tones in the nineteenth century was Paillot de Montabert, even though he did so in a manner different from early modern art theorists like Roger de Piles, who praised the Venetian painter for the interplay between the vivacity of brushstrokes and the liveliness of flesh tones. Paillot de Montabert singled out the way Titian used neighbouring colours to highlight the flesh tones. Not quite consistent with the passage quoted above, he generally praised the beauty of light skin tones and argued that the flesh tones can seem lively even if they are of one single tone. His appraisal of Titian might have been written in view of Ingres' *Valpinçon Bather*: 'he contrasted whitish flesh [*chairs*] with white sheets, and this opposition which whitened the sheets coloured the flesh. Had he refrained from white fabrics and replaced them by red the same flesh would have seemed pallid and without life'.[58] The phrasing remains vague as to whether this 'rouge' was in the fabrics or in the flesh tones, but it sounds like an attempt to evoke blood without using red pigment. This is a dissociation of the materiality of the paint from the materiality of the body, as it induces a sense of flesh through the juxtaposition of more or less pure whites.

Ingres' early critics, such as Landon and Kératry, who represented a by then conservative neoclassicism, treated Ingres like a stray student of David who made the wrong aesthetic choices while disregarding anatomy, with the effect of getting the flesh tones wrong and failing to give his painted bodies structure and proportion. In contrast, later critics were more accustomed to seeing such features as elements of the artist's aesthetic idiosyncrasy, whether they liked them or not. After the artist's return from his extended first stay in Rome in 1825, and his establishment of a studio (making him a *Chef d'école*), he was increasingly seen as a category of his own. At the occasion of the Salon of 1833 where Ingres exhibited the portraits of Madame Duvaucey and Monsieur Bertin, the term *ingriste* was coined, which identified a specific aesthetic represented by Ingres and his studio, particularly associated with portraits of women.[59] After the dramatic withdrawal of Ingres from the Salon following the critical controversy around his *Martyr de Saint Symphorien* (for once, part of the critique was the excessive muscularity of the Saint's executioners), the tendency to construct Ingres as an entity of his own amplified. It was fostered by the private exhibitions in his studio and the presentation of eleven of his works in a separate room at the exhibition at the Bazar Bonne-Nouvelle, and culminated in the retrospective at the *Exposition Universelle* of 1855.[60] While advocates and opponents of Ingres equally contributed to the fabrication of 'Monsieur Ingres', later critics, at least those benevolent to Ingres, were more prepared to appreciate the artist's flesh tones on their own terms and approved of their artificial materiality. The famous novelist and poet Théophile Gautier, for example, in his response to the 1855 Ingres retrospective, brought to life the *Grande Odalisque* in his description. He praised the 'gilded whiteness' of the shoulders and gave prominence to the flow of lines rather than that of blood, when writing of the 'soft flesh' of the back 'in which flows a delicious serpentine line'.[61] The line that, as I have argued, stands in for the skin seems to be strangely located within the body here. But it is the line, rather than the flesh, that is animate in a double sense, flowing and serpent-like.[62] In turn, Gautier imagined the flesh to be of a hybrid materiality, soft but inorganic with associations of alabaster, ivory and marble, materials similar to those evoked by Ingres in his notes for the *Venus Anadyomene*. While Gautier firmly placed the *Odalisque* in his orientalist fantasy triggered by the painting, Charles Blanc, author of an early monograph on Ingres, isolated the figure from the picture in order to admire her. Arguing that Ingres has 'modified her type in the occidental sense', he juxtaposed the 'abundant *carnations* which are the living luxury of the harem' with the 'filled and smooth' skin of this particular nude by Ingres. While using the term *carnations* in a more positive sense elsewhere in his book, in this instance the painted flesh (paint as flesh) has become vulgar and externalised as oriental. In contrast, skin is understood as pure surface which coalesces with the highly finished surface of the painting rarely showing traces of handling. Blanc frequently used the term *lisse* (smooth) for both the painted skin and the surface of the painting. With an analogy that replaces the old entanglement of flesh and paint, he thus described what more

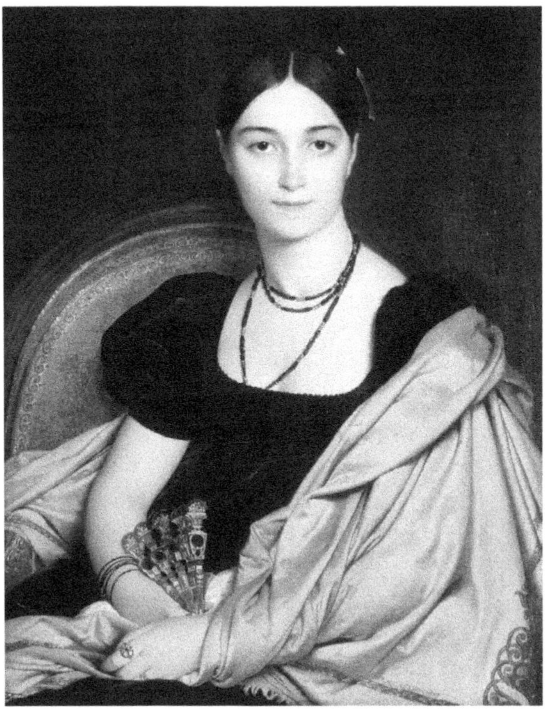

Jean-Auguste-Dominique Ingres, *Antonia Duvaucey de Nittis*, 1807, oil on canvas, 76 x 59 cm. 7.10

recent scholarship has considered to be 'a material equivalency … between the medium and the thing represented, between the breathlessly thin films of paint laid on canvas' and the depicted skin.[63]

What is more, Blanc assessed the painted skin in one of Ingres' portraits, that of Antonia Duvaucey de Nittis made 1807 in Rome (Figure 7.10), using the same words as for the *Odalisque*, praising the 'smooth skin of a brunette with light complexion [*cette peau lisse d'une brune au teint clair*]' and the 'perfection of the contour granting the curves more charm than an abundance of flesh tones [*carnations*] which would have choked, masked their elegance'.[64] Blanc, writing more than half a century after the painting was done, and, as he pointed out, after sitter and painter had died, is not interested in likeness, but in a beautiful painting in which he could admire a generic 'femme française' not entirely different from an odalisque. This streamlining of nudes and portraits would have chimed with Ingres' well-known view of himself as a *peintre d'histoire*, who works within the framework and procedures of history painting disregarding what genre he engaged with.[65] Ingres followed the procedures for history painting even when he made portraits. Unusually, preparations included working from the nude, using life models to explore poses and the situation of the figure in space. As part of his extended work for the portrait of the seated Madame Moitessier, he made drawings from the nude model to test options for the position of the sitter in the chair, only to undo it again in the painting. In the final version, all this work is covered up, making it look as if there was no body at all underneath the opulent dress.[66]

Renouncing physiognomy: Ingres' portraits of women

Despite Ingres' alignment of history painting and portraiture, sealing the skin of an idealised female nude and in a portrait commissioned by an individual sitter or by their relatives had, especially during the early decades of the nineteenth century, a different significance. The task of portraiture was at the time largely understood as rendering a likeness, and in so doing bringing out the character of an individual. At the end of the eighteenth century the *Encyclopédie méthodique* generally defined the portrait as 'the talent of imitating an individual head, & of faithfully rendering its characteristic resemblance'.[67] Lévesque, the author of the entry on portraiture, promoted the blurring of the boundaries between history and portrait painting, and insisted that portraiture is not about slavish copy, but about bringing out an individual's character by omitting detail.[68] This ultimately physiognomic paradigm of the character as the quintessence of a subject, which manifests in their features when well read, remained crucial for the understanding of portraiture throughout the nineteenth century. Paillot de Montabert equally stressed that the portraitist should seek out the 'general and permanent resemblance of the individual'.[69]

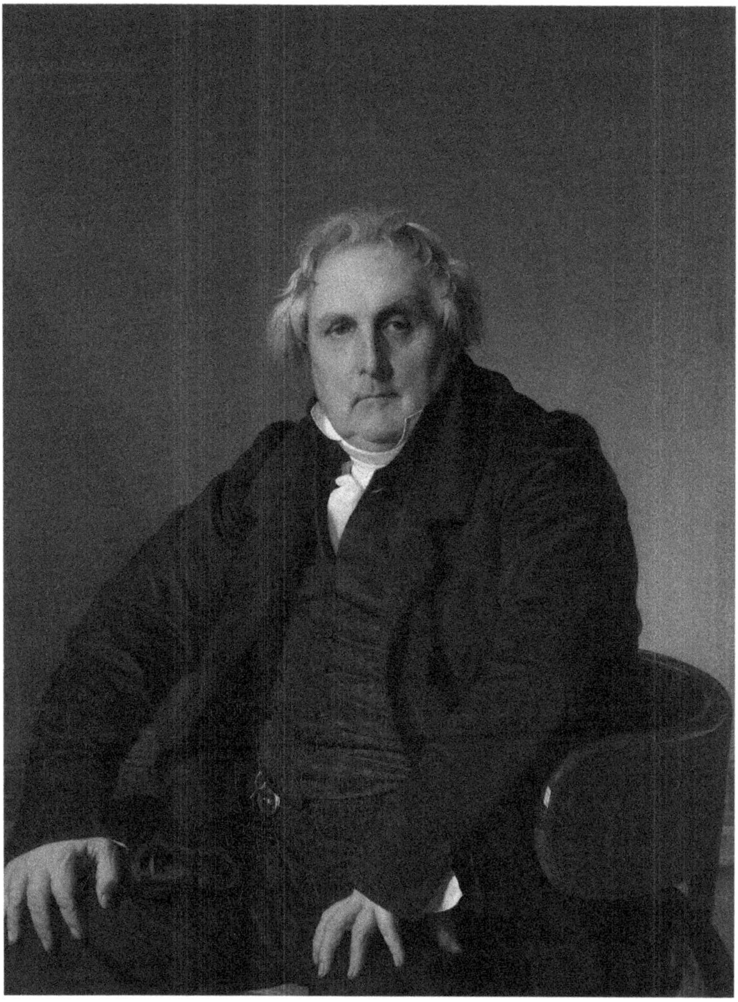

Jean-Auguste-Dominique Ingres, *Louis-François Bertin*, 1832, oil on canvas, 116 x 95 cm. 7.11

Relevant for the 'resemblance of portraits by physiognomy' were temperament and habits as well as 'mien, facial expression and character of the head'.[70] And he continued: 'what a painter should propose in offering the resemblance of an individual, is to produce a figure whose moral and physical character is sensibly manifested'.[71] To achieve this kind or resemblance, a sensibly handled 'embellishment' was favourable rather than detrimental. Nineteenth-century portraits of men especially, attempted, as Joanna Woodall has summarised, 'to reconcile a convincing characterisation of the sitter's socio-political position with depiction of the essential inner quality which was considered to justify his privileged place'.[72] Some of Ingres' images of men, notably his famous 1832 portrait of the journalist and publicist Louis-François Bertin l'Aîné, worked in this way (Figure 7.11). It became the epitome of a physiognomic and realist portrait as it captured Bertin's character along with his powerful position as spokesman and representative of the *grande bourgeoisie* in his likeness.[73] The facial features are articulated via dingy shades; folds, furrows and depressions of the fleshy skin are strongly marked in great detail. The painterly finish of *Monsieur Bertin*, however, is as smooth as in Ingres' portraits of women, and the skin tone is comparatively uniform. This is probably why some critics like Fabien Pillet bemoaned the 'cold and leaden' colouring and the lack of blood showing underneath the skin. While he appreciated *Monsieur Bertin* as one of the three best portraits of the Salon of 1833, he critiqued Ingres' 'system' of treating accessories such as clothing with the same care and accuracy 'as the truth of the flesh tones and the sensible expression of the soul'. This indifference of the brush, in the eyes of this critic, did not do justice to the rationale of a portrait and its main focus, the human face with its 'vital expressions'.[74] Others expressed sentiments of horror or observed that Monsieur Bertin looked as if made of wax, thus complementing a praise of its lifelikeness with associations of death.[75] Ingres characterised Bertin indeed merely via the relief of the facial features, and, unlike other portrait painters, refrained from suggesting any vital or emotional processes through the reddening of certain areas and from mimicking the gleam of veins underneath the epidermis via the layering of oil paint.

Be that as it may, Ingres' portraits of men and women are quite distinct from one another, as the artist was far more radical in the concealment of the painted female bodies. This was evident to the visitors of the Salon of 1833, where both the recently finished *Monsieur Bertin* and the portrait of Madame Duvaucey were displayed. In the latter portrait, painted by Ingres in 1807 while still a student in Rome, the skin, so praised by Blanc, makes no reference to the interior specification forming an even, unicoloured surface. Rather than dominating the space with an imposing gesture like Monsieur Bertin, Madame Duvaucey is fitted into the furniture in which she sits. Wrapped in the luxurious fabrics of a velvet dress and a golden-fawn Kashmir shawl, her left shoulder prolongs the curve of the chair's backrest. The adjustment of the body to the chair and picture plane leads, as many scholars have observed before, to a certain degree of anatomical distortion.[76] There is a vague sense of soft volume, but not of interior structure, and the bent arm, especially, seems devoid of any articulation. As already mentioned, this rendering of the female body to some extent complied with contemporary views of women's bodies as naturally concealed by a layer of skin which protected female anatomy from visual intrusion. If the effect was meant to be an aesthetically pleasing one, then this is tempered in the case of Ingres' portraits not only by a sense of deformation, but also by the lack of any expression of vivacity. This becomes particularly clear in a detail of an early portrait, that of Marie-Françoise Rivière (Plate 17), probably painted a year before that of her daughter Caroline.[77] While the skin is generally painted as a smooth, monochrome yellowish beige layer, the cheeks alone are distinguished by a rosy tint. The hand resting on the blue velvet cushion is so little modelled that it appears completely boneless. On the elongated fingers sit some very fine bluish-grey lines; they do not however recall those 'azure filaments' which, according to the contemporary literature on artistic anatomy, a woman's 'fine, white and translucent skin' displays.[78] They are traced in a fashion so straight that they cannot be interpreted as making reference to subcutaneous veins. They do not denote an interior, instead they refer back to an exterior in returning the colour of the velvet cushion.

Ingres' female portraits do not allow the viewer to look behind the superficial layer of the epidermis. As much as the 'forms finely rounded'[79] are illegible with regard to anatomy, the soft and non-descript materiality of women's bodies does not seem fit to express character. Nor does the face serve as a canvas on which emotions, as it was often put, 'paint themselves'. This absence of any kind of expression or allusion, in portraits of women by Ingres, and later by other artists in his circle who shared the *ingriste* aesthetics,[80] was more than just an individual or group peculiarity. It highlights the paradoxes of the female portrait in the nineteenth century. If the portrait was at the time understood as a means of bringing out a person's character, the female portrait was almost a contradiction in terms.

Jules-Antoine Castagnary, a republican who became from 1860 a friend and supporter of Gustave Courbet, included theoretical considerations on portraiture in the first of the annual salon reviews he published between 1857 and 1879. He shared the opinion that portraiture's *raison d'être* is bringing out the unique character of an individual. In a chapter entitled 'L'homme, le portrait', he puts the bourgeois philosophy of the subject in a nutshell, and declares the portrait the 'expression of individuality' in more than one sense. Any portrait should bring out the individuality in an appearance, and individuality is made the prerequisite of portraiture as such. For Castagnary, individuality is what singles out humans from other species, and differentiates them from each other, and portraiture is thus turned into a proof and manifestation of humanity. Only humans, the critic argued, 'unite the most pronounced characteristics of individuality, … delimitation and autonomy'.[81] The human is thus defined by its unity and demarcation, and so far, the neatly circumscribed female bodies in Ingres' paintings seem perfectly to comply with this intertwined notion of portraiture and individuality. Yet, for Castagnary the female portrait is a contradiction in terms. A woman's head, 'however beautiful', he elaborated,

> is of little appeal; you hasten to mentally uncover the veils that envelop the body. It is thus not individuality, the portrait, you are looking for in a woman, but the statue. Woman, this unstable being of soft and floating individuality, unites in fact none of the conditions required for a portrait, but she has all those that sculpture demands. Her purely plastic beauty, the softness of her contours, the purity of her lines, the happy harmony of her entire well balanced body, eminently take to chisel and marble.[82]

Castagnary allocated to women this paradoxical materiality many critics saw in Ingres' portraits: 'soft marble', a strange amalgam of stone and flesh – the very two materials which, as discussed in previous chapters, tended to be juxtaposed in early modern art theory when talking about the lifelike imitation of flesh tones. Castagnary in fact used the word *mollesse*, a traditional term to appraise the lifelikeness of the *carnations*, which had, in neoclassical art theory, become an attribute of the contour and had thus already moved from the flesh to the body's shape and borderlines. In their 'soft and floating individuality' women are hard to condense into a character.

Ingres' painted female skin is so uniform that it does not work as a reference to an underlying body with physiological functions, or to a bony structure which would be legible in physiognomic terms. The skin remains mute about the body structure beneath and disturbs the inside-outside relations as they are established when assuming that the body is legible. Rather than simply dismissing this petrification as a stilling of women into art, I would like to argue along the lines of Sarah Betzer, who has looked at the destabilising potential of avoiding facial and bodily expressivity. She makes this point in relation to *ingriste* images of women that hover between individual portrait and allegory. One of the examples is Amaury-Duval's portrait of the actress Rachel as Tragedy, where the statuesque quality of the portrayed has the effect of unsettling the expectations of its nineteenth-century audiences as it 'disengages the trope of the sensual Jewess'.[83] In this sense, allegorisation can be a way to escape stereotyping. Similarily, equipped with a protective layer of perfectly sealed skin, women escape the oppressive regime of physiognomy. For Baudelaire, Ingres' portraits simply do not seem to make sense in physiognomic terms. According to Lavater's system, Baudelaire suggested, the 'fingers whose narrow extremities cramp the nails', would not befit the 'ample bosom, that muscular forearm, that somewhat virile frame', a mis-match of body parts which makes this hypothetical person even illegible with regard to their gender.[84]

This hermetic closure of the skin prompted several critics to describe the experience of looking at the painted bodies as disturbing or even revolting. Lamenting – and often poking fun at – anatomical distortion continued to play a major role in these reviews, but the terms and imagery used shifted. While lack of bones, muscles and blood was still called to mind, the bodies were now more frequently explained as empty or filled with air or non-descript materials. And the negative responses to the paintings are often the most entertaining, evoking quite deftly and with a certain mocking gusto the effects of the skin sealed by paint. Théophile Silvestre, in a monographic account of the artist included in his *Histoire des artistes vivants* (1856), described the arm of Madame Duvaucey as 'inflated' and the right hand of Madame Leblanc 'as empty like a glove',[85] thus as skins without content. Baudelaire, one of the few to comment aptly and approvingly on the artist's stylistic idiosyncrasies, wrote in 1855 'that his figures look like the most correct paper-patterns, inflated with a soft, lifeless matter, and one quite alien to the human organism'.[86] These

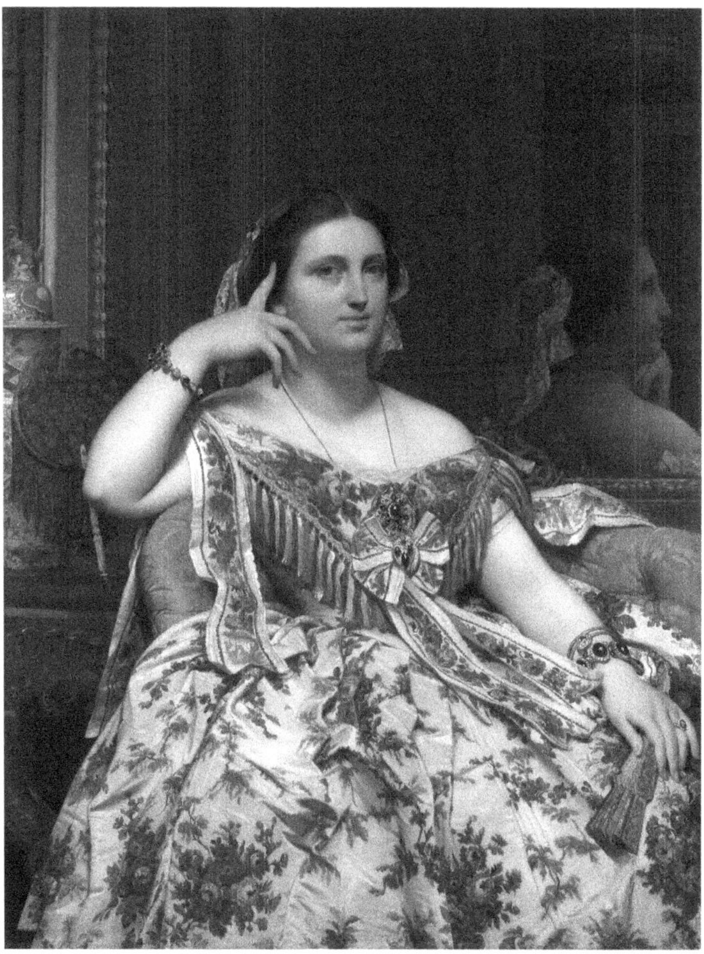

Jean-Auguste-Dominique Ingres, *Marie-Clotilde-Inès Moitessier, née de Foucauld*, 1856, oil on canvas, 120 x 92.1 cm. 7.12

bodies are empty, or at least not defined by discrete organic functionalities. Nor are they part of any reference system, a hermeneutics of the body as posited by the physiology of emotional expression. The materiality of these bodies is that of pure painted skin with nothing tangible inside. The description of the bodies as inflated, takes account of the coincidence of flatness and volume in Ingres' paintings, acknowledging that the sensuality of this skin is merely there for the eye; it is haptic as it evokes volume, but untouchable and cannot be confounded with the materiality of flesh. Painted skin might open an imaginary space, but in the end there is only the canvas behind.

This purely visual haptic appeal extends to the objects that surround the portrayed, especially in Ingres' later paintings of women of the July Monarchy's and Second Empire's aristocracy and haute bourgeoisie, such as his famous portraits of the Vicomtesse d'Haussonville and Madame Moitessier (Figure 7.12). Clad in luxurious robes and jewellery, they are surrounded by precious objects evoking the distinct materialities of porcelain, velvet, of silk spread over plush upholstery. They are encased in their interiors, very much in the manner Benjamin described it in the short section 'Louis Philippe, or the interior' of his *Arcades*: 'The interior is not just the universe of the private individual but also the étui of the private individual. To dwell means to leave traces. In the interior, these are accentuated. Coverlets and antimacassars, cases and containers are devised in abundance; in these, the traces of the most ordinary objects of use are imprinted.'[87] In Ingres' interiors though, nobody leaves traces, just like the artist leaves hardly any traces on the surface of his paintings. The heroes of the newly emerging genre of the detective novel, evoked by Benjamin in relation to those traces, would have a hard time in Ingres' interiors as would Edgar Allan Poe, 'the first physiognomist of the domestic interior'.[88] Ingres' paintings seem to resist the nineteenth-century paradigm of clues that reunited, according to Carlo Ginzburg, the detective novel, semiotic medicine, Morelli's art history, and psychoanalysis.[89] They do not open themselves up, not even through traces.

The portraits actually make a point about the closure of the pictorial space and of these interiors, as they hardly ever show doors or windows. There are only mirrors that artificially expand the space without opening it up. As with the *Baigneuse de Valpinçon*, the closure of the interior space thus corresponds with the concealment of the skin. In Ingres' paintings skin has thus separated from the early modern entanglement of skin, flesh and paint, and the materiality of the *carnations*. And yet, the human envelope remains tied to the medium: the polished skin with its very own materiality becomes a metaphor for the flatness of the painted surface. Concealing and illegible, it still evokes volume, a space ready to be filled with fantastic matter.

Notes

1 Charles-Paul Landon, 'Salon de 1819', in *Annales du Musée et de l'école moderne des beaux-arts*, vol. 1 (Paris: Imprimerie Royale, 1820), p. 29.
2 George Levitine, *The Dawn of Bohemianism: The Barbue Rebellion and Primitivism in Neoclassical France* (University Park/Penn.; London: Pennsylvania State University Press, 1978).
3 Tom Holert, *Künstlerwissen: Studien zur Semantik künstlerischer Kompetenzim Frankreich des 18. und frühen 19. Jahrhunderts* (München: Fink, 1998), pp. 119–21.
4 [Eugène Emmanuel Amaury Pineu-Duval] Amaury-Duval, *L'Atelier d'Ingres: souvenirs* (Paris: G. Charpentier 1878), p. 58. See in more detail Mechthild Fend, 'Bodily and pictorial surfaces: skin in French art and medicine, 1790–1860', *Art History*, 28 (2005), 311–39.
5 See for Ingres' early biography Vincent Pomarède, 'Élève de David', in Vincent Pomarède et al. (eds), *Ingres, 1780–1867* (Paris: Gallimard, Musée du Louvre Éditions, 2006), pp. 91–121.
6 Ibid., pp. 100–3.
7 Thomas E. Crow, *Emulation: Making Artists for Revolutionary France* (New Haven; London: Yale University Press, 1994); Abigail Solomon-Godeau, *Male Trouble: A Crisis in Representation* (London: Thames & Hudson, 1997).
8 See on Ingres' work for *Le Musée français, receuil complet des tableaux, statues et bas-reliefs, qui composent la collection nationale* (1802–12), Sarah Betzer, 'Ingres's shadows', *Art Bulletin*, 95 (2010), 78–101.
9 There is a fifth painted *académie*, today at the Musée Ingres at Montauban, but it has been suggested that it was produced earlier while Ingres was still in Toulouse. For Ingres' years as a student of David see Pomarède, 'Élève de David'.
10 Ibid., pp. 110–12.
11 See most recently ibid., p. 110.
12 This routine is mentioned at various occasions by Suvée (director of the Académie de France à Rome 1795–1807), for example, in a report from 2 December 1797, in the new *règlement* of December 1799, and in a letter written 26 September 1804. See *Correspondance des directeurs de l'Académie de France à Rome*, new series, Directorat de Suvée, 1795–1807, ed. Georges Brunel and Isabelle Julia (Rome: Edizioni dell'Elefante, 1984), vol. 2.1, pp. 94, 160; vol. 2.2, p. 558.
13 On the *envois de Rome* of 1808, Stéphane Guégan, Louis-Antoine Prat and Vincent Pomarède, 'Rome et Florence', in Pomarède et al. (eds), *Ingres*, pp. 147–231 (p. 152); Susan Siegfried, *Ingres: Painting Reimagined* (New Haven; London: Yale University Press, 2009), p. 73.
14 *Procès-verbaux de l'Académie des beaux-arts, publiés pour la Societé de l'Histoire de l'Art français*, ed. Marcel Bonnaire, vol. 3 (Paris: A. Colin, 1943), pp. 195–6. Over the course of the century the number of female nudes increased but always remained considerably lower than that of male nudes. See also Olivier Bonfait, 'Les envois de Rome et la plastique du nu', in Olivier Bonfait (ed.), *Maestà di Roma da Napoleone all'unità d'Italia. D'Ingres à Degas: les artistes français à Rome*, exh. cat. (Académie de France à Rome, 2003), pp. 177–82.

15 Solomon-Godeau, *Male Trouble*, especially pp. 46–97, 185–203.
16 Crow, *Emulation*; with regards to Ingres' relation to this tradition Sarah Betzer, *Ingres and the Studio: Women, Painting, History* (University Park/Penn.: Pennsylvania State University Press, 2012), pp. 4–10.
17 As Siegfried elaborates, the painting looked different from today's version when it was first painted and shown, as Ingres reworked it before its first public exhibition in 1827. Judging mainly from a sketch that David made of the *envois de Rome* by his students in 1809, she argues that he lowered the Sphinx to Oedipus' eye level and changed the hero's gesture. See Siegfried, *Ingres*, pp. 36–8. The Sphinx is represented according to the ways it was described at the time, see the *Dictionnaire de l'Académie française*, 5th edn 1798, entry 'Sphinx' (accessed via University of Chicago: The ARTFL Project. *Dictionnaires d'autrefois* https://artfl-project.uchicago.edu/content/dictionnaires-dautrefois).
18 For versions of the narrative popular in late eighteenth- and nineteenth-century France see Siegfried, *Ingres*, p. 28.
19 Ibid., pp. 26–35.
20 *Procès-verbaux*, ed. Bonnaire, vol. 3, p. 268.
21 Siegfried, *Ingres*, p. 75.
22 Charles-Paul Landon, 'Salon de 1822', in *Annales du Musée et de l'école moderne des beaux-arts*, vol. 1, (Paris: Imprimerie Royale, 1822), p. 93. See also Bonfait, 'Les envois de Rome et la plastique du nu', p. 180.
23 *Procès-verbaux*, ed. Bonnaire, vol. 3, pp. 267–8.
24 Linda Nochlin, 'The Imaginary Orient', *Art in America*, May 1983, 119–31, 186–91; Edward W. Said, *Orientalism* (London: Routledge and Kegan Paul, 1978).
25 Gary Tinterow and Philip Connisbee (eds), *Portraits by Ingres: Images of an Epoch* (New York: The Metropolitan Museum of Art, 1999), p. 32; Anne Lafont, 'L'orient des Capucines: une œuvre collective', conference paper, Courtauld Institute of Art, 12 June 2009. As the Couvent des Capucines was a non-institutionalised artistic site, there are barely any documents. A fictional account is Marceline Desbordes-Valmore's *La Jeunesse de Marceline: ou, L'Atelier d'un peintre* first published in 1833, discussed by Stephen Bann, 'The studio as a scene of emulation: Marceline Desbordes-Valmore's l'atelier d'un peintre', *French Studies*, 61 (2007), 26–35; see also Betzer, 'Ingres's shadows', pp. 79 and 91–2.
26 This is one of the main arguments of Melanie Ulz's book *Auf dem Schlachtfeld des Empire: Männlichkeitskonzepte in der Bildproduktion zu Napoleons Ägyptenfeldzug* (Marburg: Jonas, 2008), dealing with concepts of masculinity in images related to Napoleon's Egyptian campaign, see in particular pp. 146–51. See also Darcy Grimaldo Grigsby, *Extremities: Painting Empire in Post-Revolutionary France* (New Haven; London: Yale University Press, 2002), pp. 76–82; and more generally on the crisis of the male nude in post-revolutionary France Solomon-Godeau, *Male Trouble*.
27 For Ingres' sources see Silke Förschler, *Bilder des Harem: Medienwandel und kultureller Austausch* (Berlin: Reimer, 2010), pp. 149–54; Uwe Fleckner, *Jean-Auguste-Dominique Ingres. Das Türkische Bad: ein Klassizist auf dem Weg zur Moderne* (Frankfurt a. M.: Fischer TaschenbuchVerlag, 1996), pp. 103–19.
28 As both Siegfried, *Ingres*, p. 82, and Betzer, *Ingres and the Studio*, p. 7, have highlighted.

29 Johann Friedrich Blumenbach, *De generis humani varietate nativa* (Göttingen: Rosenbusch, 1775); see also Förschler, *Bilder des Harem*, pp. 70–3.
30 The first French translation appeared in 1763. Ingres read the letters at the latest in 1840 and took notes from his reading, see Fleckner, *Das Türkische Bad*, p. 29.
31 Mary Wortley Montagu, *Letters*, introd. Clare Brant (London: Random House, 1992), p. 169.
32 Ibid., p. 105.
33 Förschler, *Bilder des Harem*, pp. 66–7.
34 I agree with Siegfried's assessment that this piece of drapery can't clearly be identified as a specific kind of garment and that nothing indicates a movement of undressing. See Siegfried, *Ingres*, p. 76.
35 On touch and taboo see Didier Anzieu, *The Skin Ego* [1985], trans. Chris Turner (New Haven; London: Yale University Press, 1989), pp. 136–49.
36 Aileen Ribeiro, *Ingres in Fashion: Representations of Dress and Appearance in Ingres's Images of Women* (New Haven; London: Yale University Press, 1999), pp. 94–6.
37 Reported by Henri Delaborde, *Ingres, sa vie, ses travaux, sa doctrine* (Paris: Henri Plon, 1870), p. 150.
38 Robert Rosenblum, *Jean-August-Dominique Ingres* (London: Thames & Hudson, 1990); Uwe Fleckner, *Abbild und Abstraktion: die Kunst des Porträts im Werk von Jean-Auguste-Dominique Ingres* (Mainz: Philip von Zabern, 1995).
39 On Caroline Murat's role in the commissioning of the *Grande Odalisque* in particular Carol Ockman, *Ingres's Eroticized Bodies: Retracing the Serpentine Line* (New Haven: Yale University Press, 1995), pp. 33–65.
40 This Lacanian term was taken up as 'Éros morcélé' in the Ingres exhibition at the Louvre in 2006 to highlight the fact that Ingres used collage-like techniques to build up paintings such as the *Turkish Bath* and that the body part plays a role in his drawings that exceeds the usual fragmentary nature of studies. See Pomarède et al. (eds), *Ingres*, pp. 366–71.
41 See the transcription of Ingres' notes in Georges Vigne, *Dessins d'Ingres: Catalogue raisoné des dessins du musée de Montauban* (Paris: Gallimard, 1995), no. 849, p. 157.
42 Ingres stated in a letter to Mr Forrestier written 29 May 1807 that he was working on a *Venus Anadyomene*; see Vigne, *Dessins d'Ingres*, pp. 156–9.
43 Charles Blanc, *Grammaire des arts du dessin* [1867], introd. Claire Barbillon (Paris: École nationale supérieure des beaux-arts, 2000), p. 375.
44 Vigne, *Dessins d'Ingres*, pp. 158–9.
45 Ibid., no. 860, p. 159; Pomarède et al. (eds), *Ingres*, cat. no. 168, p. 368.
46 According to ancient mythology Venus was engendered without a woman, as she rose from the sea after Cronos had castrated his father Uranus and thrown his genitals into the sea. See on later nineteenth-century variations of Venus Anadyomene in relation to contemporary anxieties about male reproductive power and medical debates on reproduction Jennifer Shaw, 'The figure of Venus: rhetoric of the ideal and the Salon of 1863', in Caroline Arscott and Katie Scott (eds), *Manifestations of Venus: Art and Sexuality* (Manchester: Manchester University Press, 2000), pp. 90–108.
47 Elisabeth Bronfen, *The Knotted Subject: Hysteria and its Discontents* (Princeton/N. J.; Chichester: Princeton University Press, 1998), p. 4.
48 Mieke Bal, *Reading 'Rembrandt: Beyond the Word-Image Opposition* (Cambridge:

Cambridge University Press, 1991), p. 23, makes a similar point regarding navels in Rembrandt's paintings.

49 I am referring here in particular to Abigail Solomon-Godeau, 'The legs of the countess', *October*, 38 (1986–87), 65–108; and Lynda Nead, *The Female Nude: Art, Obscenity and Sexuality* (London; New York: Routledge, 1992).

50 Sigmund Freud, 'Fetishism' [1927], in James Strachey (ed.), *The Works of Sigmund Freud: Standard Edition*, vol. 21 (London: Hogarth Press and the Institute of Psychoanalysis, 1961), pp. 149–57.

51 Ockman, *Ingres's Eroticized Bodies*; Susan Siegfried, 'Un certain regard: Ingres, Delacroix, et l'Odalisque', in Sébastian Allard (ed.), *Paris 1820: l'affirmation de la génération romantique* (Bern: Peter Lang, 2005), pp. 61–84.

52 This remark does not occur in his critique of the *Odalisque* in Auguste-Hilarion Kératry's *Annuaire de l'École Française de Peinture ou Lettres sur le Salon de 1819* (Paris: Maradan 1820), but is mentioned in Amaury-Duval, *Atelier d'Ingres*, p. 282. See Ockman, *Ingres's Eroticized Bodies*, pp. 3 and 147, fn. 3.

53 Jean-Joseph Sue (the younger), *Élémens d'anatomie, à l'usage des peintres, des sculpteurs et des amateurs* (Paris: Méquignon, l'ainé 1788), p. 6.

54 See chapter 5, pp. 215–16.

55 Jacques-Nicolas Paillot de Montabert, *Traité complet de la peinture*, 9 vols (Paris: J.-F. Delion, 1829–51), vol. 7, pp. 422–3.

56 Kératry, *Annuaire de l'École française*, p. 107.

57 See for example Paillot de Montabert, *Traité complet de la peinture*, vol. 7, pp. 448–9. In contrast, Paillot had little appreciation for Rubens's flesh tones, see vol. 5, p. 72.

58 Ibid., vol. 7, p. 449.

59 It was first used in a critique of the Salon of 1833 by Auguste Jal and Charles Lermonant, see Betzer, *Ingres and the Studio*, pp. 11 and 83–4.

60 Andrew Carrington Shelton, *Ingres and His Critics* (Cambridge: Cambridge University Press, 2005), p. 18. See on the critical fabrication of 'Monsieur Ingres' also Adrian Rifkin, 'Ingres and the academic dictionary: an essay on ideology and stupefaction in the social formation of the "artist"', *Art History*, 6 (1983), 155–70; and *Ingres: Then, and Now* (London; New York: Routledge, 2000).

61 Théophile Gautier, *Les Beaux-Arts en Europe* (Paris, 1855), quoted in Charles Blanc, *Ingres: sa vie et ses ouvrages* (Paris: Jules Renouard, 1870), p. 27.

62 On the eroticism of the line see Ockmann, *Ingres's Eroticized Bodies*; on its feminisation in neoclassical art theory Mechthild Fend, *Grenzen der Männlichkeit: der Androgyn in der französischen Kunst und Kunsttheorie zwischen Aufklärung und Restauration* (Berlin: Reimer, 2003), pp. 34–43.

63 Susan Siegfried, 'Ingres's reading: the undoing of narrative', in Adrian Rifkin and Susan Siegfried (eds), *Fingering Ingres* (Oxford; Malden/Mass.: Blackwell Publishers, 2001), pp. 4–30, p. 26, in relation to Ingres' *Roger Freeing Angelika*, 1819.

64 Blanc, *Ingres*, p. 19.

65 This issue has been much discussed in the scholarship on Ingres, see most recently Betzer, *Ingres and the Studio*, in particular her chapter 'The *Ingriste* portrait as history'.

66 Betzer, *Ingres and the Studio*, pp. 41–61.

67 *Encyclopédie méthodique. Beaux-arts*, ed. Claude-Henri Watelet and Pierre-Charles Levesque, vol. 2 (Paris: Panckoucke, 1791), p. 205.

68 Betzer, *Ingres and the Studio*, p. 24–5.
69 Paillot de Montabert, *Traité complet de la peinture*, vol. 8, p. 352.
70 Ibid., p. 356.
71 Ibid., p. 366.
72 Joanna Woodall (ed.), *Portraiture: Facing the Subject* (Manchester; New York: Manchester University Press, 1997), p. 5.
73 See on the portrait Daniel Ternois, *Ingres: Monsieur Bertin* (Paris: Réunion des musées national; Service culturel du musée du Louvre, 1998); and for its reception as physiognomic portrait in the nineteenth century, for example Blanc, *Ingres*, p. 98. On Ingres and physiognomy see also Michael Tilby, '"Telle main veut tel pied": Balzac and the art of portraiture', in Peter Collier and Robert Lethbridge (eds), *Artistic Relations: Literature and the Visual Arts in Nineteenth-Century France* (New Haven/Conn.; London: Yale University Press, 1994), pp. 111–29.
74 F[abien], P[illet], 'Salon de 1833 (3ième article)', *Moniteur universel* (19 March 1833), pp. 763–4 (p. 764).
75 See on the comparison of Ingres' portraits with wax portraits Ockman, *Ingres's Eroticized Bodies*, pp. 97–109.
76 See for example, Fleckner, *Abbild und Abstraktion*, pp. 70–1.
77 Vincent Pomarède., 'La leçon des maîtres', in Pomarède et al. (eds), *Ingres*, pp. 122–45 (pp. 135–8).
78 Julien Fau, *Anatomie des formes extérieures du corps humain, a l'usage des peintres et des sculpteurs* (Paris: Méquignon-Marvis, 1845), p. 174.
79 Ibid.
80 Betzer, *Ingres and the Studio*.
81 Jules-Antoine Castagnary, 'Salon de 1857', in Jules-Antoine Castagnary, *Salons (1857–1870)* (Paris: Bibliothèque-Charpentier, 1892), pp. 35–6.
82 Ibid., p. 41. See on this passage by Castagnary also Fend, 'Haut wie weicher Marmor: die Frauenporträts von Jean-Auguste-Dominique Ingres', in Oliver Jehle and Sabine Slanina (eds), *Ähnlichkeit und Entstellung* (Berlin: Deutscher Kunstverlag, 2010), pp. 95–112; and Betzer, *Ingres and the Studio*, p. 226
83 Betzer, *Ingres and the Studio*, chapter 5, in particular, pp. 212–13.
84 Charles Baudelaire, 'The Exposition Universelle (1855)', in *Art in Paris, 1845–1862: Salons and Other Exhibitions*, trans. Jonathan Mayne (London: Phaidon Press, 1965), p. 133.
85 Théophile Silvestre, 'Ingres d'après nature', in Théophile Silvestre, *Histoire des artistes vivants français et étrangers: études d'après nature* (Paris: E. Blanchard, 1855–56), p. 23.
86 Baudelaire, 'The Exposition Universelle (1855)', p. 133; Charles Baudelaire, *Critique d'art*, ed. Claude Pichois (Paris: Gallimard, 1992), p. 247.
87 Walter Benjamin, *The Arcades Project*, trans. Howard Eiland and Kevin McLaughlin, prepared on the basis of the German volume edited by Rolf Tiedemann (Cambridge/Mass.; London: Belknap Press, 1999), p. 9. On 'Ingres and the Arcades', Rifkin, *Ingres*, pp. 41–71.
88 Benjamin, *The Acades Project*, p. 9.
89 Carlo Ginzburg, 'Morelli, Freud and Sherlock Holmes: clues and scientific method', *History Workshop Journal*, 9 (1980), 5–36.

8 Epilogue: segretation

As this book has shown, human nakedness imitated in colour was, over the course of the eighteenth and early nineteenth centuries, increasingly understood in terms of skin rather than flesh. For a prominent nineteenth-century French art critic and theorist, Charles Blanc, who particularly appreciated the 'smooth skin' and the 'perfection of the contour' of Ingres' nudes, skin even became a founding principle of his theories of drawing and colour. Blanc's *Grammaire des arts du dessin* is today mostly known for having introduced the Impressionists to the ideas of the chemist and colour theorist Michel-Eugène Chevreul. As director of the dye works of the Paris Gobelin factory, he dealt with the visual effects yarns of different colours had when put next to each other in a tapestry. In conjunction with this work Chevreul developed the theory of the simultaneous contrast, later so crucial to artists like Georges Seurat.[1] But despite the impact the *Grammaire* might have had on the artistic theories and uses of colour in late nineteenth-century France, Blanc cannot readily be called a colourist, and he interestingly sourced part of his own knowledge of contemporary colour theory from a student of Ingres, the painter and ceramicist Jean-Claude Ziegler.[2] His assessment of colour and drawing is rather complex, and at times contradictory. Blanc's *Grammaire* constituted one of the last attempts to provide a universal normative theory of the visual arts, which included considerations not only of architecture, sculpture and painting but also of areas like printing, metal carving and even landscape gardening. As is clear already from the book's title (it translates as 'Grammar of the arts of drawing'), drawing was for Blanc what united all these practices. He largely understood it in the multiple senses of the Italian concept of *disegno*, and followed in many ways the traditional rationale of the Académie royale de peinture et de sculpture. Blanc's views can be labelled academic in many respects, and he was, at the point of writing the book, a representative of the nineteenth-century art establishment.[3] Politically a leftist and republican throughout his life, Blanc was a member of the Académie française and of the Académie des beaux-arts, twice administrator of the École des beaux-arts and founder of the *Gazette des beaux-arts*, the journal in which both the *Grammaire des arts du dessin* and his later biography of Ingres initially appeared.[4]

While the overarching significance of drawing was a traditional view, Blanc's ways of establishing it are very much a product of the nineteenth century as many of the arguments are biologically grounded. Very eclectic in his overall approach, Blanc not only summarised scientific theory, such as Chevreul's writing on colour, but also founded his assumptions on the relationship between colour and design by associating them with presumed natural facts. For example, Blanc started his initial chapter on drawing and colour with his statement on the supremacy of drawing: 'Drawing is the masculine gender of art; colour the feminine.'[5] He thus spelled out the gendering of drawing and colour, which had remained rather implicit in early modern art theory. In so doing, he naturalised the juxtaposition and hierarchy between drawing and colour, and later described painting in sexualising terms as being engendered by the two. The initial sentence is immediately followed by his plea for the supremacy of drawing: 'Of the three principal arts that form the subject of this book: architecture, sculpture and painting, there is only one for which colour is necessary; but drawing is essential to all the three arts to such a degree that one rightly calls them the arts of drawing.'[6]

This essentialising argument for the supremacy of drawing is reinforced by the contention that the 'superiority of drawing over colour is inscribed into the very laws of nature.'[7] Human anatomy is again the point of reference here. Simply assuming that innumerable people have the same skin tone (*teint*), while their silhouettes are distinct Blanc claimed: 'All negros are black, how can we distinguish between them other than via the proportions of their limbs, their size and their gait? Nature thus employed drawing to define objects, and colour to nuance them.'[8] Treating dark skin colour indeed like the undifferentiated blackness of silhouettes, Blanc made only one particular skin colour stand in for colour here; white male supremacy and the supremacy of drawing support each other in this argument.

The assumption of the superiority of drawing does not imply however that Blanc had no appreciation for colour at all. On the contrary, he followed Georg Wilhelm Friedrich Hegel's lectures on aesthetics in his account of the historical development of different art forms in claiming that painting was the most advanced medium of the visual arts; and he agreed with Roger de Piles that colour is what defines painting. Moreover, he highly valued the art of Eugène Delacroix, an artist constructed, since the 1820s as Ingres' counterpart; the two painters were often used as examples in art critical discussions of classicism versus romanticism, line versus colour. Blanc, though, treasured both artists and famously believed that Delacroix pioneered in his painterly practice the uses of the principle of optical mixture, theorised by Chevreul. Blanc explained the technique by drawing on the example of the rose *carna-*

tions of a semi-naked woman in Delacroix's paintings for the cupola in the library of the Luxembourg Palace in Paris.

> As we were admiring the admirable freshness of this rose-tone, an artist friend of Delacroix, who had seen him at work, said smiling, 'You would be surprised if you knew what colors had produced the rosy flesh that charms you. They are tones that seen separately would seem as dull as the mud of the street.' How was this miracle wrought? By the boldness with which Delacroix had slashed the naked back of this figure with a decided green, which partly neutralized by its complement rose, forms with the rose in which it is absorbed a mixed and fresh tone apparent only at a distance, in a word a resultant color which is what is called the optical mixture.[9]

In a technique Delacroix himself called *flochetage*,[10] the painter – in Blanc's account violently – put stroke next to stroke, and miraculously transformed mud into rose-coloured flesh without mixing paint on his palette. Not made of actual matter, the fresh rose of these flesh tones is subjectively formed by the visual apparatus of those looking at them.[11] Interestingly, the new technique is introduced here via the example of the making of a woman's flesh tones. This strategy has prominent precedents Blanc was well aware of.[12] Cennini's late medieval *Libro dell'Arte*, discussed at the outset of this book, had been rediscovered and republished in the early nineteenth century, with the first French translation provided by Ingres' student Victor Mottez in 1858.[13] It explained the technique of fresco painting and the ways of putting a figure into relief via the literal incarnation – the making of flesh on the wall – of the face of the Virgin Mary. In the first half of the eighteenth century, Le Blon introduced the technique of the colour mezzotint mainly to meet the challenge of reproducing flesh tones, and took a female plaster head to be tinted as his example. In both cases however, the imitation of flesh in the respective medium was not only considered the ultimate and most difficult thing to be done with colour, but also crucially involved the physical mixing of pigments or dyes. The mixing of pigments for the imitation of flesh tones in the visual arts was tied, as I have argued, to the understanding of the human body's colours as complexion – a mixture of tones produced by a combination of saps or humours. Along with an increasingly medicalised view of skin as an organ and tissue structure since the seventeenth century, the body's colouring matter was more firmly located in an outer layer of the dermis. Still, the first medical image of the medical phenomenon of the colour of humans, which was also an early colour mezzotint – Ladmiral's illustration for Albinus's 'Dissertation on the seat and cause of the colour of Ethiopians and other humans', both isolated the colour of skin and produced it as complexion, as a mixture of dyes in primary colours. As this example aptly demonstrates, questions of skin colour and of the colour with which it is reproduced in visual media are inextricably linked, and so are, by extension, the politics and artistic procedures of colour mixture. This is also the case, and quite explicitly so, in Blanc's *Grammaire*, but the fluidity of earlier approaches is lost in his segregationism. His appreciative view of the separation of colours into individual pigments in divisionist painterly processes, and his plea for the segregation of humans of different colours go hand in hand. The latter view is expressed in the book's section on painting, where Blanc complained about the lack of appropriate models:

> Nothing is rarer than fine models, especially in France, where the mingling of races has effaced the primordial accent of creation. The fresh beauty or the integrity of primitive characters is scarcely found except among people that have not mixed their blood with that of others, like the mountaineers of Savoy and Albania, the Circassians, Ethiopians, Negroes.[14]

Without wanting to argue that divisionism as a painterly technique goes along with segregationist politics per se, I would like to point out that it does in the *Grammaire*, as Blanc aligned colour and racially defined skin colour, and does not wish the 'primitive character' of races, nor the primitive colours to physically mix. This is a far cry from Jean-Joseph Sue's 1797 *Essai sur la physiognomonie des corps vivans*. As I have shown in my chapter on skin colour, this tract, written in the aftermath of the French Revolution and during the short period of abolition of slavery (1794–1802), a state not yet re-gained in all French colonies by the time Blanc wrote his *Grammaire*, is the first artistic anatomy in France to explicitly acknowledge human variety as an important artistic concern. The then popular attempts to classify humans with skin colour as major marker of race, are foiled by the acceptance that commerce and exchange produce the mixing of people, making the majority of humans brownish in one or the other way.

Earlier on in his introductory 'Principes', Blanc turned the aspects of the human skin not having to do with colour into a foundational argument for the supremacy of drawing. He proposed the peculiar theory that the most elevated animals are monochrome, and that humankind distinguishes itself from the animal kingdom through its skin in a double sense: the human skin has only a single colour *and* it is naked; not obstructed by feathers or fur, it makes the shape of the human figure immediately visible. This might sound like evolutionary biology, but derives in fact from a mixture of German classical aesthetics and idealist philosophy, namely the classical aesthetics of Karl Philipp Moritz, Johann Wolfgang von Goethe's colour theory and Hegel's lectures on aesthetics. As the first among them, Moritz had argued that humans are singled out by their nudity. Nudity no longer carries the 'theological signature' it used to have in Christian culture,[15] but becomes a biological blessing. Unlike animals whose feathers, hair and scales obscure the visibility of their essential shape, humans are, thanks to their skin, transparent to their inner essence.[16] Blanc would have encountered elements of this theory in Goethe's *Theory of Colour* (1810) and Hegel's *Aesthetics: Lectures on Fine Art* (first published in German in 1835), both important sources for the *Grammaire*. Hegel elaborated on the human body in his section on beauty in nature, and singled out the skin, because he saw human interiority and soul shine through this semi-transparent organic envelope:

> The human body … stands in this respect at a higher stage [than the animal], since in it there is everywhere and always represented the fact that man is an ensouled and feeling unit. The skin is not hidden by plant-like unliving coverings; the pulsation of the blood shows itself over the entire surface; the beating heart of life is as it were present everywhere over the body and comes out into appearance externally as the body's own animation … Similarly the skin proves to be sensitive everywhere, and displays the *morbidezza* [delicacy], the tints of colour in flesh and veins, which are the artist's cross.[17]

The latter part of this passage highlights the colourful and animate aspects of skin – inseparable for Hegel from the organ's ability to express humanity – and is very close to Diderot's remarks on flesh tones in his *Notes on Painting* (discussed in chapter 3), a text translated into German by Goethe in 1799. While Hegel stressed the changeability of skin, Blanc took the argument of the superiority of the human envelope further. In his idiosyncratic semi-secular cosmogony he declared the monochrome human 'the work of a supreme draughtsman and not that of a colorist',[18] and set human appearance apart from nature by confining colour to the inner body:

> Inside the human body is iridescent, like nature, of a thousand colours, as the vermilion of the lips already announces, the ivory of the teeth, the blue, brown, yellow and orange hues of the iris, but, outside, the skin presents itself with only one tone the nuances of which are so fine, even in the eyes of a Titian or a Correggio, they blend from a distance into a warm and luminous unity.[19]

Flashing up from within the monochrome skin, the vivid colours at the orifices hint at the multicoloured animality of the interior. It is the sealing of the body, in the praise of skin and drawing, that affords the divide between inside and outside, skin and flesh. Georges Didi-Huberman has described this divide as the fundamental conundrum of the *incarnate*: 'One has to question oneself about this *incarnate*, beginning with this impossible division of the word. *In*, is this inside, or is it underneath? Is it not the flesh that designates the absolute sanguineous, formless [*informe*] interior of the body, in opposition to its white surface?'[20] He raises a question, but doesn't leave things entirely open, as he contrasts the formless and bloody interior with the white surface. This 'opposition', however, is not a transhistorical quality of the flesh and flesh tones, but rather a modern antagonism prompted by the concealment of the body whose skin is imagined as either a monochrome surface and screen transparent to its essence or, as in artistic anatomy, the indicator of its inner truth of bones and muscles. Just as viewers of Ingres' smooth, immaculately painted skins were provoked into fantasies about what hides inside, Blanc saw iridescent matter lurk behind the skin drawn by nature around the human body and constructed monochromy as a dividing line between humans and animals. I propose that the early modern notion of flesh tones – in its art theoretical formulations and its manifestations in visual practices – opened and opens still the possibility of not making this division between skin and flesh; it enables us to perceive of the materiality of any body as being fluid and multicoloured.

Notes

1 See among others Michael F. Zimmermann, 'Seurat, Charles Blanc, and naturalist art criticism', *Art Institute of Chicago Museum Studies*, 14 (1989), 198–209, 246–7.
2 John Gage, *Colour and Meaning: Art, Science and Symbolism* (London: Thames & Hudson, 1999), pp. 47–8.
3 Zimmermann, 'Seurat, Charles Blanc, and naturalist art criticism'.
4 See Claire Barbillon's introduction to the 2000 edition of Charles Blanc's *Grammaire des arts du dessin* [1867] (Paris: École nationale supérieure des beaux-arts), pp. 17–18. The English translation of the *Grammaire* first published in 1874 skips large parts of the original, namely the more general opening 'Principes' and the chapter on sculpture.
5 Blanc, *Grammaire*, p. 53. On the gendering of colour in the *Grammaire*, see MonikaWagner, 'Linie – Farbe – Material: Kunsttheorie und Geschlechterkampf', in Barbara Hüttel et al. (eds), *Re-Visonen: zur Aktualität der Kunstgeschichte* (Berlin: Akademie Verlag, 2002), pp. 195–207; Georges Roque, 'Portrait de la couleur en femme fatale', *Art&Fact. Revue des historiens de l'art de l'université de Liège*, 10 (1991), 4–10, and for the early modern period Partricia L. Reilly, 'Writing out color in Renaissance art theory', *Genders*, 12 (1991), 78–99.
6 Blanc, *Grammaire*, p. 53.
7 Ibid.
8 Ibid.
9 Charles Blanc, *Grammar of Painting and Engraving*, trans. Kate Newell Doggett (New York; Cambridge/Mass.: Hurd & Houghton, 1874), p. 162; *Grammaire*, p. 537; on Blanc and Delacroix see Gage, *Colour and Meaning*, pp. 47–8, 199–200. Blanc does not explicitly label this forceful manner of painting as male, but – while colour kept its connotation as female – French art critique of the second half of the nineteenth century often considered the handling of paint, especially in impasto, as a virile activity. See Matthias Krüger, *Das Relief der Farbe: Pastose Malerei in der französischen Kunstkritik 1850–1890* (München; Berlin: Deutscher Kunstverlag, 2007).
10 Max Imdahl, *Farbe: kunsttheoretische Reflexionen in Frankreich* (München: Fink, 1987), pp. 89–90.

11 On subjective vision see Jonathan Crary, *Techniques of the Observer: On Vision and Modernity in the Nineteenth Century* (Cambridge/Mass.; London: MIT Press, 1990).
12 Blanc cites both Cennini and Le Blon in his *Grammaire*, pp. 549, 614.
13 Cennini, *Traité de la peinture de Cennino Cennini, mis en lumière pour la première fois avec des notes par le chevalier G. Tambroni, traduit par Victor Mottez* (Paris: Vve J. Renouard, 1858). See also Betzer, *Ingres and the Studio*, pp. 109 and 255, fn. 41.
14 Blanc, *Grammar*, pp. 109–10; *Grammaire*, p. 515.
15 Giorgio Agamben, *Nudities* [2009], trans. David Kishik and Stefan Pedatella (Stanford/Cal.: Stanford University Press, 2011), p. 57.
16 Karl Philipp Moritz, '[Die Signatur des Schönen] Inwiefern Kunstwerke beschrieben werden können' [1788], in Gottfried Boehm and Norbert Miller (eds), *Bibliothek der Kunstliteratur*, vol. 3: *Klassik und Klassizismus* (Frankfurt a. M.: Deutscher Kunstverlag, 1995), pp. 372–83 (pp. 375–6); Johann Wolfgang Friedrich von Goethe, 'Farbenlehre' [1810], ed. Manfred Wenzel, in *Sämtliche Werke*, vol. 23/1 (Frankfurt: Suhrkamp, 1991), pp. 204–19.
17 Georg Wilhelm Friedrich Hegel, *Aesthetics: Lectures on Fine Art* [1835], trans. Malcom Knox, vol. 1 (Oxford: Clarendon Press, 1975), p. 146; see on Hegel and flesh tones Annik Pietsch, 'Der "glanzlose Seelenduft der Fleischfarbe": Schlesingers Hegel-Porträt', in Daniela Bohde and Mechthild Fend (eds), *Weder Haut noch Fleisch: das Inkarnat in der Kunstgeschichte* (Berlin: Gebr. Mann, 2007), pp. 133–58; Georges Didi-Huberman, *La peinture incarnée: suivi de Le chef-d'œuvre inconnu par Honoré de Balzac* (Paris: Les Éditions de Minuit, 1985), pp. 27–8.
18 Blanc, *Grammaire*, p. 61. See on biological concepts in Blanc's *Grammaire* also Matthias Krüger, 'Der Begriff des *disegno* im Zeitalter der Evolutionstheorie: biologische Konzepte in Charles Blancs *Grammaire des Arts du Dessin*', in Matthias Krüger, Christine Ott and Ulrich Pfisterer (eds), *Die Biologie der Kreativität* (Zürich; Berlin: diaphanes, 2013), pp. 75–90, in particular, p. 79.
19 Blanc, *Grammaire*, p. 62.
20 Didi-Huberman, *La peinture incarnée*, p. 22.

Select bibliography

Agamben, Giorgio, *Nudities* [2009], trans. David Kishik and Stefan Pedatella (Stanford/Cal.: Stanford University Press, 2011).

Alberti, Leon Battista, *On the Art of Building in Ten Books*, trans. Joseph Rykwert, Neil Leach and Robert Tavernor (Cambridge/Mass.; London: MIT Press, 1988).

Albinus, Bernhard Siegfried, *Dissertatio secunda de sede et caussa coloris Aethiopum et caeterorum hominum* (Leiden: Theodorum Haak; Amsterdam: Jacobum Graall & Henricum de Leth, 1737).

— *Tabulae sceleti et musculorum corporis humani* (Leiden: Prostant apud Joannem & Hermannum Verbeek, 1747).

Alibert, Jean-Louis-Marie, *Description des maladies de la peau observées à l'hôpital Saint Louis* (Paris: chez Barrois l'ainé et fils, 1806).

Amaury-Duval [Eugène Emmanuel Amaury Pineu-Duval], *L'Atelier d'Ingres: souvenirs* (Paris: G. Charpentier 1878).

Anzieu, Didier, *The Skin Ego* [1985], trans. Chris Turner (New Haven; London: Yale University Press, 1989).

Arasse, Daniel, *The Guillotine and the Terror* [1987], trans. Christopher Miller (London: Lane, 1989).

Baecque, Antoine de, *The Body Politic: Corporeal Metaphor in Revolutionary France, 1770–1800* [1993], trans. Charlotte Mandell (Stanford/Cal.: Stanford University Press, 1997).

Bakhtin, Michael, *Rabelais and His World*, trans. Helene Iswolsky (Cambridge/Mass.: MIT Press, 1968).

Bann, Stephen, 'The studio as a scene of emulation: Marceline Desbordes-Valmore's l'atelier d'un peintre', *French Studies*, 61 (2007), 26–35.

Barthes, Roland, *The Semiotic Challenge* [1985], trans. Richard Howard (Berkeley: University of California Press, 1994).

Bartholin, Thomas, *Anatomia reformata* (Leiden: Apud Franciscus Hackium, 1651).

Baudelaire, Charles, *Art in Paris, 1845–1862: Salons and Other Exhibitions*, trans. Jonathan Mayne (London: Phaidon Press, 1965).

— *Critique d'art*, ed. Claude Pichois (Paris: Gallimard, 1992).

Baudino, Isabelle (ed.), *Lumières*, 14 (2009), Special issue: L'invention et la représentation des races au XVIIIe siècle.

Baxandall, Michael, *Patterns of Intention: On the Historical Explanation of Pictures* (New Haven; London: Yale University Press, 1985).

— *Shadows and Enlightenment* (New Haven; London: Yale University Press, 1995).
Bellenger, Sylvain (ed.), *Girodet 1767–1824* (Paris: Gallimard; Musée du Louvre Éditions,).
Benjamin, Walter, *The Arcades Project*, trans. Howard Eiland and Kevin McLaughlin, prepared on the basis of the German volume edited by Rolf Tiedemann (Cambridge/Mass.; London: Belknap Press, 1999).
Benthien, Claudia, *Skin: On the Cultural Border Between Self and the World* [1999], trans. Thomas Dunlap (New York; Chichester: Columbia University Press, 2002).
Bernier, François, 'Nouvelle division de la terre, par les differentes espèces ou races d'homme qui l'habitent', *Journal des sçavans*, April 1684, 133–40.
Bertoloni Meli, Domenico, *Mechanism, Experiment, Disease: Marcello Malpighi and Seventeenth-Century Anatomy* (Baltimore: Johns Hopkins University Press, 2011).
Betzer, Sarah, 'Ingres's shadows', *Art Bulletin*, 95 (2010), 78–101.
— *Ingres and the Studio: Women, Painting, History* (University Park/Penn.: Pennsylvania State University Press, 2012).
Bhabha, Homi K., *The Location of Culture* [1994] (London; New York: Routledge, 2004).
Bichat, Xavier, *Traité des membranes en général et de diverses membranes en particulier* (Paris: Richard, Caillé et Ravier, 1799).
— *Recherches physiologiques sur la vie et la mort* (Paris: Brosson, Gabon et Cie, 1800).
— *Anatomie générale, appliquée à la physiologie et à la médecine*. 4 vols (Paris: Brosson, Gabon et Cie, 1801).
— *Physiological Researches upon Life and Death*, trans. Tobias Watkins (Philadelphia: Smith and Maxwell, 1809).
— *A Treatise on the Membranes in General, and on Different Membranes in Particular*, trans. John G. Coffin (Boston: Cummings and Hilliard; Cambridge/Mass.: Hilliard & Metcalf, 1813).
— *General Anatomy, applied to Physiology and the Practice of Medicine*, trans. Constant Coffyn. Revised and corrected by George Calvert. 2 vols (London: Printed for the Translator, 1824).
— *Traité d'anatomie descriptive*. New edn, revised and corrected. 5 vols (Paris: Gabon, 1829).
Bidloo, Govard, *Anatomia humani corporis, centum & quinque tabulis, per artificiosiss. G. de Lairesse ad vivum delineatis* (Amsterdam: for the widow of Joannes van Someren, the heirs of Joannes van Dyk, Henry Boom and widow of Theodore Boom, 1685).
— *Ontleding des menschelyken lichaams* (Amsterdam: by de weduwe van Joannes van Someren, de erfgenaamen van Joannes van Dyk, Hendrik en de weduwe van Dirk Boom, 1690).
Bindman, David, *Ape to Apollo: Aesthetics and the Idea of Race in the 18th Century* (Ithaca/New York: Cornell University Press, 2002).
— and Henry Louis Gates (eds), *The Image of the Black in Western Art*. 5 vols (Cambridge/Mass.: Belkap Press, 2010–14).
Binet, Étienne [René François], *Essay des merveilles de nature et des plus nobles artifices* (Rouen: R. de Beauvais, 1621).

Blanc, Charles, *Ingres: sa vie et ses ouvrages* (Paris: Jules Renouard, 1870).
— *Grammar of Painting and Engraving*, trans. Kate Newell Doggett (New York; Cambridge/Mass.: Hurd & Houghton, 1874).
— *Grammaire des arts du dessin* [1867], introd. Claire Barbillon (Paris: École nationale supérieure des beaux-arts, 2000).
Blanckaert, Claude, 'Of monstrous Métis? Hybridity, fear of misrecognition, and patriotism from Buffon to Paul Broca', in Sue Peabody and Tyler Edward Stovall (eds), *The Color of Liberty: Histories of Race in France* (Durham/N.C.; London: Duke University Press, 2003), pp. 42–65.
— 'La classification des races au XVIIIe siècle: l'anthropologie naturaliste entre méthode et anti-méthode', *Lumières*, 14 (2009), 3–41, Special issue: *L'invention et la répresentation des races au XVIIIe siècle.*
Bloch, Marc, *The Royal Touch: Sacred Monarchy and Scrofula in England and France* [1961], trans. J. E. Anderson (London: Routledge and Kegan Paul, 1973).
Blumenbach, Johann Friedrich, *De generis humani varietate nativa* (Göttingen: Rosenbusch, 1775).
Blumenfeld, Carol, *Une facétie de Fragonard: les révélations d'un dessin retrouvé* (Montreuil: Gourcuff Gradenigo, 2013).
Bohde, Daniela, *Haut, Fleisch und Farbe: Körperlichkeit und Materialität in den Gemälden Tizians* (Emstetten: Edition Imorde, 2002).
— 'Skin and the search for the interior: the representation of flaying in the art and anatomy of the cinquecento', in Florike Egmond and Robert Zwijnenberg (eds), *Bodily Extremities: Preoccupations with the Human Body in Early Modern European Culture* (Aldershot: Ashgate, 2003), pp. 10–47.
— 'Pellis Memoriae Peccatorum: die Moralisierung der Haut in Frontispizen und Anatomietheatern der Niederlande im 17. Jahrhundert: ein blinder Flecken in der Medizingeschichte nach 1945', in Albert Schirrmeister (ed.), *Zergliederungen: Anatomie und Wahrnehmung in der Frühen Neuzeit* (Frankfurt a. M.: Vittorio Klostermann, 2005), pp. 327–58.
— '"Le tinte delle carni": zur Begrifflichkeit von Haut und Fleisch in italienischen Kunsttraktaten des 15.–17. Jahrhunderts', in Daniela Bohde and Mechthild Fend (eds), *Weder Haut noch Fleisch: das Inkarnat in der Kunstgeschichte* (Berlin: Gebr. Mann, 2007), pp. 41–63.
— *Kunstgeschichte als physiognomische Wissenschaft: Kritik einer Denkfigur der 1920er bis 1940er Jahre* (Berlin: Akademie Verlag, 2012).
— and Mechthild Fend (eds), *Weder Haut noch Fleisch: das Inkarnat in der Kunstgeschichte* (Berlin: Gebr. Mann, 2007).
Bonfait, Olivier, 'Les envois de Rome et la plastique du nu', in Olivier Bonfait (ed.), *Maestà di Roma da Napoleone all'unità d'Italia. D'Ingres à Degas: les artistes français à Rome*, exh. cat. (Académie de France à Rome, 2003), pp. 177–82.
Bordes, Philippe and Régis Michel, *Aux Armes et aux Arts! Les arts et la Revolution 1789–1799* (Paris: A. Biro, 1988).
Bordeu, Théophile, *Recherches anatomiques sur la position des glandes et sur leur action* (Paris: chez G. F. Quillau, 1751).
— *Recherches sur le pouls, par rapport aux crises* (Paris: De Bure l'aîné, 1756).

— *Inquiries Concerning the Varieties of the Pulse, And the Particular Crisis Each more Especially Indicates* (London: T. Lewis and G. Kearsly, 1764).

Bouchardon, Edme, *L'anatomie nécessaire pour l'usage du dessein* (Paris, chez Chereau et Joubert, 1741).

Boulle, Pierre H., 'François Bernier and the origins of the modern concept of race', in Sue Peabody and Tyler Stovall (eds), *The Color of Liberty: Histories of Race in France* (Durham/N.C.; London: Duke University Press, 2003), pp. 11–41.

Bourgery, Jean-Baptiste Marc and Nicolas-Henri Jacob, *Traité complet de l'anatomie de l'homme, comprenant la médecine opératoire.* 8 vols (Paris: C. A. Delaunay, 1831–54).

Boury, Dominique, 'Bordeu et Barthez: le malentendu "vitaliste"', *La lettre de la Maison française d'Oxford*, 14 (2001), 71–84.

Brepohl, Erhard, *Theophilus Presbyter und das mittelalterliche Kunsthandwerk: Gesamtausgabe der Schrift* De diversis artibus. 2 vols (Köln: Böhlau, 1999).

Brockliss, Laurence and Colin Jones, *The Medical World of Early Modern France* (Oxford: Clarendon Press, 1997).

Bronfen, Elisabeth, *The Knotted Subject: Hysteria and its Discontents* (Princeton/N.J.; Chichester: Princeton University Press, 1998).

Bruhn, Matthias, 'Beyond the icons of knowledge: artistic styles and the art history of scientific imagery', in Horst Bredekamp, Birgit Schneider and Vera Dünkel (eds), *The Technical Image: A History of Scientific Imagery* [2008] (Chicago: University of Chicago Press, 2015), pp. 36–45.

Brunello, Franco (ed.), *De arte illuminandi e altri trattati sulla tecnica della miniatura medievale* (Vincenza: N. Pozza, 1975).

Bryson, Norman, *Tradition and Desire: From David to Delacroix* (Cambridge: Cambridge University Press, 1984).

Buffon, Georges-Louis Leclerc, Comte de, *Histoire naturelle, générale et particulière, avec la description du Cabinet du Roy*. 15 vols (Paris: Imprimerie Royale, 1749–67).

Buschhaus, Markus, *Über den Körper im Bilde sein: eine Medienarchäologie anatomischen Wissens* (Bielefeld: transcript Verlag, 2005).

Butler, Judith, *The Psychic Life of Power: Theories in Subjection* (Stanford/Cal.: Stanford University Press, 1997).

Cabanis, Pierre-Jean-Georges, *Rapports du physique et du moral de l'homme*. 2 vols (Paris: Crapart, Caille et Ravier, 1802).

— *Œuvres philosophiques de Cabanis*, ed. and introd. Claude Lehec and Jean Cazneuve. 2 vols (Paris: Presses universitaires de France, 1956).

Callen, Anthea, 'The body and difference: anatomy training at the École des beaux-arts in Paris in the later nineteenth century', *Art History*, 20 (1997), 23–60.

— 'Degas's *Bathers*: hygiene and dirt – gaze and touch', in Richard Kendall and Griselda Pollock (eds), *Dealing with Degas: Representations of Women and the Politics of Vision* (New York: Universe, 1992), pp. 159–85.

Camper, Petrus, *Dissertation physique de Mr. Pierre Camper, sur les différences réelles que présentent les traits du visage chez les hommes de différents pays et de différents ages; sur le beau qui caractèrise les statues antiques et les pierres gravées*, trans. from the Dutch by Denis Bernard Quatremere D'Isjonval (Utrecht: B. Wild & J. Altheer, 1792).

— *The works of the late Professor Camper on the Connexion between the Science of Anatomy and the Arts of Drawing, Painting, Statuary, in two books*, trans. T. Cogan (London: C. Dilly, 1794).
— *Oeuvres qui ont pour object l'histoire naturelle, la physiologie et l'anatomie comparée*. 3 vols (Paris: H.-J. Hansen, 1803).
Canguilhem, George, *Knowledge of Life* [1963], ed. Paola Marrati and Todd Meyers, trans. Stefanos Geroulanos and Daniela Ginsburg (Ashland/Ohio: Fordham University Press, 2008).
Carastro, Marcello, 'La notion de *khrôs* chez Homère: éléments pour une anthropologie de la couleur en Grèce ancienne', in Marcello Carastro (ed.), *L'Antiquité en couleurs: catégories, pratiques, représentations* (Grenoble: Jérôme Millon, 2009), pp. 301–13.
Carr, J. L., 'Pygmalion and the philosophes: the animated statue in eighteenth-century France', *Journal of the Warburg and Courtauld Institutes*, 23 (1960), 239–55.
Castagnary, Jules-Antoine, *Salons (1857–1870)* (Paris: Bibliothèque-Charpentier, 1892).
Caylus, Comte de, *Vies d'Artistes du XVIIIe siècle. Discours sur la Peinture: Salons*, ed. André Fontaine (Paris: Librairie Renard, H. Laurens, Éditeur, 1910).
Cennini, Cennino d'Andrea, *Traité de la peinture de Cennino Cennini, mis en lumière pour la première fois avec des notes par le chevalier G. Tambroni, traduit par Victor Mottez* (Paris: Vve J. Renouard, 1858).
— *The Craftmen's Handbook: The Italian 'Il libro dell'Arte'*, trans. Daniel V. Thomspon, Jnr. [1933 Yale University Press] (New York: Dover Publications, 1960).
Chamayou, Grégoire, 'La querelle des têtes tranchées: les médecins, la guillotine et l'anatomie de la conscience au lendemain de la Terreur', *Revue d'histoire des sciences*, 61 (2008), 333–65.
Choulant, Ludwig and Mortimer Frank, *History and Bibliography of Anatomic Illustration* [1852] (New York: Hafner, 1945).
Clark, Timothy J., '"Gross David with the swoln cheek": an essay on self-portraiture', in Michael S. Roth (ed.), *Rediscovering History: Culture, Politics, and the Psyche* (Stanford/Cal.: Stanford University Press, 1994), pp. 243–307, 483–93.
Cloquet, Jules, *Anatomie de l'homme, ou Description et figures lithographiées de toutes les parties du corps humaine*. 8 vols (Paris: Impr. de C. de Lasteyrie, 1821–31).
Comar, Philippe (ed.), *Figures du corps: une leçon d'anatomie à l'École des beaux-arts* (Paris: Beaux-arts de Paris, 2008).
Condillac, Étienne Bonnot, Abbé de, 'A treatise on the sensations', in *Philosophical Writings of Étienne Bonnot, Abbé de Condillac*, trans. Franklin Philip with the collaboration of Harlan Lane (Hillsdale, N.J.: Lawrence Erlbaum, 1982), pp. 1–415.
— *Traité des Sensations* [1754] (Paris: Librairie Arthème Fayard, 1984).
Les conférences de l'Académie royale de la peinture et de sculpture, ed. Jacqueline Lichtenstein and Christian Michel. 5 vols (Paris: École nationale supérieure des Beaux-Arts, 2007–12).
Connor, Steven, *The Book of Skin* (London: Reaktion Books, 2004).
Correspondance des directeurs de l'Académie de France à Rome, new series, ed. Georges Brunel and Isabelle Julia (Rome: Edizioni dell'Elefante, 1979–).
Correspondance littéraire, philosophique et critique, ed. Friedrich Melchior Baron

von Grimm et al. Revised from the original by Maurice Tourneux. 16 vols (Paris: Garnier Frères 1877–82).
Crary, Jonathan, *Techniques of the Observer: On Vision and Modernity in the Nineteenth Century* (Cambridge/Mass.; London: MIT Press, 1990).
Critchell, Samantha, 'What colour is "nude"? Fashion debates a loaded term', *Associated Press*, 17 May 2010, www.nola.com/fashion/index.ssf/2010/05/what_color_is_nude_fashion_deb.html
Crow, Thomas E., *Painters and Public Life in Eighteenth-Century Paris* (New Haven; London: Yale University Press, 1985).
— *Emulation: Making Artists for Revolutionary France* (New Haven; London: Yale University Press, 1994).
Cunningham, Andrew, *The Anatomist Anatomis'd: An Experimental Discipline in Enlightenment Europe* (Farnham; Burlington/Vt.: Ashgate, 2010).
Curran, Andrew S., *The Anatomy of Blackness: Science and Slavery in an Age of Enlightenment* (Baltimore: Johns Hopkins University Press, 2011).
Cuyer, Édouard and Mathias Duval, *Histoire de l'anatomie plastique: les maîtres, les livres et les écorchés* (Paris: Picard & Kaan, 1898).
Dandré-Bardon, Michel-François, *Traité de peinture suivi d'un essai sur la sculpture* (Paris: Saillant, 1765).
Daston, Lorraine and Peter Galison, *Objectivity* (New York: Zone Books, 2007).
Davis, John W., 'The Molyneux problem', *Journal of the History of Ideas*, 21 (1960), 392–408.
Davis, Whitney, 'The renunciation of reaction in Girodet's Sleep of Endymion', in Norman Bryson, Michael Ann Holly and Keith Moxey (eds), *Visual Culture: Images and Interpretations* (Hanover; London: University Press of New England [for] Wesleyan University Press, 1994), pp. 168–201.
— 'Winckelmann divided: mourning the death of art history', *Journal of Homosexuality*, 27 (1994), 141–59.
Debord, Jean-François, 'De l'anatomie artistique à la morphologie', in Jean Clair (ed.), *L'âme au corps: art et sciences (1793–1993)*, exh. cat. (Paris: Réunion des musées nationaux, Gallimard, 1993/94), pp. 102–17.
Décultot, Élisabeth, *Johann Joachim Winckelmann: enquète sur la genèse de l'histoire de l'art* (Paris: Presses Universitaires de Frances, 2000).
Degenaar, Marjolein, *Molyneux's Problem: Three Centuries of Discussion on the Perception of Forms* (Dordrecht; Boston; London: Kluwer Academic, 1996).
Delaborde, Henri, *Ingres, sa vie, ses travaux, sa doctrine* (Paris: Henri Plon, 1870).
Deleuze, Gilles and Felix Guattari, *A Thousand Plateaux: Capitalism and Schizoprhenia*, trans. Brian Massumi (Minneapolis, Minn.: University of Minnesota Press, 1987).
De Man, Paul, *Allegories of Reading: Figural Language in Rousseau, Nietzsche, Rilke and Proust* (New Haven; London: Yale University Press, 1979).
Denk, Claudia, *Artiste, Citoyen & Philosophe: der Künstler und sein Bildnis im Zeitalter der französischen Aufklärung* (München: Fink, 1998).
Derrida, Jacques, *Memoirs of the Blind: The Self-portrait and Other Ruins* [1991], trans. Pascale-Anne Brault and Michael Naas (Chicago: University of Chicago Press, 1993).

— 'A silkworm of one's own', in Hélène Cixous and Jacques Derrida, *Veils*, trans. Geoffrey Bennington (Stanford/Cal.: Stanford University Press, 2001, pp. 17–108.
— *On Touching: Jean-Luc Nancy* [2000], trans. Christine Irizarry (Stanford/Cal.: Standford University Press, 2005).
Descartes, René, *Œuvres*, ed. Charles Adam and Paul Tannery, vol. 11 (Paris: J. Vrin, 1996).
Dictionnaire culturel en langue française, ed. Alain Rey. 4 vols (Paris: Dictionnaires le Robert, 2005).
Dictionnaire de l'Académie française, 1st edn (1694), 4th edn (1762) 5th edn 1798, 6th edn (1832–35) (accessed via University of Chicago: The ARTFL Project. *Dictionnaires d'autrefois* https://artfl-project.uchicago.edu/content/dictionnaires-dautrefois)
Nouveau dictionnaire de l'Académie française, 2nd edn (Paris: J. B. Coignard, 1718).
Dictionnaire des sciences médicales, par une societé de médecins et de chirurgiens. 58 vols (Paris: Panckoucke, 1812–22).
Dictionnaire universel de médecine, trans. M James et al. Revised, corrected and augmented by Julien Busson, Docteur-Régent de la Faculté de Medecine de Paris. 5 vols (Paris: chez Briasson, David, Durand, 1746–48).
Diderot, Denis, *Dialogues by Denis Diderot*, trans. and introd. Francis Birrell (London: Routledge, 1927).
— *Œuvres complètes*, ed. Herbert Dieckmann and Jean Varloot. 33 vols (Paris: Herrmann, 1975–).
— *Diderot on Art*, trans. John Goodman, introd. Thomas Crow. 2 vols (New Haven; London: Yale University Press, 1995).
— *Thoughts on the Interpretation of Nature and Other Philosophical Works*. Introduced and annotated by David Adams (Manchester: Clinamen Press, 1999).
Didi-Huberman, Georges, *La peinture incarnée: suivi de Le chef-d'œuvre inconnu par Honoré de Balzac* (Paris: Les Éditions de Minuit, 1985).
— 'La couleur de la chair ou le paradoxe de Tertullien', *Nouvelle revue de la psychanalyse*, 35 (1987), Special issue: *Le champ visuel*, 9–49.
Dorlin, Elsa, *La matrice de la race: généalogie sexuelle et coloniale de la Nation française* (Paris: La Découverte, 2006).
Douglas, Mary, *Purity and Danger: An Analysis of Concepts of Pollution and Taboo* (London: Routledge and Kegan Paul, 1966).
Ducci, Annamaria, '"Leur chair chante des Marseillaises": la main dans les écrits sur l'art en France, repères pour un parcours', in Mariacarla Gadebusch Bondio (ed.), *Die Hand: Elemente einer Medizin- und Kulturgeschichte* (Berlin: LIT, 2010), pp. 239–64.
Duden, Barbara, *The Woman Beneath the Skin: A Doctor's Patients in Eighteenth-century Germany* [1987], trans. Thomas Dunlap (Cambridge/Mass.: Harvard University Press, 1991).
Dumaître, Paule, *La curieuse destinée des planches anatomiques de Gérard de Lairesse, peintre en Hollande: Lairesse, Bidloo, Cowper* (Amsterdam: Rodopi, 1982).
Duverney [also Du Verney], Joseph-Guichard, *Œuvres anatomiques* (Paris: C. A. Jombert, 1761).
Elias, Norbert, *The Civilizing Process: The History of Manners* [1939] (Oxford: Blackwell, 1978).

Encyclopédie méthodique. Beaux-arts, ed. Claude-Henri Watelet and Pierre-Charles Lévesque. 2 vols (Paris: Panckoucke, 1788–91).

Encyclopédie ou dictionnaire raisonné des sciences, des arts et des metiers, ed. Denis Diderot and Jean le Rond d'Alembert. 17 vols, 1751–65, and 11 vols plates, 1762–72 (accessed via University of Chicago: ARTFL Encyclopédie Projet (winter 2008 edn), ed. Robert Morrissey, http://encyclopedie.uchicago.edu/).

Fau, Julien, *Explication d'un nouvel écorché à l'usage des artistes* (Paris: Méquignon-Marvis, 1844).

— *Anatomie des formes extérieures du corps humain, a l'usage des peintres et des sculpteurs* (Paris: Méquignon-Marvis, 1845).

— *The Anatomy of the External Forms of Man, intended for the use of artists, painters and sculptors*, trans. Robert Knox (London: Bailliere, 1849).

Felfe, Robert, '*Naer het leven*: eine sprachliche Formel zwischen bildgenerierenden Übertragungsvorgängen und ästhetischer Vermittlung', in Claudia Fritzsche, Karen Leonhard and Gregor J. M. Weber (eds), *Ad Fontes: Niederländische Kunst des siebzehnten Jahrhunderts in Quellen* (Petersberg: Michael Imhof Verlag, 2013), pp. 165–95.

Félibien, André, *Des Principes de l'architecture, de la sculpture, de la peinture et des autres arts qui en dépendent* (Paris: J. B. Coignard, 1676).

Fend, Mechthild, 'Zeichen in der Oberfläche: Valie Exports body sign action', *Psychoanalyse im Widerspruch*, 15:29 (2003), 51–9.

— *Grenzen der Männlichkeit: Der Androgyn in der französischen Kunst und Kunsttheorie zwischen Aufklärung und Restauration* (Berlin: Reimer, 2003). Translated as: *Les limites de la masculinité: l'androgyne dans l'art et la théorie de l'art en France (1750–1830)* (Paris: La Decouverte, 2011).

— '"Körpersehen": über das Haptische bei Alois Riegl', in Andreas Mayer and Alexandre Métraux (eds), *Kunstmaschinen: Spielräume des Sehens zwischen Wissenschaft und Kunst* (Frankfurt a. M.: Fischer, 2005), pp. 166–202.

— 'Bodily and pictorial surfaces: skin in French art and medicine, 1790–1860', *Art History*, 28 (2005), 311–39.

— 'Die Substanz der Oberfläche: Haut und Fleisch in der französischen Kunst und Kunsttheorie des 17.bis 19. Jahrhunderts', in Daniela Bohde and Mechthild Fend (eds), *Weder Haut noch Fleisch: Das Inkarnat in der Kunstgeschichte* (Berlin: Gebr. Mann, 2007), pp. 87–104.

— 'Haut wie weicher Marmor: die Frauenporträts von Jean-Auguste-Dominique Ingres', in Oliver Jehle and Sabine Slanina (eds), Ähnlichkeit und Entstellung (Berlin: Deutscher Kunstverlag, 2010), pp. 95–112.

— 'Portraying skin disease: Robert Carswell's dermatological watercolours', in Kevin Siena and Jonathan Reinarz (eds), *A Medical History of Skin* (London: Pickering and Chatto, 2013), pp. 147–64.

— 'Flesh-tones, skin-color and the eighteenth-century color print', in Felix Ensslin and Charlotte Klink (eds), *Aesthetics of the Flesh* (Berlin: Sternberg Press, 2014), pp. 203–27.

— 'Marie-Guillemine Benoist's *Portrait d'une Négresse* and the visibility of skin colour', in Caroline Rosenthal and Dirk Vanderbeke (eds), *Probing the Skin* (Cambridge: Cambridge Scholars Publishing, 2015), pp. 192–210.

Ferrier, Morvenna et al., 'The trouble with nudity in fashion', *Guardian*, 10 May 2010, www.theguardian.com/lifeandstyle/2010/may/20/fashion-colour-nude-racist
Fischel, Angela, 'Sehen, Darstellen, Beschreiben: mikroskopische Beobachtung in den Kupferstichen der Micrographia', *kunsttexte.de* 1.2002, http://edoc.hu-berlin.de/kunsttexte/download/bwt/fischel.pdf
Fleckner, Uwe, *Abbild und Abstraktion: die Kunst des Porträts im Werk von Jean-Auguste-Dominique Ingres* (Mainz: Philip von Zabern, 1995).
— '"Pourquoi une belle esquisse nous plaît-elle plus qu'un beau tableau?": Fragonard, Diderot et l'éloquence du pinceau dans quelques portraits du XVIIIe siècle', in Thomas W. Gaethgens et al. (eds), *L'art et les normes sociales au 18ième siècle* (Paris: Éditions de la Maison des sciences de l'homme, 2001), pp. 509–33.
Flourens, Pierre, 'Recherches anatomiques sur le corps muqueux, ou appareil pigmental de la peau, dans l'Indien Charrua, le nègre et le mulatre' *Comte rendu hebdomodaire des séances de l'Académie des sciences*, 3 (1836), 700–6.
Forrester, John, 'The homoeomerous parts and their replacement by Bichat's Tissues', *Medical History*, 38 (1994), 444–58.
Förschler, Silke, *Bilder des Harem: Medienwandel und kultureller Austausch* (Berlin: Reimer, 2010).
Foucault, Michel, *The Order of Things: An Archaeology of the Human Sciences* [1966], trans. A. M. Sheridan Smith (London: Tavistock 1970).
— *The Birth of the Clinic: An Archaeology of Medical Perception* [1963], trans. A. M. Sheridan Smith (London: Tavistock, 1973).
— 'Technologies of the self', in Paul Rabinow (ed.), *Michel Foucault.Ethics, Subjectivity and Truth: Essential Works of Foucault 1954–1984*, vol. 1 (London: Tavistock, 1988), pp. 223–51.
Fournier, Marian, *The Fabric of Life: Microscopy in the Seventeenth Century* (Baltimore; London: Johns Hopkins University Press, 1996).
Freund, Amy, *Portraiture and Politics in Revolutionary France* (University Park/Penn.: Pennsylvania State University Press, 2014).
Gaethgens, Thomas, 'La doctrine académique: histoire d'une fiction', in *Les conférences de l'Académie royale de la peinture et de sculpture*, ed. Jacqueline Lichtenstein and Christian Michel, vol. 1 (Paris: École nationale supérieure des Beaux-Arts, 2007), pp. 13–23.
Gage, John, *Colour and Culture: Practice and Meaning from Antiquity to Abstraction* (London: Thames & Hudson, 1993).
— 'Colour words in the high Middle Ages', in Erma Hermens (ed.), *Looking Through Paintings: The Study of Painting Techniques and Materials in Support of Art Historical Research* (Baarn: de Prom; London: Archetype publication, 1998), pp. 35–48.
— *Colour and Meaning: Art, Science and Symbolism* (London: Thames & Hudson, 1999).
Garb, Tamar, *The Painted Face: Portraits of Women in France 1814–1914* (New Haven; London: Yale University Press, 2007).
Gaultier, Gabriel-Antoine, *Recherches sur l'organisation de la peau de l'homme et sur les causes de sa coloration* (Paris: chez Gabon, 1809).
Gavrylenko, Valeria, 'The body without skin', in Manfred Horstmanshoff, Helen King

and Claus Zittel (eds), *Blood, Sweat and Tears: The Changing Concepts of Physiology from Antiquity into Early Modern Europe* (Leiden: Brill, 2012), pp. 481–502.
Gerdy, Pierre-Nicolas, *Anatomie des formes extérieures du corps humain, appliquée à la peinture, à la sculpture et à la chirurgie* (Paris: Bechet jeune, 1829).
— *Anatomie des peintres. Atlas* (Paris: Bechet jeune, 1829).
— *Physiologie médicale didactique et critique* (Paris: Crochard, 1832).
Germer, Stefan, *Kunst, Macht, Diskurs: die intellektuelle Karriere des André Félibien im Frankreich von Louis XIV* (München: Fink, 1997).
Ginzburg, Carlo, 'Morelli, Freud and Sherlock Holmes: clues and scientific method', *History Workshop Journal*, 9 (1980), 5–36.
Goethe, Johann Wolfgang Friedrich von, 'Farbenlehre' [1810], ed. Manfred Wenzel, in *Sämtliche Werke*, vol. 23/1 (Frankfurt: Suhrkamp, 1991).
Goldstein, Jan, *The Post-Revolutionary Self: Politics and Psyche in France, 1750–1850* (Cambridge/Mass.; London: Harvard University Press, 2005).
Goodden, Angelica, *Diderot and the Body* (Oxford: Legenda, 2001).
Goodman, Dena, *The Republic of Letters: A Cultural History of the Enlightenment* (Ithaca; London: Cornell University Press, 1994).
Grand-Clément, Adeline, *La fabrique des couleurs: histoire du paysage des Grecs anciens* (Paris: de Broccard, 2011).
Grew, Nehemia, *The Anatomy of Plants: With an Idea of a Philosophical History of Plants* (London: W. Rawlins, for the Author, 1682).
— *Anatomie des Plantes: Qui contient une Description exacte de leurs parties & de leurs usages, et qui fait voir comment elles se forment, & comment elles croissent* (Leiden: Pierre Vander, 1685).
Grimaldo Grigsby, Darcy, *Extremities: Painting Empire in Post-Revolutionary France* (New Haven; London: Yale University Press, 2002).
Grindle, Nicholas, 'Our own imperfect knowledge: Petrus Camper and the search for the "Ideal Form"', *RES: Anthropology and Aesthetics*, no. 31 (spring 1997), 139–48.
Grivel, Charles, 'Der siderale Körper: zum Prinzip des Kommunikation', in J. Hörisch and M. Wenzel (eds), *Armaturen der Sinne: literarische und technische Medien 1870 bis 1920* (München: Fink, 1990), pp. 177–99.
Groebner, Valentin, '*Complexio*/complexion: categorizing individual natures, 1250–1600', in Lorraine Daston and Fernando Vidal (eds), *The Moral Authority of Nature* (Chicago; London: University of Chicago Press, 2004), pp. 361–83.
Guédron, Martial, *Peaux d'âmes: l'interprétation physiognomonique des œuvres d'art* (Paris: Éditions Kimé, 2001).
— *De chair et de marbre: imiter et exprimer le nu en France (1745–1815)* (Paris: Éditions Champion, 2003).
— *L'art de la grimace: cinq siècles d'excès de visage* (Paris: Hazan, 2011).
Haigh, Elizabeth, *Xavier Bichat and the Medical Theory of the Eighteenth Century* (London: Wellcome Institute for the History of Medicine, 1984).
Hallam, Elizabeth, 'Articulating bones: an epilogue', *Journal of Material Culture*, 15 (2010), 465–92.
Haller, Albrecht von, *Dissertation sur les parties irritables et sensibles des animaux*, trans. Samuel-Auguste-David Tissot (Lausanne: Marc-Michel Bousquet, 1755).

— *A Dissertation on the Sensible and Irritable Parts of Animals*, trans. Samuel-Auguste-David Tissot (London: J. Nourse, 1755).
— *Elementa physiologiæ corporis humani*. 8 vols (Lugduni Batavorum: Apud Cornel Haak, 1757–66).
— *Élémens de physiologie, ou Traité de la structure et des usages des différentes parties du corps humain*, trans. Pierre Tarin and Toussaint Bordenave (Paris: chez Prault fils, 1769).
Halliday, Tony, *Facing the Public: Portraiture in the Aftermath of the French Revolution* (Manchester; New York: Manchester University Press, 1999).
— *The Temperamental Nude: Class, Medicine and Representation in eighteenth-century France* (Oxford: Voltaire Foundation, 2010).
Hannaway, Caroline and Ann La Berge (eds), *Constructing Paris Medicine* (Amsterdam; Atlanta: Rodopi, 1998).
Harvey, Elizabeth D. (ed.), *Sensible Flesh: On Touch in Early Modern Culture* (Philadelphia: University of Pennsylvania Press, 2003).
Haskell, Francis and Nicholas Penny, *Taste and the Antique: The Lure of Classical Sculpture, 1500–1900* (New Haven; London: Yale University Press, 1981).
Hegel, Georg Wilhelm Friedrich, *Aesthetics: Lectures on Fine Art* [1835], trans. Malcom Knox. 2 vols (Oxford: Clarendon Press, 1975).
Heinen, Ulrich, 'Haut und Knochen – Fleisch und Blut: Rubens' Affektmalerei', in Ulrich Heinen and Andreas Thielemann (eds), *Rubens Passioni: Kultur der Leidenschaften im Barock* (Göttingen: Vandenhoeck & Ruprecht, 2001), pp. 70–109.
— 'Peter Paul Rubens: Barocke Leidenschaften', in Nils Büttner and Ulrich Heinen (eds), *Rubens: Barocke Leidenschaften*, exh. cat. Herzog Anton Ulrich Museum Braunschweig (Braunschweig; München: Hirmer, 2004), pp. 28–38.
Held, Jutta, *Französische Kunsttheorie des 17. Jahrhunderts und der absolutistische Staat: Le Brun und die ersten acht Vorlesungen an der königlichen Akademie* (Berlin: Reimer, 2001).
Heller-Roazen, Daniel, *The Inner Touch: Archaeology of a Sensation* (New York: Zone Books, 2007).
Hendriksen, Marieke, *Elegant Anatomy: The Eighteenth-Century Leiden Anatomical Collections* (Leiden; Boston: Brill, 2015).
Hennepe, Mienekete, *Depicting Skin: Visual Culture in Nineteenth-Century Medicine* (Wageningen: Ponsen & Looijen, 2007).
— 'Of the fisherman's net and skin pores: reframing conceptions of the skin in medicine 1572–1714', in Manfred Horstmanshoff, Helen King and Claus Zittel (eds), *Blood, Sweat and Tears: Changing Concepts of Physiology from Antiquity into Early Modern Europe* (Leiden: Brill, 2012), pp. 524–48.
Herding, Klaus, *Pierre Puget: Das bildnerische Werk* (Berlin: Gebr. Mann, 1970).
— 'Schwindender Heroismus – gesteigerte Sinnlichkeit: Pugets *Milon von Kroton* als Ausdruck einer Krise der Männlichkeit im absolutistischen Zeitalter', in Mechthild Fend and Marianne Koos (eds), *Männlichkeit im Blick: visuelle Inszenierungen in der Kunst seit der Frühen Neuzeit* (Köln; Weimar; Wien: Böhlau, 2004), pp. 137–59.
Hogarth, William, *The Analysis of Beauty* (London: J. Reeves, 1753).
Holert, Tom, *Künstlerwissen: Studien zur Semantik künstlerischer Kompetenz im*

Frankreich des 18. und frühen 19. Jahrhunderts (München: Fink, 1998).
Honegger, Claudia, *Die Ordnung der Geschlechter: die Wissenschaften vom Menschen und das Weib, 1750–1850* (Frankfurt a. M.; New York: Campus, 1991).
Hooke, Robert, *Micrographia: or some Physiological Descriptions of Minute Bodies made by Magnifying Glasses* (London: Jo. Martyn and Ja. Allestry, 1665).
— 'A General Scheme, or Idea of the Present State of Natural Philosophy', in *The Posthumous Works of Robert Hooke* (London: Richard Weller, 1705).
Hunter, Matthew, *Wicked Intelligence: Visual Art and the Science of Experiment in Restoration London* (Chicago; London: University of Chicago Press, 2013).
Hyde, Melissa, *Making Up the Rococo: François Boucher and his Critics* (Los Angeles/ Cal.: Getty Publications, 2006).
Imdahl, Max, *Farbe: kunsttheoretische Reflexionen in Frankreich* (München: Fink, 1987).
Jahn, Ilse (ed.), *Geschichte der Biologie*, 3rd edn (Berlin: Spektrum, 2000).
Johnson, Dorothy, *Jacques-Louis David: Art in Metamorphosis* (Princeton/N.J.; Chichester: Princeton University Press, 1993).
— 'Mythologie et anatomie: science et création dans l'art français autour de 1800', in Anne Lafont (ed.), *L'artiste savant à la conquête du monde moderne* (Strasbourg: Presses universitaires de Strasbourg, 2010), pp. 33–42.
— *David to Delacroix: The Rise of Romantic Mythology* (Chapel Hill/N.C.: University of North Carolina Press, 2011).
Johnson, James H., 'Versailles, meet Les Halles: masks, carnival, and the French Revolution', *Representations*, 73 (winter 2001), 89–116.
Jollet, Étienne, 'Les rapports entre les sciences et les beaux-arts dans les écrits de C.-H. Watelet', *Revue du dix-huitième siècle*, 31 (1999), 217–31.
Joly, Morvenna, 'L'obsession du "dessous": Diderot et l'image anatomique', *Recherches sur Diderot et sur l'Encyclopédie*, 43 (2008), 57–70.
Jordanova, Ludmilla, *Sexual Visions: Images of Gender in Sciences and Medicine between the Eighteenth and Twentieth Centuries* (New York; London: Harvester Wheatsheaf, 1989).
— *Nature Displayed: Gender, Science and Medicine, 1760–1820* (London; New York: Longman, 1999).
Kemp, Martin and Marina Wallace, *Spectacular Bodies: The Art and Science of the Human Body from Leonardo to Now* (London: Hayward Gallery; Los Angeles: University of California Press, 2000).
Kilgour, Frederick G., *The Evolution of the Book* (New York; Oxford: Oxford University Press, 1998).
Klaus, Sidney, 'A history of the science of pigmentation', in James J. Nordlund (ed.), *The Pigmentary System: Physiology and Pathophysiology* (Oxford: Blackwell, 2006), pp. 5–10.
Körner, Hans, '"Die Epidermis der Statue": Oberflächen der Skulptur vom späten 17. bis zum frühen 19. Jahrhundert', in Daniela Bohde and Mechthild Fend (eds), *Weder Haut noch Fleisch. Das Inkarnat in der Kunstgeschichte* (Berlin: Gebr. Mann, 2007), pp. 105–32.
Koos, Marianne, 'Haut als mediale Metapher in der Malerei von Caravaggio', in Daniela Bohde and Mechthild Fend (eds), *Weder Haut noch Fleisch: das Inkarnat*

in der Kunstgeschichte (Berlin: Gebr. Mann, 2007), pp. 65–85.
— *Haut, Farbe und Medialität: Oberfläche im Werk von Jean-Étienne Liotard (1702–1789)* (Paderborn: Fink, 2014).
Koschorke, Albrecht, *Körperströme und Schriftverkehr: Mediologie des 18.Jahrhunderts* (München: Fink, 1999).
Krüger, Matthias, *Das Relief der Farbe: Pastose Malerei in der französischen Kunstkritik 1850–1890* (München; Berlin: Deutscher Kunstverlag, 2007).
— 'Der Begriff des *disegno* im Zeitalter der Evolutionstheorie: biologische Konzepte in Charles Blancs *Grammaire des Arts du Dessin*', in Matthias Krüger, Christine Ott and Ulrich Pfisterer (eds), *Die Biologie der Kreativität* (Zürich; Berlin: diaphanes, 2013), pp. 75–90.
Krüger-Fürhoff, Irmela Marei, *Der versehrte Körper: Revisionen des klassizistischen Schönheitsideals* (Göttingen: Wallstein, 2001).
Kruse, Christiane, 'Fleisch werden – Fleisch malen: Malerei als "incarnazione". Mediale Verfahren des Bildwerdens in Cennino Cenninis Libro dell'Arte', *Zeitschrift für Kunstgeschichte*, 63 (2000), 305–26.
— *Wozu Menschen malen: historische Begründungen eines Bildmediums* (München: Fink, 2003).
Lafont, Anne, 'Les rencontres hypothétiques du peintre et de son modèle: clefs sociales dans l'interprétation du tableau', and 'Un portrait entre cliché racial et émancipation sociale', in Anne-Lise Desmas (ed.), *Les portraits du pouvoir: actes du colloque organisé par Olivier Bonfait et Brigitte Marin* (Paris: Somogy, 2003), pp. 115–25; pp. 110–13.
— 'Étrange étrangeté: la science au cœur de la répresentation de l'Africain', in Anne Lafont (ed.), *L'artiste savant à la conquête du monde moderne* (Strasbourg: Presses Universitaires de Strasbourg, 2010), pp. 141–56.
Lagrave, Jean-Paul (ed.), *Madame Helvétius et la Société d'Auteuil* (Oxford: Voltaire Foundation, 1999).
Lajer-Burcharth, Ewa, *Necklines: The Art of Jacques-Louis David after the Terror* (New Haven; London: Yale University Press, 1999).
— 'Pompadour's touch: difference in representation', *Representations*, 73 (2001), 54–88.
— 'The self in exile: David's *Portrait of Emmanuel-Joseph Sieyès*', in Mark Ledbury (ed.), *David after David: Essays on the Later Work* (Williamstown/Mass.: Sterling and Francine Clark Institute and New Haven; London: Yale University Press, 2007), pp. 232–51.
Lanoë, Catherine, *La poudre et le fard: une histoire des cosmétiques de la Renaissance aux Lumières* (Seyssel: Champ Vallon, 2008).
Lapauze, Henry, *Les dessins de J.-A.-D. Ingres du Musée de Montauban* (Paris: J.-E. Bulloz, 1901).
— *Ingres, sa vie et son œuvre (1780–1867), d'après les documents inédits* (Paris: J.-E. Bulloz, 1911).
Lavater, Johann Heinrich, *Élémens anatomiques d'ostéologie et de myologie à l'usage des peintres et des sculpteurs*, trans. Gauthier de la Peyronie (Paris: Ziegler, 1797).
Lavater, Johann Kaspar, *Physiognomische Fragemente zur Beförderung der Menschenkenntnis*. 4 vols (Leipzig: Winterthur 1775–78).

— *L'art de connaître les hommes par la physionomie*, trans., ed. and augmented by Jacques-Louis Moreau de la Sarthe. 10 vols (Paris: L. Prudhomme 1806).

Le Blon, Jacob Christoph, *Coloritto; or the Harmony of Colouring in Painting: Reduced to Mechanical Practice, under Easy Preceps, and Infallible Rules* [London, 1725].

Le Blond de la Tour, Antoine, *Lettre du Sieur Le Blond de La Tour, à un de ses amis, contenant quelques instructions touchant la Peinture* (Bordeaux: P. Du Coq, 1669).

Le Cat, Claude-Nicolas, *Traité des sens* (Rouen [*s.n.*], 1740).

— *Traité de la couleur de la peau humaine en général, de celle des negres en particulier et de la métamorphose d'une de ces couleurs en l'autre, soit de naissance, soit accidentellement* (Amsterdam [*s.n.*], 1765).

Lehmann, Ann-Sophie, 'Jan van Eyck und die Entdeckung der Leibfarbe', in Daniela Bohde and Mechthild Fend (eds), *Weder Haut noch Fleisch: das Inkarnat in der Kunstgeschichte* (Berlin: Gebr. Mann, 2007), pp. 21–40.

— 'Fleshing out the body: the "colours of the naked" in workshop practice and art theory, 1400-1600', in Ann-Sophie Lehmann and Herman Roodenburg (eds), *Body and Embodiment in Netherlandish Art. Neederlands Kunsthistorisch Jaarboek* 58 (Zwolle: Wanders, 2008), pp. 86–109.

— 'The matter of the medium: some tools for an art theoretical interpretation of materials', in Christy Anderson et al. (eds), *The Matter of Art: Materials, Practices, Cultural Logics, c. 1250–1750* (Manchester: Manchester University Press, 2015), pp. 21–41.

Leighton, John, *Jacques-Louis David: Portrait of Jacobus Blauw* (London: National Gallery Publications, 1987).

Leonhard, Karin, *Bildfelder: Stilleben und Naturstücke des 17. Jahrhunderts* (Berlin: Akademie Verlag, 2013).

Lepik-Kopaczyńska, Wilhemina, 'Das antike Inkarnat in der Überlieferung der mittelalterlichen Humanisten', in Johannes Irmscher (ed.), *Renaissance und Humanismus in Mittel- und Osteuropa* (Berlin: Akademie Verlag, 1962), pp. 76–83.

— *Die antike Malerei* (Berlin: Akademie Verlag, 1963).

Levitine, George, *The Sculpture of Falconet*, with a translation from the French of Falconet's *Réflexions sur la sculpture* by Eda Mezer Levitine (Greenwich/Conn.: New York Graphic Society, 1972).

— *The Dawn of Bohemianism: The Barbue Rebellion and Primitivism in Neoclassical France* (University Park/Penn.; London: Pennsylvania State University Press, 1978).

Libby, Susan H., 'The color of Frenchness: racial identity and visuality in French anti-slavery imagery, 1788–94', in Adrienne L. Childs and Susan H. Libby (eds), *Blacks and Blackness in European Art of the Long Nineteenth Century* (Farnham; Burlington/Vt.: Ashgate, 2014), pp. 19–45.

Lichtenstein, Jacqueline, *The Eloquence of Colour* (Berkeley: University of California Press, 1993).

— and Christian Michel, 'La réflexion artistique des academicians', in, *Les conférences de l'Académie royale de peinture et de sculpture*, ed. Jacqueline Lichtenstein and Christian Michel, vol. 1 (Paris: École nationale supérieure des beaux-arts, 2008), pp. 25–42.

Lifchez, Raymond, 'Jean-Galbert Salvage and his *Anatomie du gladiateur combattant*: art and patronage in post-revolutionary France', *Metropolitan Museum Journal*, 44 (2009), pp. 163–84.

Lilien, Otto M., *Jacob Christoph Le Blon 1667–1741: Inventor of Three and Four Colour Printing* (Stuttgart: Hiersemann, 1985).

Lilti, Antoine, 'Sociabilité et mondanité: les hommes de lettres dans les salons parisiens au XVIIIe siècle', *French Historical Studies*, 28 (2005), 415–45.

Linnaeus, Carl, *Systema naturae sive regna tria naturae systematice propostia per classes, ordines, genera, & species*, 1st edn (Leiden: Theodorum Haak, 1735); 10th edn (Stockholm: Salvi, 1758).

Littré, Alexis, ['De la structure de la peau'], in *Histoire de l'Académie Royale des Sciences*, Année MDCCII (Paris: chez Gabr. Martin, Jean-Bapt. Coignard, et les Frères Guerin, 1743).

Loh, Maria, *Titian Remade: Repetition and the Transformation of Early Modern Italian Art* (Los Angeles/Cal.: Getty Publications, 2007).

Lorry, Anne-Charles, *Tractatus de morbis cutaneis* (Paris: Guillemin Cavelier, 1777).

Ludwig, Christianus Gottlieb, respondente F. Grützmacher, 'De humore cutem inungente pro loco', [Leipzig, 1748], in Albrecht von Haller (ed.), *Disputationum anatomicarum selectarum*, vol. 7, pars 2 (Göttingen: Vandenhoek, 1751), pp. 33–64.

Macsotay, Tomas, 'Suffering bodies, sensible artists: vitalist medicine and the visualizing of corporeal life in Diderot', in Manfred Horstmanshoff, Helen King and Claus Zittel (eds), *Blood, Sweat and Tears: Changing Concepts of Physiology from Antiquity into Early Modern Europe* (Leiden: Brill, 2012), pp. 267–91.

Malcolmson, Cristina, *Studies of Skin Color in the Early Royal Society: Boyle, Cavendish, Swift* (Farnham: Ashgate, 2013).

Malpighi, Marcello, *Opera Omnia. Tomis duobus comprehensa* (London: Prostant apud Robertum Scott, 1686).

— *Opere scelte di Marcello Malpighi*, ed. Luigi Bellori (Torino: Unione Tipograpico-editrice Torinese, 1967).

Margócsy, Dániel, *Commercial Visions: Science, Trade, and Visual Culture in the Dutch Golden Age* (Chicago: University of Chicago Press, 2014).

Marks, Laura, *The Skin of the Film: Intercultural Cinema, Embodiment, and the Senses* (Durham/N.C.; London: Duke University Press, 2000).

— *Touch: Sensous Theory and Multisensory Media* (Minneapolis; London: University of Minnesota Press, 2002).

Massing, Ann, 'French painting technique in the seventeenth and early eighteenth centuries and De La Fontaine's *Académie de la peinture* (Paris 1679)', in Erma Hermens (ed.), *Looking Through Paintings: A Study of Painting Techniques and Materials in Support of Art Historical Research* (Baarn: de Prom, 1998), pp. 319–90.

Mazzolini, Renato, 'Anatomische Untersuchungen über die Haut der Schwarzen (1700–1800)', in Gunter Mann and Franz Dumont (eds), *Die Natur des Menschen: Probleme der physischen Anthropologie und Rassenkunde (1750–1850)*(Stuttgart: Gustav Fischer 1990), pp. 169–87.

— 'Las castas: interracial crossing and social structure, 1770–1835', in Staffan Müller-Wille and Hans-Jörg Rheinberger (eds), *Heredity Produced: At the Crossroads of Biology, Politics, and Culture, 1500–1870* (Cambridge/Mass.; London: MIT Press, 2007), pp. 349–73.

A Medicinal Dictionary, Including Physic, Surgery, Anatomy, Chymistry, and Botany, in all their Branches Relative to Medicine, by R. James. 3 vols (London: T. Osborne, 1743–45).

Meijer, Miriam Claude, *Race and Aesthetics in the Anthropology of Petrus Camper (1722–1789)* (Amsterdam: Rodopi, 1999).

Merrifield, Mary P., *Medieval and Renaissance Treatises on the Arts of Painting: Original Texts with English Translations* (Mineola/N.Y.: Dover Publications, 1999).

Michel, Christian, *Charles-Nicolas Cochin et l'art des Lumières* (Rome: École française de Rome, 1993).

— 'Deutsche Ästhetik und französische Kunsttheorie am Ende des Ancien Régime: die "Encyclopédie méthodique. Beaux-Arts"', in Uwe Fleckner et al. (eds), *Jenseits der Grenzen: französische und deutsche Kunst vom Ancien Régime bis zur Gegenwart* (Köln: DuMont, 2000), pp. 329–44.

— *L'Académie royale de peinture et de sculpture (1648–1793): la naissance de l'école française* (Genève: Droz, 2012).

Miller, Christopher, *The French Atlantic Triangle: Literature and Culture of the Slave Trade* (Durham/N.C.; London: Duke University Press, 2008).

Montagu, Jennifer, *The Expression of the Passions: The Origin and Influence of Charles Le Brun's Conférence sur l'expression générale et particulière* (New Haven; London: Yale University Press, 1994).

— 'The quarrel of drawing and colour in the French Academy', in Victoria v. Flemming and Sebastian Schütze (eds), *Ars naturam adiuvans: Festschrift für Matthias Winner* (Mainz: Philipp von Zabern, 1996), pp. 548–56.

Montagu, Mary Wortley, *Letters*, introd. Clare Brant (London: Random House, 1992).

Moravia, Sergio, 'From *homme machine* to *homme sensible*: changing eighteenth-century models of man's image', *Journal of the History of Ideas*, 39 (1978), 45–60.

Mülder-Bach, Inka, *Im Zeichen Pygmalions: das Modell der Statue und die Entdeckung der 'Darstellung' im 18. Jahrhundert* (München: Fink 1998).

Nead, Lynda, *The Female Nude: Art, Obscenity and Sexuality* (London; New York: Routledge, 1992).

Nicot, Jean, *Le Thresor de la langue françoise, tant ancienne que moderne* (Paris: David Douceur, 1606).

Nochlin, Linda, 'The imaginary Orient', *Art in America*, May 1983, 119–31, 186–91.

Ockman, Carol, *Ingres's Eroticized Bodies: Retracing the Serpentine Line* (New Haven: Yale University Press, 1995).

Oppenheimer, Margaret A., 'Three newly identified paintings by Marie-Guillemine Benoist', *Metropolitan Museum Journal*, 31 (1996), 143–50.

— '"The charming spectacle of a cadaver": anatomical and life study by women artists in Paris, 1775–1815', *Nineteenth-Century Art Worldwide*, 6 (2007), www.19thc-artworldwide.org/spring07/46-spring07/spring07article/142-qthe-charming-spectacle-of-a-cadaverq-anqthe-charming-spectacle-of-a-cadaverq-anatomical-and-life-study-by-women-artists-in-paris-17751815

Otis, Laura, *Membranes: Metaphors of Invasion in Nineteenth-Century Literature, Science, and Politics* (Baltimore; London: Johns Hopkins University Press, 1999).

Outram, Dorinda, *The Body and the French Revolution: Sex, Class and Political Culture* (New Haven: Yale University Press, 1989).

Paillot de Montabert, Jacques-Nicolas, *Traité complet de la peinture.* 9 vols (Paris: J.-F. Delion, 1829–51).

Paré, Alex, 'Peindre la chair. Rendu des carnations et image du corps dans la peinture française des années 1680–1740' (MA dissertation, École du Louvre, Paris, 2009).

Park, Katharine, *Secrets of Women: Gender, Generation, and the Origins of Human Dissection* (New York: Zone Books, 2006).

Peabody, Sue, *'There Are No Slaves in France': The Political Culture of Slavery in the Ancien Regime* (New York; Oxford: Oxford University Press, 1996).

— and Tyler Stovall (eds): *The Color of Liberty: Histories of Race in France* (Durham/N.C.; London: Duke University Press, 2003).

Percival, Melissa, *The Appearance of Character: Physiognomy and Facial Expression in Eighteenth-Century France* (Leeds: Modern Humanities Research Association, 1999).

— *Fragonard and the Fantasy Figure: Painting the Imagination* (Farnham; Burlington/Vt.: Ashgate, 2012).

— and Graeme Tytler (eds): *Physiognomy in Profile: Lavater's Impact on European Culture* (Newark/Del.: University of Delaware Press, 2005).

Pernety, Antoine-Joseph, *Dictionnaire portatif de peinture, sculpture et gravure* (Paris: Bauche, 1757).

— *Discours sur la physionomie, et les avantages des connoissances physionomiques* (Berlin: Georges Jacques Decker, 1769).

Pickstone, John, 'Bureaucracy, liberalism and the body in post-revolutionary France: Bichat's physiology and the Paris School of Medicine', *History of Science*, 19 (1981), 115–42.

Pietsch, Annik, 'Der "glanzlose Seelenduft der Fleischfarbe": Schlesingers Hegel-Porträt', in Daniela Bohde and Mechthild Fend (eds), *Weder Haut noch Fleisch: das Inkarnat in der Kunstgeschichte* (Berlin: Gebr. Mann, 2007), pp. 133–58.

Piles, Roger de, *L'art de peinture de C.A. Du Fresnoy. Enrichie de remarques, & augmenté d'un Dialogue sur le coloris* (Paris: Nicolas Langlois, 1668).

— *Dialogue sur le coloris* (Paris: Nicolas Langlois, 1673).

— *Conversations sur la connoissance de la peinture et sur le jugement qu'on doit faire des tableaux. Où par occassion il est parlé de Rubens* (Paris: Nicolas Langlois, 1677).

— *Les premiers éléments de la peinture pratique* (Paris: chez Nicolas Langlois, 1684).

— *Cours de peinture par principes* (Paris: chez Jacques Estienne, 1708).

— *Dialogue upon Colouring*, trans. Mr. Ozell (London: printed for Daniel Brown and Bernard Lintott, 1711).

P[illet], F[abien], 'Salon de 1833 (3ième article)', *Moniteur universel* (19 March 1833), pp. 763–4.

Pinault Sørensen, Madeleine, 'La peau de l'homme noir', *Lumières*, 14 (2009): Special issue: *L'invention et la représentation des races au 18ème siècle*, 101–14.

Pollock, Griselda, *Differencing the Canon: Feminist Desires and the Writing of Art's Histories* (London; New York: Routledge, 1999).

Pomarède, Vincent et al. (eds), *Ingres, 1780–1867* (Paris: Gallimard; Musée du Louvre Éditions, 2006).

Pommier, Édouard, 'Winckelmann et la vision de l'Antiquité classique dans la France des Lumières et de la Révolution', *Revue de l'art*, 83 (1989), 9–20.

Popkin, Jeremy, *You Are All Free: The Haitian Revolution and the Abolition of Slavery* (Cambridge: Cambridge University Press, 2010).
— *A Concise History of the Haitian Revolution* (Malden/Mass.: Wiley-Blackwell, 2012).
Potts, Alex, *Flesh and the Ideal: Winckelmann and the Origins of Art History* (New Haven; London: Yale University Press, 1994).
Procès-verbaux de l'Académie royale de peinture et de sculpture, 1648–1793 ed. Anatole de Montaiglon. 10 vols (Paris: Société de l'histoire de l'art Français, 1875–92).
Procès-verbaux de l'Académie des beaux-arts, publiés pour la Societé de l'Histoire de l'Art français, ed. Marcel Bonnaire. 3 vols (Paris: A. Colin, 1937–43).
Puttfarken, Thomas, *Roger de Piles' Theory of Art* (New Haven; London: Yale University Press, 1985).
— 'Composition, perspective and presence: observations on early academic theory in France', in John Onians (ed.), *Sight and Insight: Essays on Art and Culture in Honour of E. H. Gombrich at 85* (London: Phaidon Press, 1994).
— *The Discovery of Pictorial Composition: Theories of Visual Order in Painting 1400–1800* (New Haven; London: Yale University Press, 2000).
Quilley, Geoff and Kay Dian Kriz (eds), *An Economy of Colour: Visual Culture and the Atlantic World, 1660–1830* (Manchester; New York: Manchester University Press, 2003).
Reilly, Partricia L., 'Writing out color in Renaissance art theory', *Genders*, 12 (1991), 78–99.
Reuter, Astrid, *Marie-Guilhelmine Benoist: Gestaltungsräume einer Künstlerin um 1800* (Berlin: Lukas Verlag, 2002).
Rey, Roselyne, *Naissance et développement du vitalisme en France de la deuxième moitié du XVIII*ème *siècle à la fin du premier Empire* (Oxford: Voltaire Fondation, 2000).
Ribeiro, Aileen, *Ingres in Fashion: Representations of Dress and Appearance in Ingres's Images of Women* (New Haven; London: Yale University Press, 1999).
Riegl, Alois, *Historical Grammar of the Visual Arts* [1966], trans. Jacqueline E. Jung (New York: Zone Books, 2004).
Rifkin, Adrian, 'Ingres and the academic dictionary: an essay on ideology and stupefaction in the social formation of the "artist"', *Art History*, 6 (1983), 155–70.
— *Ingres: Then, and Now* (London; New York: Routledge, 2000).
Rifkin, Benjamin A., *Human Anatomy: From the Renaissance to the Digital Age* (New York: Abrams, 2006).
Riolan, Jean (the younger), *Anthropographia ex propriis et novis observationibus collecta, concinnata* (Paris: Ex officina Plantiniana, apud H. Peter, 1618).
— *Œuvres anatomiques*, trans. Pierre Constant (Paris: Denys Moreau, 1629).
— *Encheiridium anatomicum, et pathologicum, in quo ex naturali constitutione partium, recessus a naturali statu demonstratur* (Leyden: A. Wyngaerden, 1649).
— *A Sure Guide; or, the Best and Nearest Way to Physick and Chyrurery … Being an Anatomical Description of the Whol Body of Man, and its Parts, with their Respective Diseases*, trans. Nich. Culpeper (London: Peter Cole, 1657).
— *Manuel anatomique et pathologique: ou, abrégé de toute l'anatomie, & des usages que l'on en peut tirer pour la connoissance, & pour la guerison des maladies* (Paris: Gaspard Meturas, 1661).

Roberts, K. B. and J. D. W. Thomlinson, *The Fabric of the Body: European Traditions of Anatomical Illustrations* (Oxford; New York: Clarendon Press, 1992).
Rodari, Florian (ed.), *Anatomie de la couleur: l'invention de l'estampe en couleurs* (Paris: Bibliothèque nationale de France, 1996).
Roque, Georges, 'Portrait de la couleur en femme fatale', *Art & fact. Revue des historiens de l'art de l'université de Liège*, 10 (1991), 4–10.
— *Art et sciences de la couleur: Chevreul et les peintres de Delacroix à l'abstraction* (Nîmes: Jacqueline Chambon, 1997).
Rosenberg, Pierre (ed.), *Fragonard*, exh. cat., Paris, Grand Palais; New York, Metropolitan Museum (Paris: Réunion des musées nationaux, 1987).
Rosenblum, Robert, *Jean-August-Dominique Ingres* (London: Thames & Hudson, 1990).
Rosenthal, Angela, 'Visceral culture: blushing and the legibility of whiteness in eighteenth-century British portraiture', *Art History*, 27 (2004), 563–92.
Said, Edward W., *Orientalism* (London: Routledge and Kegan Paul, 1978).
Salvage, Jean-Galbert, *Anatomie du Gladiateur combattant, applicable aux beaux-arts, ou, traité des os, des muscles, du mécanisme des mouvemens, des proportions et des caractères du corps humain* (Paris: chez l'auteur, 1812).
Sarasin, Philipp, *Reizbare Maschinen: eine Geschichte des Körpers 1765–1914* (Frankfurt a. M.: Suhrkamp, 2001).
— 'The body as medium: nineteenth-century European hygiene discourse', *Grey Room*, 29 (2007), 48–65.
Sawday, Jonathan, *The Body Emblazoned: Dissection and the Human Body in Renaissance Culture* (London; New York: Routledge, 1995).
Schiebinger, Londa, *Nature's Body: Gender in the Making of Modern Science* (New Brunswick/N. J.: Rutgers University Press, 2004).
Schilder, Paul, *The Image and Appearance of the Human Body: Studies in the Constructive Energies of the Psyche* (London: Kegan Paul, Trench, Trubner, 1935).
Schmidt-Linsenhoff, Viktoria, 'Male alterity in the French Revolution: two paintings by Anne-Louis Girodet at the Salon of 1798', in Ida Blohm, Karen Hagemann and Catherine Hall (eds), *Gendered Nations: Nationalism and Gender Order in the Long Nineteenth Century* (Oxford; New York: Berg, 2000), pp. 81–105.
— 'Klassizismus und Slaverei: zum Funktionswandel kultureller Differenz in A. L. Girodets *Portrait du Citoyen Belley* und M. G. Benoists *Portrait d'une Négresse*', in Hansjörg Bay and Kai Merten (eds), *Die Ordnung der Kulturen: zur Konstruktion ethnischer, nationaler und zivilisatorischer Differenzen 1750–1850* (Würzburg: Könighausen & Neumann, 2006), pp. 173–93.
— *Ästhetik der Differenz: Postkoloniale Perspektiven vom 16.–21. Jahrhundert*. 2 vols (Marburg: Jonas Verlag, 2010).
— 'Who is the subject? Marie-Guilhelmine Benoist's *Portrait d'une Négresse*', in Agnes Lugo-Ortiz and Angela Rosenthal (eds), *Slave Portraiture in the Atlantic World* (Cambridge: Cambridge University Press, 2013), pp. 315–43.
Schmuhl, Yvonne, 'Das Inkarnat in der griechischen Malerei', *RIHA Journal* 0061, 26 November 2012, www.riha-journal.org/articles/2012/2012–oct-dec/schmuhl-inkarnat

Schnapper, Antoine and Arlette Sérullaz, *Jacques-Louis David: 1748–1825*, exh. cat., Musée du Louvre (Paris: Réunion des musées nationaux, 1989).

Schwartz, Fredric J., *Blind Spots: Critical Theory and the History of Art in Twentieth-Century Germany* (New Haven; London: Yale University Press, 2005).

Scott, Katie, 'Invention and privilege in early modern France: the case of colour', in Liliane Hiliare-Pérez and Anne-Françoise Garçon (eds), *Les chemins de la nouveauté: innover, inventer au regard de l'histoire* (Paris: Éditions du CTHS, 2003), pp. 167–86.

Shaw, Jennifer, 'The figure of Venus: rhetoric of the ideal and the Salon of 1863', in Caroline Arscott and Katie Scott (eds), *Manifestations of Venus: Art and Sexuality* (Manchester: Manchester University Press, 2000), pp. 90–108.

Shell, Hanna Rose: 'Casting life, recasting experience: Bernard Palissy's occupation between maker and nature', *Configurations*, 12 (2004), 1–40.

Shelton, Andrew Carrington, *Ingres and His Critics* (Cambridge: Cambridge University Press, 2005).

Sheriff, Mary D., 'Invention, resemblance, Fragonard's *Portraits de Fantaisie*', *Art Bulletin*, 49 (1987), 77–87.

— *Fragonard: Art and Eroticism* (Chicago; London: University of Chicago Press, 1990).

— *Moved by Love: Inspired Artists and Deviant Women in Eighteenth-Century France* (Chicago; London: University of Chicago Press, 2004).

Sidlauskas, Susan, *Cézanne's Other: The Portraits of Hortense* (Berkeley; Los Angeles; London: University of California Press, 2009).

Siegfried, Susan, 'Ingres's reading: the undoing of narrative', in Adrian Rifkin and Susan Siegfried (eds), *Fingering Ingres* (Oxford; Malden/Mass.: Blackwell Publishers, 2001), pp. 4–30.

— 'Un certain regard: Ingres, Delacroix, et l'Odalisque', in Sébastian Allard (ed.), *Paris 1820: l'affirmation de la génération romantique* (Bern: Peter Lang, 2005), pp. 61–84.

— *Ingres: Painting Reimagined* (New Haven; London: Yale University Press, 2009).

Silvestre, Théophile, *Histoire des artistes vivants français et étrangers: études d'après nature* (Paris: E. Blanchard, 1855–56).

Smalls, James, 'Slavery is a woman: "race", gender and visuality in Marie Benoist's *Portrait d'une négresse* (1800)', *Nineteenth-Century Art Worldwide*, 3:1 (2004).

Smith, Pamela, 'Vermilion, mercury, blood, and lizards: matter and meaning in metal-working', in Ursula Klein and Emma Spary (eds), *Materials and Expertise in Early Modern Europe: Between Market and Laboratory* (Chicago; London: University of Chicago Press, 2009), pp. 29–49.

Solomon-Godeau, Abigail, 'The legs of the countess', *October*, 39 (1986/87), 65–108.

— *Male Trouble: A Crisis in Representation* (London: Thames & Hudson, 1997).

Spary, Emma, *Utopia's Garden: French Natural History from Old Regime to Revolution* (Chicago; London: University of Chicago Press, 2000).

Stafford, Barbara Maria, *Body Criticism: Imaging the Unseen in Enlightenment Art and Medecine* (Cambridge/Mass.; London: MIT Press, 1991).

Starobinski, Jean, *Jean-Jacques Rousseau: Transparency and Obstruction* [1957], trans. Arthur Goldhammer (Chicago; London: University of Chicago Press, 1988).

Steinke, Hubert, 'Haller's concept of irritability and sensibility and its reception in France', *La lettre de la Maison française d'Oxford*, 14 (2001), 37–69.

— *Irritating Experiments: Haller's Concept and the European Controversy on Irritability and Sensibility, 1750–90* (Amsterdam: Rodopi, 2005).

Stoichita, Victor, *The Self-Aware Image: An Insight into Early Modern Meta-Painting* [1993] (Cambridge: Cambridge University Press, 1997).

— 'L'inconscient iconographique de George Wilhelm Friedrich Hegel: la rose et les raisins', in Hubert Locher and Peter Schneemann (eds), *Grammatik der Kunstgeschichte. Sprachprobleme und Regelwerk im 'Bilddiskurs': Oskar Bätschmann zum 65. Geburtstag* (Emstetten; Berlin: Edition Imorde, 2008), pp. 162–77.

— 'Michelangelos Haut', in Hans-Georg Arburg et al. (eds), *Mehr als Schein: Ästhetik der Oberfläche in Film, Kunst, Literatur und Theater* (Zürich; Berlin: diaphanes, 2008), pp. 34–51.

— *The Pygmalion Effect: From Ovid to Hitchcock* (Chicago; London: University of Chicago Press, 2008).

— *L'image de l'Autre: Noirs, Juifs, Musulmans et 'Gitans' dans l'art occidental des Temps modernes 1453–1789* (Paris: Hazan and Musée du Louvre, 2014).

Stuurmann, Stiep, 'François Bernier and the invention of racial classification', *History Workshop Journal*, 50 (2000), 1–21.

Sue, Jean-Joseph (the elder), *Anthropotomie, ou l'art d'injecter, de dissequer, d'embaumer et de conserver les parties du corps humain* (Paris: chez l'auteur, & chez Cavellier au Lis d'or, 1765).

Sue, Jean-Joseph (the younger), *Élémens d'anatomie, à l'usage des peintres, des sculpteurs et des amateurs* (Paris: Méquignon, l'ainé 1788).

— *Essai sur la physiognomonie des corps vivans, considérée depuis l'homme jusqu'à la plante* (Paris: l'auteur, 1797).

— *Recherches physiologiques, et expériences sur la vitalité* (Paris: chez l'auteur, An VI [1797]).

Swan, Claudia, '"Ad vivum", "naer het leven", "from the life": considerations on a mode of representation', *Word and Image*, 11 (1995), 353–72.

Taws, Richard, *The Politics of the Provisional: Art and Ephemera in Revolutionary France* (University Park/Penn.: Pennsylvania State University Press, 2013).

Ternois, Daniel, *Ingres: Monsieur Bertin* (Paris: Réunion des musées national; Service culturel du musée du Louvre, 1998).

Thomson, Ann, 'Mechanistic materialism vs vitalistic materialism', *La lettre de la Maison française d'Oxford*, 14 (2001), 21–36.

Tilby, Michael, '"Telle main veut tel pied": Balzac and the art of portraiture', in Peter Collier and Robert Lethbridge (eds), *Artistic Relations: Literature and the Visual Arts in Nineteenth-Century France* (New Haven; London: Yale University Press, 1994), pp. 111–29.

Tinterow, Gary and Philip Connisbee (eds), *Portraits by Ingres: Images of an Epoch* (New York: The Metropolitan Museum of Art, 1999).

Theophilus Presbyter, *De diversis artibus*, ed. and trans. C. R. Dodwell (Oxford: Clarendon Press, 1961).

Tocqué, Louis, 'Reflexions sur la peinture et particulièrement sur le genre du portrait' [1750], in Arnauld Doria (ed.), *Le discours de Tocqué sur le genre du portrait* (Paris: Jean Schemit, 1930), pp. 1–40.

Tortebat, François [and Roger de Piles], *Abrégé d'anatomie accommodé aux arts de peinture et de sculpture* (Paris: chez ledit Tortebat, 1667–68).

Ulz, Melanie, *Auf dem Schlachtfeld des Empire: Männlichkeitskonzepte in der Bildproduktion zu Napoleons Ägyptenfeldzug* (Marburg: Jonas, 2008).

Valerius, Gudrun, *Académie Royale de Peinture et de Sculpture 1648–1793: Geschichte. Organisation. Mitglieder* (Norderstedt: Books on Demand, 2010).

Vidal, Mary, 'The "other atelier": Jacques-Louis David's female students', in Melissa Hyde and Jennifer Milam (eds), *Women, Art, and the Politics of Identity in Eighteenth-Century Europe* (Aldershot; Burlington/Vt.: Ashgate, 2003), pp. 237–61.

Vigarello, George, *Concepts of Cleanliness: Changing Attitudes in France since the Middle Ages* [1987], trans. Jean Birell (Cambridge: Cambridge University Press, 1988).

— *Le sentiment de soi: histoire de la perception du corps* (Paris: Éditions du Seuil, 2014).

Vigée-Lebrun, Elisabeth, *Souvenirs de Madame Louise-Elisabeth Vigée-Lebrun*. 3 vols (Paris: Librairie de H. Fournier, 1835–37).

Vigne, Georges, *Dessins d'Ingres: catalogue raisoné des dessins du musée de Montauban* (Paris: Gallimard, 1995).

Vila, Anne C., *Enlightenment and Pathology: Sensibility in the Literature and Medicine of Eighteenth-century France* (Baltimore; London: Johns Hopkins University Press, 1998).

— (ed.), *A Cultural History of the Senses in the Age of Enlightenment* (London: Bloomsbury Academic, 2014).

Voltaire, François-Marie Arouet de, *Œuvres complètes de Voltaire*, new edn, ed. Louis Moland. 54 vols (Paris: Garnier frères, 1877–85).

Vries, Lyckle de, *Gerard de Lairesse: An Artist between Stage and Studio* (Amsterdam: Amsterdam University Press, 1999).

Wagner, Monika, 'Linie – Farbe – Material: Kunsttheorie und Geschlechterkampf', in Barbara Hüttel et al. (eds), *Re-Visonen: zur Aktualität der Kunstgeschichte* (Berlin: Akademie Verlag, 2002), pp. 195–207.

Wegenstein, Bernadette, *Getting Under the Skin: The Body and Media Theory* (Cambridge/Mass.: MIT Press, 2006).

Weston, Helen, 'Representing the right to represent: the portrait of citizen Belley, ex-representative of the colonies by A.-L. Girodet', *RES: Anthropology and Aesthetics*, no. 26 (autumn 1994), 83–99.

— 'Girodet's *Portrait of C. Belley. Ex-Representative of the Colonies*: in remembrance of "Things Sublime"', in Adrian Forty and Susanne Küchler (eds), *The Art of Forgetting* (Oxford: Berg, 1999), pp. 75–92.

— '"The cook, the thief, his wife and her lover": La Ville-Leroulx's *Portrait de Négresse* and the signs of misrecognition', in Valerie Mainz and Griselda Pollock (eds), *Work and the Image* (Aldershot: Ashgate, 2000), pp. 53–73.

Wheeler, Roxanne, *The Complexion of Race: Categories of Difference in Eighteenth-Century British Culture* (Philadelphia: University of Pennsylvania Press, 2000).

Wildenstein, Daniel, *Documents complémentaire au catalogue de l'œuvre de Louis David* (Paris: Fondation Wildenstein, 1973).

Williams, Hannah, *Académie Royale: A History in Portraits* (Farnham; Burlington/Vt.: Ashgate, 2015).

Wilson, Michael, 'A new acquisition for the National Gallery: David's Portrait of Jacobus Blauw', *Burlington Magazine*, 126 (1984), 694–8.

Winckelmann, Johann Joachim, *Reflections on the Paintings and Sculptures of the Greeks*, trans. Henry Fuseli (London: the translator, 1765).

— 'Gedanken über die Nachahmung der Griechischen Werke in der Mahlerey und Bildhauerkunst' [1755], in *Kleine Schriften, Vorreden, Entwürfe* (Berlin: de Gruyter, 1968).

— *Schriften und Nachlaß*, ed. Akademie der Wissenschaften und der Literatur, Mainz; Akademie der gemeinnützigen Schriften zu Erfurt; Winckelmann-Gesellschaft (Mainz: Philipp von Zabern, 1996).

— *History of Ancient Art* (New York: F. Ungar Publishing Co., 1969).

— *History of the Art of Antiquity*, trans. Harry Francis Mallgrave, introd. Alex Potts (Los Angeles/Cal.: Getty Research Institute, 2006).

Wipfler, Esther Pia (ed.), *Kunsttechnik und Kunstgeschichte: das Inkarnat in der Malerei des Mittelalters* (München: Zentralinstitut für Kunstgeschichte, 2012).

Wolfe, Charles T., 'The allure of the flesh and the vitality of materialism: aporias of embodiment', in Felix Ensslin and Charlotte Klink (eds), *Aesthetics of the Flesh* (Berlin: Sternberg Press, 2014), pp. 83–106.

— and Motoichi Terada, 'The animal economy as object and program in Montpellier vitalism', *Science in Context*, 21 (2008), 537–79.

Wolff, Katja, 'Schwarz-Weiß-Malerei: Beobachtungen zum Inkarnat in Bildnissen mit Mohrenpagen', in Annegret Friedrich (ed.), *Die Freiheit der Anderen: Festschrift für Viktoria Schmidt-Linsenhoff zum 21. August 2004* (Marburg: Jonas Verlag, 2004), pp. 137–44.

Woodall, Joanna (ed.), *Portraiture: Facing the Subject* (Manchester; New York: Manchester University Press, 1997).

— 'Wtewael's *Perseus and Andromeda*: looking for love in early seventeenth-century Dutch painting', in Caroline Arscott and Katie Scott (eds), *Manifestations of Venus: Art and Sexuality* (Manchester; New York: Manchester University Press, 2000), pp. 39–68.

Wrigley, Richard, *The Origins of French Art Criticism: From the Ancien Régime to the Restoration* (Oxford; New York: Oxford University Press, 1993).

Zeuch, Ulrike (ed.), *Verborgen im Buch. Verborgen im Körper: Haut zwischen 1500 und 1800*, exh. cat. Herzog Anton August Bibliothek Wolfenbüttel (Wiesbaden: Harrowitz, 2003).

Ziegler, Joseph, 'Skin and character in medieval and early Renaissance physiognomy', *Micrologus. Nature, Sciences and Medieval Societies*, 13 (2005), 511–35, Special issue: *The Human Skin*.

Zimmermann, Michael F., 'Seurat, Charles Blanc, and naturalist art criticism', *Art Institute of Chicago Museum Studies*, 14 (1989), 198–209, 246–7.

Index

Note: Art works and texts can be found under authors' names.

EU authorised representative for GPSR:
Easy Access System Europe, Mustamäe tee 50,
10621 Tallinn, Estonia
gpsr.requests@easproject.com

www.ingramcontent.com/pod-product-compliance
Ingram Content Group UK Ltd.
Pitfield, Milton Keynes, MK11 3LW, UK
UKHW061933100926
8556IPUK00007B/905

* 9 7 8 0 7 1 9 0 8 7 9 6 7 *